The Care of Strangers

THE CARE
OF STRANGERS

The Rise of America's
Hospital System

Charles E. Rosenberg

Basic Books, Inc., Publishers   *New York*

Library of Congress Cataloging-in-Publication Data

Rosenberg, Charles E.
  The care of strangers.

  Bibliography: p.353
  1. Hospitals—United States—History—19th century.
  2. Hospitals—United States—History—20th century.
  3. Medicine—United States—History—19th century.
  4. Medicine—United States—History—20th century.
  I. Title.
  RA981.A2R59 1987   362.1'1'0973   87–47421
  ISBN 0–465–00877–1

For Drew

Contents

Contents

Illustrations follow page 182

Acknowledgments

I have been working on this book for almost two decades, much of that time inadvertently, as I studied other aspects of American medical history. It was not until the past decade that I seriously considered writing a book on hospitals. It took shape as I came gradually to realize that the history of twentieth-century medicine, the medical profession, and medical care could not be explained without an understanding of the hospital's origins—and that this history was a revealing microcosm of the changes that have transformed society more generally during the past two centuries. The current debate on hospital policy only sharpened my interest.

During these years I have benefited from the help and suggestions of dozens of friends and colleagues. Perhaps most important have been the thoughtful efforts of librarians and archivists; Adele A. Lerner, of the Medical Archives, New York Hospital–Cornell Medical Center; Richard J. Wolfe, of the Francis A. Countway Library of Medicine; Caroline Morris, of Pennsylvania Hospital; Nancy McCall of the Alan Mason Chesney Medical Archives, the Johns Hopkins Medical Institutions; Allen H. Stokes of the University of South Carolina's South Caroliniana Library; and Lisabeth M. Holloway, Ellen Gartrell, Christine Ruggere, and Thomas Horrocks of the Historical Collections of the College of Physicians of Philadelphia have been particularly helpful. The reference notes reflect my indebtedness to these institutions and many other archives, medical libraries, hospitals, and historical societies. During the same years I have learned much from my own students who have written research papers and dissertations relevant to the development of American hospitals. I would like to thank Bonnie Blustein, Priscilla Ferguson Clement, Gail Farr, Vanessa Gamble, Lindsay Granshaw, Carole Haber, Joel Howell, Edward Morman, Leo O'Hara, Naomi Rogers, Nancy Tomes, and Karen Wilkerson; they have all helped in ways that might not be apparent from a reading of specific reference notes, but have in sum made this a better book. The Institute for Advanced Study at Princeton (where I drafted the first section in 1979–80) and the Center for Advanced Study in the Behavioral Sciences at Stanford (where I drafted the central chapters during the academic year 1983–84) proved ideal places to learn and work.

Barbara Bates, Muriel Bell, Bruce Kuklick, Susan Reverby, Barbara Rosenkrantz, and Rosemary Stevens have read large or small portions of the manuscript and their comments have helped make this a clearer and more accessible book. Steve Fraser, my editor at Basic Books, read each chapter as I drafted it and then the entire manuscript when completed. His suggestions for revision were invariably relevant and incisive. Mary Fissel checked the text and especially the reference notes for accuracy and consistency. Most important, Drew Faust read every chapter—some several times; she provided an acute editorial conscience and an example of level-headed commitment to scholarship that made it impossible not to finish this project or to do less than my best.

The Care of Strangers

Introduction

Suddenly, it seemed in the late 1960s, the American hospital became a problem. It has remained one. Depending on the critic's temperament, politics, or pocketbook, the hospital appeared a source of uncontrolled inflationary pressure, an instrument of class and sexual oppression, or an impersonal monolith, managing in its several ways to dehumanize rich and poor at once, if not alike. To many such detractors, it seemed the stronghold of a profession jealous of its prerogatives and little concerned with needs that could not be measured, probed, or irradiated. Meanwhile, hospital costs mounted inexorably.

In the 1980s, hospitals became the center of a rather differently focused sense of crisis, but of crisis nevertheless. Today, the debate turns on questions of bureaucratic control and the hospital as marketplace actor. Physicians in both the academic world and private practice—villains in the critique of the late 1960s and 1970s—now perceive themselves as beset by government on the one hand and corporate medicine on the other. The foci of debate over medical policy have shifted, yet the hospital remains at the center of controversy.

This is hardly surprising. The hospital is in some ways peculiarly characteristic of our society. Within the walls of a single building, high technology, bureaucracy, and professionalism are juxtaposed with the most fundamental and unchanging of human experiences—birth, death, pain. It is no accident that both black comedy and soap opera should have found the hospital a natural setting. It is an institution clothed with an almost mystical power, yet suffused with a relentless impersonality and a forbidding aura of technical complexity. Like the ship of fools that symbolized man's ineradicable frailties in early modern Europe, the hospital can be seen as a late twentieth-century symbol of the gap between human aspirations and necessary human failings—displayed not in the confines of a ship adrift upon the sea, but in an institution that reproduces values and social relationships of the wider world yet manages at the same time to remain isolated in its particular way from the society that created and supports it.

The development of the hospital over time has similarly reproduced in microcosm the history of a larger society. In 1800, the hospital was still an insignificant aspect of American medical care. No gentleman of property or standing would have found himself in a hospital unless stricken with insanity or felled by epidemic or accident in a strange city. When respectable persons or members of their family fell ill, they would be treated at home. If we define "hospital" as an institution dedicated exclusively to inpatient care of the sick, then there were only two hospitals in America: Philadelphia's Pennsylvania Hospital and the New York Hospital.

If too sick to be cared for at home, urban workers were most likely to find themselves in an almshouse, not a hospital. Although envisioned as a "receptacle" for the dependent and indigent, the almshouse had by the late eighteenth century become in part a municipal hospital in function if not in name. Growing numbers of sick in the almshouses of America's seaport cities required the development of separate wards for their care—separate, that is, from the simply destitute, the orphaned, the marginally criminal, and the permanently incapacitated who also populated this warehouse for the dependent. In smaller communities, the few chronically ill, handicapped, or aged individuals in the local almshouse hardly justified a separate wing or building; instead a local physician might call several times a week, and the more severely ill patients were simply placed together in a few wardlike rooms.

By the Civil War, the situation was largely unchanged. Several dozen hospitals had been founded by private groups, but county and municipal institutions were still the major providers of inpatient care—and even in the largest cities and among the working poor, dispensaries and hospital outpatient departments treated a far greater number than were ever admitted to inpatient beds. In our country, as a mid-nineteenth-century New Yorker put it, "the people who repair to hospitals are mostly very poor, and seldom go into them until driven to do so from a severe stress of circumstances."[1] In 1873, the first American hospital survey located only 178, including mental institutions; they contained a total of less than fifty thousand beds.[2] Only a few of these were integrated with medical school instruction, while none regarded research as an explicit commitment. Obligatory residency and internship programs, like hospital certification, lay several generations in the future.

Not only did the hospital play a small role in the provision of medical care before the Civil War, it was in its internal structure a very different institution from that we know in the late twentieth century. It was not directed by a bureaucracy of credentialed administrators; it was certainly not dominated by the medical profession and its needs. Lay trustees still felt it their duty to oversee every aspect of hospital routine. The hospital was very much a mirror of the society that populated and supported it, a society rooted in deference and hierarchy, a society in which traditional attitudes toward the responsibility of wealth were very much alive. Medical men needed and used the hospital; they could not control it.

The hospital was not yet dominated and justified, as it has come to be, by an intimidating arsenal of tools and techniques. Aside from a handful of surgical procedures, there was little in the way of medical capability in 1800 that could not be made easily available outside the hospital's walls—at least in homes of the middle class and the wealthy. Physicians could ordinarily do little to alter the course of a patient's illness and almost as little to monitor quality of life on the ward. Contemporary therapeutics offered few procedures that could not be understood and evaluated by a well-informed layman. Much of household medicine was, in fact, identical with hospital treatment; indeed something of the social efficacy of early nineteenth-century therapeutics may well have rested on this very community of understanding.[3] The hospital in early national America was defined primarily by need and dependency, not by the existence of specialized technical resources.

Much of this had changed by the first decade of the twentieth century. The hospital had become far more central, both in the provision of medical care and in the careers of ambitious physicians. In 1909, a census of American hospitals located 4,359 with 421,065 beds (a total that did not include mental or chronic disease hospitals such as tuberculosis sanitariums).[4] Not only had the hospital spread widely in the United States, it had become a potential recourse for a much larger proportion of Americans; the prosperous and respectable as well as the indigent were now treated in hospitals, frequently by their regular physicians.

And treated in ways that seemed increasingly arcane and impressive. Few laymen presumed an understanding of the disease concepts, the therapeutics, the diagnostic tests, and the surgical procedures that justified the hospital's newly prominent role in medical care. Knowledge, like every kind of work within the hospital, had become increasingly specialized. So too had the hospital as physical artifact. Early nineteenth-century hospitals were architecturally little different from other large public buildings, but by 1900 the hospital had assumed a characteristic physical form, its internal spaces defined by their functions and those functions understood in technical and bureaucratic terms.

The hospital had become easily recognizable to twentieth-century eyes. It had grown in size, had become more formal and bureaucratic, and increasingly unified in authority, consistently reflecting medical needs and perceptions. All of this had come about without dramatic conflict, without formal planning or even informal concert, but within a set of social perceptions, economic relationships, ongoing technical innovations, and professional values—all of which interacted to dictate a pattern of development as precise as anything that might have resulted from formal planning. By the First World War, the shape of the hospital's late twentieth-century descendant was apparent in its already vigorous and expansive predecessor.

Indeed, by 1920 almost all those criticisms of the hospital so familiar to us in the past two decades were already being articulated by critics both within and outside the medical profession. Concerned observers of the hospital pointed toward a growing coldness and impersonality; they deprecated an increasing concern with acute ailments and a parallel neglect of the aged, of chronic illness, of the convalescent, of the simply routine. They warned of a socially insensitive and economically dysfunctional obsession with inpatient at the expense of outpatient and community-oriented care. An understanding of the patient's social and family environment, such Progressive Era critics contended, was necessary to a full understanding both of the cause of sickness and appropriate therapeutics. Medicine had to be brought out of the hospital and into the community—insofar as possible into the home. But such views were not to prevail. Those aspects of early twentieth-century institutional medicine not centered on the hospital's wards—the independent dispensary, the public health nurse and physician, the hospital's own outpatient facilities—actually decreased in significance as the hospital and its inpatient service grew ever more prominent in the culture of medicine.

The "culture of medicine" is not simply an ornamental phrase; there is such a culture, one accepted and assimilated in generation-specific form by every physician. And it was a formative element in the shaping of the modern hospital. If the creation of the hospital as a quintessentially modern institution is a central theme of the pages that follow, another is the way in which the perceptions, the values and rewards, the career patterns, and, increasingly, the specific knowledge of physicians have structured this development. The evolution of the hospital has reflected a clear and consistently understood vision. That vision looked inward toward the needs and priorities of the medical profession, inward toward the administrative and financial needs of the individual hospital, inward toward the body as a mechanism opaque to all but those with medical training—and away from that of patient as social being and family member. It was a vision, moreover, so deeply felt as to preclude conscious planning, replacing it instead with a series of seemingly necessary actions.[5]

The decisions that shaped the modern hospital have been consistently guided by the world of medical ideas and values. I refer not simply to specific insights such as the germ theory or the new diagnostic and curative tools provided by the x-ray and immunology, but more generally to the attitudes and aspirations that gave the profession its peculiar identity. It has become fashionable in recent years to interpret medical self-conceptions as best explicable in marketplace terms, and obviously economic realities do explain a good deal of that which we see in past medical behavior; individuals do not ordinarily act in ways contrary to their perceived economic interest. But interest cannot be understood in economic terms alone. The honor accorded innovation, the satisfaction of intellectual competence in a world of pervasive mediocrity, for example, are meaningful compensations, if perhaps ultimately no more transcendent than dollars and cents (and possibly more self-deluding). One can hardly understand the evolution of the hospital without some understanding of the power of ideas, of the allure of innovation, of the promised amelioration of painful and incapacitating symptoms through an increasingly effective hospital-based technology.

The ethos of the medical profession elicited change as it defined behavior. The germ theory, antiseptic surgery, clinical pathology, and the x-ray were evidence of that change and seeming proof of the value of medical aspirations. That there could be conflict between aspects—and achievements—of the medical culture and other needs of human beings only occasionally occurred to those physicians who dominated hospital medicine. Given the long-standing unwillingness of federal authority to intrude in the delivery of medical care, the needs and outlooks of medical men coupled with the social attitudes and financial decisions of lay trustees and local governments shaped the modern hospital.

American communities had grown proud of their hospitals; ethnic and religious groups saw their institutions as symbols of community identity and respectability. Small towns saw them as badges of energy and modernity. Initiated in the late eighteenth and early nineteenth centuries as a welfare institution framed and motivated by the responsibilities of Christian stewardship, the twentieth-century American hospital has tended to see itself as a necessary response to scientific understanding and the hope of secular healing. In neither era was it easily subjected to marketplace discipline or balanced considerations of public interest. The hospital conformed to a rationality, but it was a rationality shaped by lay expectations and given specific form by the interests and perceptions of those who worked within it.

The modern hospital is a unique institution. At the same time it has shared the history and displayed many of the characteristics of other large institutions, such as corporate enterprises, urban public schools, and welfare departments. Bureaucratic organization and administration by a stratum of the credentialed, for example, have come to characterize all of these organizations. In this sense, the hospital has to be seen as but one aspect of a new social structure in which a range of functions—education, welfare, and work as well as health care—were moving from the home to institutional sites. By the 1880s, Americans were well aware that many of them no longer lived in small, face-to-face settings; communities would simply have to adjust to these new realities. Families would come increasingly to depend on strangers for care at times of sickness and approaching death.

The patient's experience of that care would evolve as well. Perhaps the most important single element in reshaping the day-to-day texture of hospital life was the professionalization of nursing. In

1800, as today, nurses were the most important single factor determining ward and room environment. Nursing, like professional hospital administration and changed modes of hospital financing, has played a key role in shaping the modern hospital.

Each one of these elements might well deserve more detailed treatment. Yet I have made all somewhat subordinate to the role of the medical profession. I do not mean to imply that physicians alone were responsible for the shape of the modern hospital; this is obviously not the case. But their role was a particularly dynamic one. I am convinced that the history of American hospitals can best be made comprehensible by focusing on the physician's role in eliciting and shaping change.

Unlike most laymen connected with the hospital, physicians felt a keen motivation to impose their will on its internal order. They knew what they wanted and assumed that an inevitably increasing store of knowledge would define and redefine the institutional options they saw as legitimate and desirable. Medical men provided a specific content and public rationale for the institution; an arsenal of specific procedures seemed increasingly to constitute and justify the hospital enterprise. A key aspect of the hospital's history is the precise integration of medical careers, ideas, and, somewhat later, practice patterns into the growing institution.

By the First World War, the hospital had grown markedly different from its antebellum predecessors, just as American society itself had changed. Those traditional ties of deference, patronage, and social responsibility that had created an implicit structure for the hospital in Federalist America had faded by the end of the nineteenth century. Oversight by pious and paternalistic laymen had been largely replaced by the seemingly impersonal and neutral categories of medical diagnosis and the self-confident management of professional administrators and aspiring physicians. To many physicians and increasing numbers of laymen, the hospital had become the only appropriate place to practice medicine of the highest quality. The hospital had already assumed its modern shape.

Much of this evolution took place in the half century between 1870 and 1920. Changes in the American hospital between the end of World War II and the present have certainly been dramatic—the assumption of a key federal role, for example, the development and spread of third-party payment, the integration of an ever-more complex technology into the hospital's therapeutic repertoire. Nevertheless, the modern hospital's basic shape had been established by 1920. It had become central to medical education and was well integrated into the career patterns of regular physicians; in urban areas it had already replaced the family as the site for treating serious illness and managing death. Perhaps most important, it had already been clothed with a legitimating aura of science and almost boundless social expectation.

The organization of this book reflects this chronological emphasis. The first three chapters describe the modest beginnings of the hospital in the years before the Civil War, emphasizing especially its effect on the patients who inhabited it and the hospital's meaning to the lay trustees and physicians who nominally controlled it. A fourth chapter sketches the motivations and social sources of support for a budding midcentury hospital expansion and reform. The bulk of the book is then arranged topically and concerns itself with the pivotal half century of change between 1870 and 1920. Chapters five through twelve deal with issues such as the coming of scientific medicine to the hospital, medical careers and education, the impact of professional nursing, authority patterns, the arrival of private patients, and the altered texture of life on the ward. Chapter 13 describes the early twentieth-century hospital and efforts to make it a more flexible and humane institution, underlining the longevity and tenacity of problems we have come to see in the last quarter century as peculiarly contemporary. A final chapter looks to events in the past half century and emphasizes ways in which the past has imposed itself on the present.

To most observers, the twentieth-century hospital seems an inevitable, if perhaps imperfect, institution, one that grew unavoidably out of the interaction between social necessity and an emerging technical capacity. Despite this aura of inevitability, however, both logic and history emphasize that the American hospital's development has been contingent. Its history reflects a mixture of policy and drift, of change that grew out of the complex interaction between technical innovation, social attitudes, demographic and economic realities, and, finally, the crystallizing aspirations and values of an increasingly self-conscious medical profession. The hospital's functions and boundaries were negotiated in the past and are being renegotiated today; its history reflects choices not made as well as those pursued.

In writing this book, I have been particularly concerned with the perspective of the men and women who lived and worked in the hospital. I hope not to have ignored their perceptions or reduced them to data in some schematized model of change. With the exception of a minority of publicists for the new scientific medicine, actors in the hospital's past did not see themselves as part of a necessary evolution. Physicians evaluated their careers and made choices about their relationship to the hospital; trustees saw their role in quite a different way while responding to the social assumptions and moral imperatives of their particular generation. To nurses, orderlies, and cooks, the hospital was a place to work, and, through most of the nineteenth century, to live. To most patients, the hospital was an episode, though a particularly trying and perhaps final one. All these actors brought with them particular beliefs and preconceptions, ideas about the nature of social responsibility, the cause and cure of disease, the appropriate relationships between men and women and among the social classes. I hope in part to recreate this meaning, to see the hospital and medicine through their eyes while at the same time understanding it as a microcosm of more general social realities.[6]

The hospital is both more and less than a creature of twentieth-century technology and bureaucracy; it is both alike and fundamentally different from a factory, public school, or corporate headquarters. In discussing the impersonal and highly technical aspects of the twentieth-century hospital, I hope not to have endorsed the romantic impulse that contrasts a hypothetical world of past social unity and emotional support with an emotionally sterile modernity. Although the late twentieth-century hospital may often assume a bleak and dehumanizing aspect, hospitals have never been ideal places in which to receive care. Traditional hospitals offered little in the way of therapeutics, minimal creature comforts, and the ambiguous benefits of an energetic paternalism; late twentieth-century hospitals offer the hope of healing, but at enormous economic and often emotional cost. The traditional hospital illustrates the deprivation and brutalization of the ordinary working man's life; the modern hospital demonstrates the intractable frailties of humankind and the ultimate difficulty of any belief system—whether it be traditional religion and the humoral pathology of 1800 or the new faith embodied in computer-guided scanners and organ transplants—in the unyielding face of pain and death.

PART I

A Traditional Institution, 1800–1850

CHAPTER 1

To Heal the Sick: The Antebellum Hospital and Society

In October of 1810, Ezra Stiles Ely, a newly ordained Presbyterian minister, began to preach in New York City's almshouse hospital. Few other emissaries from New York's church-going and servant-employing classes had ever set foot in its bleak corridors. Yet each year a thousand new patients were admitted to the hospital, Ely explained in his diary, and two hundred died without religious consolation.[1]

The very existence of the almshouse and its poverty-stricken inhabitants dramatized the insecurity of life for most New Yorkers. It underlined as well the enormous gap that separated social classes in this still deferential early nineteenth-century city. The young hospital chaplain entered the almshouse with much the same bravado and anxiety as if he had been undertaking a ministry in Burma or the Gold Coast. Although it was in fact the largest hospital in a thriving port city (its private competitor, the New York Hospital, was far smaller) the internal logic of the almshouse allied it more closely to the hospice of the Middle Ages than to the twentieth-century hospital. It housed the insane, the blind and crippled, the aged, the alcoholic and syphilitic, as well as the ordinary working man suffering with an extended siege of rheumatism, bronchitis, or pleurisy. Few who entered the almshouse did so voluntarily; it was a last resort for the city's most helpless and deprived.

To Ely, the hospital was filled with the "depraved and miserable of our race." Perhaps most shocking, it was a "grand receptacle of blasted, withered, dying, females," prostitutes that is, ignorant of religion yet willing to mock his pious words, even from the "beds of disease, planted with thorns" upon which they lay.² It took a strong stomach and high seriousness of purpose for the young man to enter this nest of moral and physical decay. The smells accumulating from "bodies stowed in as thick as they could lie" was almost overpowering. Patients had to share beds; on one such pallet he found two "abandoned" girls, thirteen and fifteen. A victim of typhus fever in another room had been allowed to lie dead for a full day among his fellow patients before being removed. In still another ward, the liberal use of vinegar and burning linen could not, as it was hoped, disguise the overpowering odor of impending death; without "aromatics" Ely would have been moved to "vomition." The stiffness of the young man's diction expressed the alienation he must have felt. Physical contact with the patients was more than Ely could endure; and on at least one occasion he drew back as a woman reached out to touch him in an unexpected gesture of warmth.³

Ely could never bridge the abyss that separated him from the almshouse patients. Occasionally, however, he would meet an inmate who had clearly seen better days, and the moment of identification brought a thrill of horror and empathy. One such unfortunate was an aged Presbyterian clergyman; in the turmoil of American society no one could feel safe from sickness, age, and ultimately the almshouse. Although they were clearly a small minority among the patients, Ely could not well have avoided noticing once-respectable citizens in the hospital wards; in this society the signs of class identity were unmistakable. One fever victim, for example, was clearly a man of "more than common parts, for every article of his dress, and every word of his language, indicates him to be of a respectable family and education."⁴ Few such found their way into any hospital, and Ely was always surprised to come upon a "Christian" as he passed through the wards. Self-respecting New Yorkers were naturally ashamed to find themselves in such surroundings; it meant their abandonment by family, by employers, even by congregations if they were churchgoers. For in this small society, community membership implied responsibility—in families, among members of the same congregation, between employer and employee. No responsible master of a servant would allow even a hired member of his or her "family" to be cared for by strangers.

Ely's sense of distance from his charges reflected the vast difference between the culture into which he had grown to manhood and that which ruled in the wards. Many of the hospital's inmates were immigrants, and even the Presbyterian Scots spoke a broad dialect, which the young clergyman could barely understand. The far larger number of Irish patients presented an even greater challenge to Ely's forbearance; he detested their alcoholism, their "superstitions," their faith in oil and wafers, and in unintelligible Latin ritual. Sailors seemed to live in their own world of masculine bravado. Blacks, too, even if superficially deferential and overtly Christian, might harbor belief in visions and the ability of witchcraft to cause disease. Ely found few spiritual allies within the hospital. Nurses and attendants were almost always recruited from recovered patients and differed little in background from their charges. It was only natural that a lady from one of New York's "most respectable families" should have chided Ely for publishing his almshouse journal: it was, as she saw it, "nothing but a history of ****** and beggars."[5]

If the good society was ordered and predictable, the hospital Ely experienced in the years between 1810 and 1813 was a microcosm of antithetical disorder. Cooking and foraging were each ward's responsibility and meant confusion and agitation three times a day. The rooms were too crowded for the sexes to be segregated—and Ely predicted the generation of another crop of paupers. Children circulated restlessly through the almshouse; they could not be kept to themselves, nor could the many young prostitutes be kept from "all intercourse with wicked men."[6] Despite some efforts at classification, most wards were a hodgepodge of ages and sexes, of disabilities and ailments.

But Ely discerned a moral logic that transcended the suffering and filth of the almshouse hospital. Certainly, age and disease might on occasion strike even the virtuous, yet most of the hospital's inmates were victims of their own immorality or imprudence. "In nine cases out of ten," he explained, "premature sickness comes in consequence of making a god of animal appetite." Even the insane had almost always become demented as a result of habitual indulgence in some base passion (while the idiot, although personally blameless, embodied the physical consequence of Adam's fall and millennia of subsequent sin).[7] Ely shared with most physicians of his day a belief in the role of volition in causing disease. Certainly, the prostitutes and alcoholics who cluttered the almshouse hospital provided living proof that God chastised sin immediately and inevitably through the body's own mechanisms; one need not await the hereafter to encounter punishment for spiritual transgression. Therapeutics, as well, illustrated the precise moral order designed into

God's material world; it seemed no more than appropriate to Ely that mercury, the only accepted remedy for syphilis, should induce suffering and disfigurement almost as severe as that caused by the disease itself.[8]

Ely persisted for several years in this taxing chaplaincy. His sense of spiritual vocation demanded that he devote what energies he possessed to regeneration of the potentially savable among the almshouse inhabitants. Similarly, the men of substance who founded, supported, and governed America's first voluntary hospitals felt called upon to use their wealth and leisure in ameliorating the lot of their less fortunate brethren. The worthy among the helpless sick deserved better than a bundle of straw in an almshouse medical ward.

A Vision of Mercy

In 1800, America's population was 5,308,483. Only 322,000 lived in communities larger than twenty-five hundred.[9] A person who felt sick was ordinarily treated by a neighbor or relative. If the illness persisted, he or she would consult a physician, whose credentials were usually limited to apprenticeship with a local practitioner, but who normally knew his patients personally and treated them in their homes.

Most Americans in 1800 had probably heard that such things as hospitals existed, but only a minority would have ever had occasion to see one. Philadelphia's Pennsylvania Hospital had been founded in 1752; New York Hospital, although organized in 1771, did not receive patients until the 1790s; and Boston's Massachusetts General Hospital did not open until 1821. If few Americans had encountered one of these institutions—or visited the hospital wards of an almshouse—fewer still would have been treated in one. Most hospital patients were urban workers or seamen; only occasionally did the member of a prosperous and respectable family find his or her way into a hospital bed. The great majority of such unfortunates were victims of accident or insanity. Even among the working poor, sickness and dependence meant, as Ezra Stiles Ely discovered, institutional care in an almshouse ward.[10] The hospital was little more than an embryo in the era of Adams and Jefferson. And though hospitals increased in scale and numbers with the growth of America's urban population, they remained and were to remain insignificant in the provision of medical care in antebellum America. Yet to that handful of elite urban physicians who staffed them and those philanthropists who supported and administered them, these pioneer hospitals were significant indeed.

The origins of the American hospital began as much with ideas of dependence and class as with the unavoidable incidence of sickness and accident. If most philanthropists were a trifle uncertain about the internal working of a hospital, they knew with certainty what they did not want. And that was an almshouse. One of the fundamental motivations in founding America's first hospitals was an unquestioned distinction between the worthy and unworthy poor, between the prudent and industrious objects of a benign stewardship and those less deserving Americans whose own failings justified their almshouse incarceration. Thus, it was only natural that the Pennsylvania Hospital should, in the late eighteenth century, have demanded a written testimonial from a "respectable" person attesting to the moral worth of an applicant before he or she could be admitted to a bed.[11] Philadelphia's Lying-In Charity hospital assured potential supporters in 1834, for example, that great care would be taken to

discriminate between the deserving and the undeserving. . . . Our object is not to encourage inactivity and improvidence, but to mitigate the unavoidable suffering incident by nature to the feebler portion of the human family, and to furnish some of the cheering comforts required, and which the individual cannot possibly procure.[12]

In every city there were young men adrift from family and community, mechanics and hard-working artisans stricken with incapacitating illness or aged widows of irreproachable character who had spent a lifetime in piety and hard work. There were the insane as well, helpless by definition and drawn—as did not seem to be the case with most other ills—from every social class. To help such unfortunates was no less than demanded by the responsibilities of Christian stewardship. "It is unnecessary to urge the propriety and even obligation of succouring the poor in sickness," advocates of a Boston hospital argued in 1810. "The wealthy inhabitants of the town of Boston have always evinced that they consider themselves as 'treasurers of God's bounty'; and in Christian countries, in countries where Christianity is practiced, it must always be considered the first of duties to visit and heal the sick."[13]

The hospital was something Americans of the better sort did for their less fortunate countrymen; it was hardly a refuge they contemplated entering themselves. Nevertheless, as all conceded, the hospital's benefits extended well beyond the immediate recipients of its care. The hospital's wards and amphitheater would serve as a school of clinical medicine, and some physicians at least would have the advantage of seeing and treating a broad variety of patients. And although a few American medical schools had come into being by 1810—Pennsylvania, Harvard, Dartmouth and New York's College of Physicians—their formal curriculum was entirely didactic: a three-to-four-month term of formal lectures repeated without change each year. The aspiring medical student was required to sit through two "courses" of such lectures before becoming eligible for his degree. Clinical training was no part of the medical school's responsibilities—insofar as the student learned such skills, it would be at the side of his preceptor. Yet as thoughtful observers had been aware for at least a century, not even the busiest doctor could boast a practice approximating the number and variety of cases a young man would see in the hospital's wards.

Advocates of America's first hospitals all emphasized the institution's educational function. It was an argument that appealed to municipal pride as well. To found a hospital was to keep one's eager and ambitious young physicians at home for their training. To Philadelphians in mideighteenth century, it meant avoiding the expense, moral temptation, and danger of an ocean voyage and residence in London or Edinburgh; to New Yorkers and Bostonians, somewhat later, it meant that their ablest young men would not have to voyage south to rival Philadelphia for clinical experience. The alliance of medical school and hospital, the governors of New York Hospital boasted in 1809, "promise to afford all those means of improvement in medical science that have so long been desired for the honor and advantage of the State."[14]

The advantages of hospital work for established clinicians were even more immediate. To the prominent physicians and surgeons who walked its wards and treated its patients, hospital appointments meant both honor and profit. The hospital was from its very origins inextricably linked to the careers of successful and ambitious medical men. Christianity, intellectual curiosity, and a laudable ambition were consistent in underlining the centrality of the hospital to such leaders of the medical community. It is hardly surprising that prominent clinicians played a pivotal role in the founding of all our early voluntary hospitals. The Quaker physician Thomas Bond enlisted Benjamin Franklin in lobbying for establishment of the Pennsylvania Hospital, while a similar role was played by Samuel Bard in New York and James C. Jackson and John Collins Warren in Boston. It was a pattern to be followed in American cities both large and small throughout the nineteenth century.

The benefits of the hospital would, its advocates contended, be distributed among every social class. The worthy poor would find an opportunity to recover outside the almshouse's demeaning walls, while society would profit from the productive skills of each worker restored to health. The insane of every class would find an appropriate haven and perhaps in time clarity of mind. The established urban physician would be allowed to exercise his benevolence and clinical acumen, while younger clinicians could hone those skills that might eventually allow them to replace their teachers as leaders in their city's medical profession. Those of the better sort who supported and assumed ultimate responsibility for these pioneer hospitals would be fulfilled in their responsibility as Christians, while society in general would profit from having more skillful practitioners at its command. It is to our benefit that "those physicians," as Massachusetts General Hospital (MGH) trustees put it in 1822, "to whom necessity compels us to entrust the lives of our wives and children, do not witness patients for the first time in our chambers nor apply their first remedies to those whose health is so precious to us."[15] The "us" who were potential contributors to the hospital were clearly not those who would be treated in its wards.

Its most energetic antebellum advocates never envisioned the hospital as central to medical care; even for the urban working class, the hospital was seen as a last resort. It was expensive; it was unnatural; it was potentially demoralizing. (Throughout the nineteenth century, American philanthropists were haunted by the specter of "pauperization"—the fear that provision of aid in any form would inevitably sap the moral capacity of those receiving it.) Ordinarily a home atmosphere and the nursing of family members provided the ideal conditions for restoring health. Only the most crowded and filthy dwellings were inferior to the hospital's impersonal ward, and only in a minority of cases could hospital medicine provide skills and techniques not available outside its walls. Thus, it was natural for early nineteenth-century philanthropists to have supported dispensary and outpatient medicine enthusiastically; it was always preferable to treat a patient in his or her own home. Perhaps most important, the great majority of Americans in the early nineteenth century assumed that their nation's exuberant economy would never produce the enormous number of hospital patients that filled old world institutions. "In our country," as prominent MGH physicians James Jackson and John Collins Warren put it in 1822, "there are few persons, few men at least, who would ever stand in need of public or private charity, after their entrance into active life, if they were uniformly virtuous and industrious."[16]

Although charity was always a potential menace to its recipients, the hospital's patients were seen as genuinely needy almost by definition and less likely than recipients of free food or fuel to be impostors, for none but the ill and desperate would willingly seek the dubious comforts of a hospital ward. The hospital, moreover, was usually pictured by its antebellum advocates as an island of morally improving decorum in the stressful and disordered life of its patients. But such hopes were not to become realities. Life inside the hospital's walls was never entirely under the control of those earnest Americans who bore legal and financial responsibility for it.

Life on the Ward

Hospital reality began with admissions. Formal criteria in all the early voluntary hospitals were similar. None admitted contagious or chronic ills. The former endangered the hospital's staff and patients, the latter undermined its limited ability to provide beds for the potentially curable. As the chronicler of Philadelphia's Pennsylvania Hospital explained in 1831, the institution was not intended to be an asylum for "poverty and decrepitude." No incurable cases would be admitted. The editor of the *Boston Medical and Surgical Journal* defended a similar policy of the Massachusetts General Hospital:

For our own part we cannot conceive why any one should suppose it an act of *inhumanity* to reject patients of this description. The reception of them into an institution designed for the cure of diseases which are within the power of medical and surgical skill, would be the surest of all modes of defeating the objects of such an establishment.

Both hospitals had only a limited number of free beds. If chronic cases were admitted, MGH attending physician James Jackson argued, these beds would be soon filled and "the hospital would become an asylum for the sick poor, like an almshouse, instead of being a place for the relief of disease."[17]

Similarly, private hospitals sought to admit only the morally worthy. The prostitute and alcoholic like the victim of typhus fever or smallpox (assumed to be contagious) or cancer (acknowledged to be incurable) would be excluded and left to the almshouse, that residuary legatee of a city's misery. Thus lying-in (maternity) patients were often admitted to private charities if married, rebuffed if unwed. Some institutions would admit an unmarried woman with her first pregnancy, but reject her subsequent indiscretions. Such moral strictures could not well be applied to paying patients; the early hospitals were too hard-pressed for income. The Pennsylvania Hospital, for example, would admit incurable cases if they paid their way—and venereal, alcoholic, and contagious cases as well if they could afford care. The rate for smallpox victims was five dollars a week in the 1840s, for venereal and alcoholic cases four dollars.[18]

But no matter how poor they might be, it was hoped that no curable patients of good character need ever find themselves in an almshouse. One of the universal anxieties of respectable Americans throughout the nineteenth century lay in the fear of social decline and the polluting mixture of classes. When the New York Dispensary found itself in need of larger quarters, for example, it could appeal by invoking the vision of its one room, "where those who are still respectable, but by misfortune are reduced to the necessity of asking for relief of this charity, are obliged to mingle with the most loathsome objects of wretchedness."[19] Similar motives lay behind the establishment of New York's Society for the Asylum for Lying-In Women. When the New York Hospital closed its lying-in ward, the society's managers explained:

There now remained no refuge for patients of this class but the Almshouse, where the virtuous and the vicious were indiscriminately treated. The visitors [of the Society] could not conscientiously advise a virtuous wife, to seek a home and companionship among *degraded, unmarried mothers.* And it was found, that, worthy females would suffer want, and even hazard life, before subjecting themselves to such association.[20]

This was a world of social assumption in which the worthy and unworthy were categorically distinct and easily distinguishable.

The admissions process was no simple exercise in differential diagnosis. Nor was it entirely controlled by medical men and medical criteria. Throughout the first half of the nineteenth century, the laymen who bore ultimate legal and moral responsibility for American hospitals sought to maintain practical control of admissions. (This was true of both voluntary and municipal hospitals. In almshouse hospitals, salaried agents of the governing board normally admitted the sick as they did the indigent in general.) Inevitably, particular decisions reflected both medical and social criteria. In the early years of the Massachusetts General Hospital, for example, patients had at first to make written application, then be seen by a physician, then be approved by the visiting committee of the Board of Trustees (who also set an appropriate rate of board in individual cases or secured a local citizen or Massachusetts township as guarantor). Cases of "sudden accident" could be admitted at any time, but even such trauma cases had to be approved retroactively by formal action of the lay board's subcommittee. No physician could unilaterally control access to even the beds he himself attended. Even the eminent Benjamin Rush could assure a friend only that he would appear before the Pennsylvania Hospital's visiting committee and plead the case of a prospective candidate for admission, but he could not simply admit him even though Rush served as an attending physician at the hospital.[21] Significantly, in none of these early nineteenth-century hospitals was there a special place for the examination of prospective patients; the process of admission took place as much in social as in physical space. "A place is required for the reception of persons who wish to enter the hospital—a receiving room," an MGH medical staff committee argued in 1833. Prospective patients "now remain in the apothecary's room to the great inconvenience of those who have duties to perform there; and sometimes also, to the annoyance of the persons themselves who are waiting."[22]

In most cases, voluntary hospital admission reflected the patient's place in a network of deference and social relationships. Membership in a particular church, long service to a particular family, an appropriate demeanor—all served to separate the worthy sheep from the almshouse-bound goats. As late as 1853, for example, a prominent Philadelphia medical man was pleased to recommend a

Mrs. Milne for Pennsylvania Hospital admission. She was the wife of a skillful, but alcoholic, ladies' shoemaker.

I have known Mrs. Milne since four or five years: and she is well known to Mrs. Jackson, my sister Mrs. Henry, to Mrs. [Buckley], and to many other ladies. I believe we can all testify that she is deserving, industrious, well-behaved and respectable.[23]

Especially in the early years of the century such personal ties often dictated admission decisions. In some institutions, no patient could be received without the "recommendation" of a subscriber. In out-patient dispensaries, similarly, a signed certificate from a contributor might be necessary before a poor man could receive medical attention. At the New York Dispensary, for example, annual subscribers of five dollars had the privilege of "recommending" two patients at a time; anyone donating fifty dollars was awarded the privilege for life. No patient was to be treated without a certificate from one such subscriber. Where individual philanthropists supported free inpatient beds, they often retained the right to approve the beds' occupants.[24] Such personal control of access to hospital beds embodied in a concrete way the ties between client and patron fundamental to a deferential and ordered society; the hospital was meant to implement, not supplant, such ties.

But a word of clarification. Lay control of antebellum hospital admissions was never absolute. A medical examination was always required; laymen could not well decide whether a disease was curable or incurable, contagious or noncontagious, or provide a prognosis of its course. Throughout the first half of the century, medical decisions grew increasingly important, and by the time of the Civil War lay control over the number of available free beds served as the most significant everyday constraint within which physicians decided to admit or reject a particular applicant.

From the patient's point of view, admission was quite a different matter. Most prospective patients shared certain of the social attitudes of their betters: accepting any charity was humiliating. Only the destitute and friendless would look to a hospital for relief from pain and want. Few entertained a twentieth-century faith in the necessary efficacy of medicine, while surgery inspired a well-founded horror. Before anesthesia or antisepsis, only trauma, impending blindness, or the excruciating and incapacitating pain of a bladder stone, hernia, or occasional superficial tumor would induce anyone to face the surgeon's knife voluntarily. A chronicler of the Lowell Hospital expressed the attitude of that mill town's operatives when he recalled the

. . . deep and general prejudice prevailing among those who come here for employment, in whose minds the very idea of a hospital has been associated with scenes of anguish and terror; and whose reluctance to become inmates of one is increased by a feeling of independence and a repugnance to submit to such restraint and control as they imagine may be required.[25]

It was not until after midcentury that such prejudices were overcome, the chronicler continued, and even highly contagious cases were often removed from boarding houses only by force. Popular fears of experimentation and the perhaps well-meaning but inexperienced ministrations of youthful house officers helped make the hospital ordinarily more threat than haven to the respectable mechanic or widow.

In a period still dominated by the incursions of acute infectious disease, moreover, many potential patients would die or recover before the hospital could become an option. A disproportionate number of hospital cases were thus chronic or lingering ills—rheumatism, dysentery, bronchitis, heart or kidney ailments. Sufferers from such ailments did not ordinarily die, but neither did they get well. And in many cases even the crude meals and shelter provided by the antebellum hospital were an improvement over the patient's normal environment. Hester Carey, for example, a forty-five-year-old "Maiden Lady," was admitted to the Cincinnati Hospital on April 11, 1838. She had already been treated by a private practitioner for rheumatism and was still troubled by pain and stiffness.

She complains also of a variety of other ailments: weakness in the breast, great palpitations of the heart, on making much exertion, general debility of the system, want of appetite, and costiveness. Gave her cathartic to remove costiveness, and prescribed camphor and opium for rheumatism. . . . Patient left the house about 16th of June very much improved.[26]

Such cases provided the bulk of hospital admissions in antebellum America; both diagnosis and symptom-oriented treatment were typical of the day-to-day routine of hospital medicine (as was the vagueness of criteria for discharge and in this case even the date).

Rest, warmth, and a nourishing diet were fundamental aspects of hospital care—and accepted as such by laymen and physicians alike.

Inevitably, the patient populations at both private and public hospitals had a good deal in common. Suffering from semichronic ills, they tended to remain in the hospital for weeks or months. At the Philadelphia Almshouse, for example, the average length of stay for patients identified in an 1807 census was a year in the general wards, three to five in the "incurable" wards. Of 702 women attended in the lying-in ward at the Pennsylvania Hospital between 1807 and 1831, the average stay was almost fifty-two days; indigence, not difficult pregnancies or deliveries, dictated such extended hospital care. At the Pennsylvania Hospital, a youthful house physician could complain in 1808 that the inpatients were so routine, chronic, and uninteresting that his duties would be intellectually barren without the variety provided by outpatient work. A half century later, MGH house physicians could complain in similar terms of the chronic patients who filled their wards. Experienced hospital physicians contended in the fall of 1834 that the Philadelphia Almshouse was ill-suited to clinical teaching because "few acute cases are introduced into the Almshouse; they are generally old chronic cases, owing to the general disinclination to go to an almshouse."[27]

Thus the patient's hospital experience was determined, first, by his or her location in society, which defined the likelihood of applying for admission; and second, by the natural course of the illness from which he or she suffered. Most patients were simply not that sick; the critically ill could not be kept alive by "extraordinary means" and most antebellum hospital patients were, in fact, not even bedridden. The Inspection Committee at MGH could, for example, report after visiting every patient on October 27, 1826, that they found them all "comfortable not one very sick: Marcus Jones had walked out; and John Battiste gone home." Later in the century, in a similar vein, a Philadelphia General Hospital (PGH) resident could, in describing a typical day, note that "most of the beds are now unoccupied, because many of the patients are convalescent and are out in the yard sitting, smoking, or reading."[28]

This was no acute-care facility. Although it may have meant pain and long-term disability or discomfort, the patient's reality was determined, in addition to those social factors we have discussed, more by his physical sensations and his attitude toward those feelings, than by the intrusions of medicine. Historians have painted a conventional picture of relentless purging and bleeding throughout the antebellum years, of a therapeutics that killed as frequently as it cured. But such views are much exaggerated. There were indeed physicians, in the first quarter of the century especially, who bled aggressively and tinkered ruthlessly with bowels and digestive tracts. Yet such activism was atypical. Hospital records indicate that bleeding was not universally prescribed during most of the antebellum years, but routine only in certain well-demarcated conditions, the first few days of a severe fever, for example. By the late 1830s and 1840s, shifts in therapeutic views pointed toward an ever more lenient regimen: one emphasizing diet, rest, and the healing power of nature in place of the violent purges and emetics that had been more fashionable in the century's first quarter.

Even surgery was limited largely to the setting of fractures, the reducing of dislocations, and, most commonly, the treatment of superficial ulcers and abscesses, conditions not life-threatening but implying lengthy hospitalization. (At PGH in the 1840s, hospital committee minutes indicate that there was always at least one "ulcer ward.") At every institution there were many surgical admissions, but few operations. This pattern was not immediately altered by the availability of anesthesia. In October of 1858, for example, a dozen years after the introduction of ether in 1846, New York Hospital's First Surgical Division saw 109 patients treated but only 8 operations performed. Three of these were for compound fractures of the skull (presumably desperate and perfunctory procedures on moribund accident victims).[29] The management, that is, of most "surgical conditions" was largely expectant, based on diet and rest, the regular changing of dressings, and the healing power of nature.

The relatively brief but highly intrusive surgical procedures that have come to figure so prominently in the twentieth-century hospital were almost unknown. Major operations were infrequent and constituted something of an event—often advertised well ahead of time so that they might be observed by interested students and local practitioners. But even in those cases in which surgery was unavoidable, most respectable Americans preferred to be cared for in their homes (or hotels or boarding houses if they came to the city for treatment) rather than in the hospital. Only the conjunction of poverty with a handful of then-operable surgical conditions defined an individual as an appropriate subject for voluntary surgery in an antebellum hospital. It was only natural that hospital patients in America should have been referred to as boarders and the fees of paying patients as board; it accurately reflected the less than central role of therapeutics in shaping the patients' hospital experience.

The line between sickness and dependency was consistently ill defined. Within the almshouse itself, the vagueness of these categories was exemplified in the loose way in which inmates were shifted from working wards to sick wards "if they were *much* indisposed" and then back, depending both on their health and conditions of crowding in the several areas. Almshouse ward designations reflected ability to work as much as diagnosis (healthy and convalescent inmates were, of course, expected to work, partially to defray the cost of their care, but, even more important, as a deterrent to pauperism). In 1835, for example, Philadelphia's Board of Guardians for the Poor suggested the following arrangement of women's wards in the almshouse:[30]

1. aged and helpless women in bad health
2. aged and helpless women who can sew and knit
3. aged and helpless women who are good sewers
4. spinners

In cases of venereal disease or alcoholism, the line between sickness and dependence was confused by still another variable; here treatment and punishment were also inextricably related. It was only natural that in those hospitals that did treat venereal cases—the females prostitutes and the males ordinarily sailors or laborers—such convalescents should have been expected to work long enough to help pay for their hospitalization. (And, as we have seen, conventional mercury treatment left patients in a painful and debilitated condition.) If admitted as paying patients in voluntary hospitals, venereal cases were frequently charged a higher rate of board; in revealingly parallel incidents at the Massachusetts General and Pennsylvania hospitals, patients originally admitted as venereal had their weekly charges reduced when attending physicians found that they had mistaken their original diagnoses.[31] Alcoholics were treated with a punitiveness similar to that shown sufferers from syphilis and gonorrhea. The managers of the Pennsylvania Hospital, for example, decided that any patient admitted as a consequence of the intemperate use of strong drink should be denied "free intercourse" and the "privileges of the house," including the use of pen and ink and the receiving of visitors without express permission from one of the attending managers or physicians.[32]

Discharge as well as admission reflected social criteria. Again and again authorities complained that they could not in conscience discharge patients without homes to provide care. Occasionally, they paid for the return of convalescents or chronic patients to family or friends away from the city; in other cases, they provided fresh clothing or even small sums of money. In 1828, for example, the MGH Visiting Committee authorized the superintendent to pay the passage of one Eliza Nichols to Salem, "she being about to be discharged well, and being very destitute."[33] In municipal hospitals, of course, the payment of travel costs to recuperating patients seemed no more than prudent; such individuals would then burden the taxpayers of their native town or county were they to fall ill again. The lay managers of both private and public hospitals did not see the inmates of their institutions in narrowly clinical terms, but as social, economic, and, most important, moral beings. Not surprisingly, this broad and intrusively conceived paternalism implied an appropriately hierarchical control of every person within the hospital and of every aspect of its administration.

A Not-So-Ordered Institution

This unified vision could not create a similarly ordered and hierarchical institution. The antebellum hospital's reality defied the neat social and administrative assumptions of its founders. Neither biology nor human nature could so easily be brought to heel. Contemporary prognostic abilities, to cite one example, were hardly adequate to the differentiation of curable and incurable ills. Ultimately, length of stay served in practice to differentiate the chronic from the acute; and just as the almshouse would transfer patients from hospital wards to "outwards," so the voluntary hospital would transfer its incurable or undesirable patients to the almshouse hospital. Contagion too presented a challenge to both benevolence and clinical acumen. Contemporaries agreed that influenza, smallpox, and venereal disease were certainly communicable, typhus and dysentery probably so (especially in crowded circumstances). The dilemma posed by contagion did not end with the process of admission. Fevers and outbreaks of wound infection, childbed fever, and erysipelas might suddenly flare up inside the hospital, even if patients had not exhibited symptoms of contagious ailments when they were admitted. What was to be done with such patients?

Far less dramatic realities presented administrators with a recurring maze of ad hoc decisions. Incurable patients were not to be admitted—but what of the victims of trauma or of sickness too ill to recover but too sick to be turned away? It might seem cruel to dismiss a particularly worthy and grateful older woman even if she had overstayed the statutory limit of residence and no sign of cure had become evident. Rates of pay might have to be adjusted again and again as weeks grew into months, and patients found themselves unable to meet their agreed-upon board bills. Such problems plagued trustees as they sought to balance humanitarianism against available financial resources.

Even in the best run hospitals, chronically straitened budgets dictated that patients would find no frills or luxuries. Early in the nineteenth century especially, crowded rooms and eighteenth-century sensibilities meant that operations would ordinarily be performed in the common ward; similarly, patients might die and be placed in coffins within sight and smell of the surviving patients. Screens to curtain such terminally ill patients seemed a costly innovation in New York Hospital in 1818, and the trustees ignored attending physician David Hosack's request that they be provided. As late as 1859, a Philadelphia Almshouse hospital surgeon could still complain that dead bodies were often left in the wards and placed directly in coffins while the surviving patients looked on. Many contemporaries still saw no need to isolate the reality of working-class death from the presumably blunted sensibilities of working-class life. Examining rooms too were an amenity assumed as necessary only later in the century; the ward remained the center for diagnosis and therapeutics, for every aspect of life and death until the last third of the nineteenth century.[34] Such "luxuries" as tables and stands had also to wait until after the Civil War. At New York Hospital, for example, the few chairs in each ward were used for storing vials, bowls, cups and the like, while hospital sanitation was often a problem both for its inmates and for the institution's unfortunate neighbors. There were rarely proper places to wash and dry bedding in even the best run hospitals. Passersby were assailed not only with the stench from hospital privies, but the sight of tattered sheets and blankets waving from windows and makeshift lines. In 1842, the vestry of Christ Church complained to the New York Hospital's Board of Governors that parishioners going and coming to church on the Sabbath had to pass "sheets in a condition too filthy to be beheld by any one without loathing and disgust."[35] And this was the comparatively well-endowed and responsibly-administered New York Hospital.

Almshouse conditions were far worse. The Charleston almshouse hospital, for example, was beset in the decades before 1861 with a recurring incidence of scurvy, although the dietary origin of that ailment had been known for a century. In the 1840s, a chief resident physician at the Philadelphia Almshouse had complained of enormous overcrowding; there had not been a bed unoccupied for several years, and even with bedsteads filling the corridors, some patients still had to sleep on the floor. Supplies were always inadequate and nurses were forced to tear up threadbare sheets and blankets to serve as bandages.[36]

A Minority of Paying Patients

Not all antebellum hospital patients endured such conditions; the minority of voluntary hospital patients who paid for their "board" lived rather more comfortably. Although it does not fit easily into a traditional view of the early nineteenth-century hospital as refuge for only the most dependent, pay or part-pay patients were always a part of the American hospital. Slim endowments and less than generous state and municipal support made their presence a necessity. The presence of paying patients was in fact the most significant difference between America's private hospitals and their English models and predecessors. In the United Kingdom, patients did not pay in voluntary hospitals (although a small guarantee for possible burial costs might be demanded).[37] Though settled and respectable Americans did not ordinarily patronize hospitals, there were always some potential paying patients in large cities: for example, bachelors, travelers, and merchants without local domestic arrangements. Small shopkeepers and skilled artisans could pay some small amount for board (while their wives or other family members often had to keep working and were thus unable to nurse them). Of 58,508 patients treated at the Pennsylvania Hospital during its first century (1752 to 1854), 24,659 paid all or part of their board.[38] But despite such numbers, the hospital's fundamental paternalism remained unquestioned, for many of these paying patients were either sailors or mental patients, deprived by class or mental condition of truly autonomous status.

A substantial portion of private hospital income throughout the antebellum period came from the board of seamen. As early as 1798, need and English precedent had led to the creation of an insurance fund to underwrite medical care for sailors on American vessels. Merchant seamen were required to contribute twenty cents a month and thus help prepay the costs of possible hospitalization.[39] The collector of the appropriate port arranged for payment with a local hospital, and, though these arrangements were not without friction, they continued through most of the nineteenth century in New York, Philadelphia, and a number of other ports. In New Haven, for example, roughly one-half of the New Haven Hospital's patients between its opening in 1833 and 1850 were merchant seamen paid for by the Collector of the Port of New Haven. At New York Hospital in one typical year, 1845, of $36,865.34 in income, $16,-337.31 was realized from payments for the care of seamen.[40] (In Boston, a marine hospital had been built by the national government before the Massachusetts General Hospital came into existence; thus seamen in the Boston area did not provide a similarly large proportion of private hospital patients.) But sailors were not the most docile of supplicants, and collectors at the various ports tended to be no less intractable in their willingness to provide prompt and adequate payment. Despite the income that it provided, many hospital administrators felt that their role as drydock for incapacitated sailors was far more trouble than it was worth. Although technically classified as paying patients, sailors were not accorded the ordinary pay patient's amenities and respect; the simple fact of third-party payment could not redefine their social identity.

Limited income and a continued marginality to medical care meant that voluntary hospital policies and priorities could change little in the antebellum years. The only major shift came in regard to the insane. Care of the "deranged" was a primary goal in the founding of America's two eighteenth-century hospitals. At the Pennsylvania Hospital, such patients played a prominent role until 1841, when a building to provide care for the insane exclusively was opened in a then bucolic area some miles west of the city. New York Hospital was even less sanguine about the problems created by insane patients in a building dedicated primarily to care of the physically ill. As early as 1808, the Board of Governors constructed a separate building on the hospital's grounds for their "lunatics." This ultimately evolved into a hospital in an entirely different part of the city, the Bloomingdale Asylum.

In the early decades of the nineteenth century, attitudes toward the institutional care of the insane began to shift markedly, and by the mid-1820s, special hospitals had become a much-discussed and increasingly plausible way to deal with this troublesome category of patient. Americans had come to accept the notion that mental patients deserved a very special sort of hospital environment, while decades of experience at the Pennsylvania Hospital had demonstrated how disruptive such patients could be to the routine of a general hospital.[41] The early history of the Massachusetts General Hospital demonstrates this shift in attitude with convenient precision. The earliest appeals for the creation of a general hospital in Boston came immediately before the War of 1812 and emphasized its potential role in caring for the insane. Appeals after the war emphasized that donations for the new institution could be earmarked either for care of the insane or the physically ill, implying that the two tasks were separable.[42] And the psychiatric division of the Massachusetts General, then and now known as the McLean Hospital, was opened not only in a different location, but in 1818, almost four years before the general hospital admitted its first patient. As asylums became more widely accepted in the nineteenth century, care of the insane ceased to be a concern for voluntary hospitals. None of the important private hospitals founded in the decades after the Massachusetts General considered the care of "lunatics" an appropriate concern; indeed, most explicitly placed insanity among those conditions ineligible for admission. It was difficult enough to maintain a due order and healing atmosphere in wards for the indigent sick and injured without the disquieting presence of chronically insane patients.[43]

A Desired Order

Order was a word almost sacred in the terminology of those pious gentlemen who wrote the bylaws, raised the funds, and sat on the boards of America's first hospitals. They regarded all the hospital's inmates as moral minors—the house physicians, nurses, and domestics as well as the patients. Again and again, hospital bylaws casually lumped "patients, servants, and attendants" into the same category, and in almost every case, the particular regulations were aimed at controlling behavior.

The internal routine of both municipal and voluntary hospitals was as paternalistic and ordered as their managers could devise. Spiritual as well as material healing was part of the institution's assumed responsibility. In the New York Hospital, for example, Bibles were placed in every ward. (Though in 1811 the Board of Governor's Visiting Committee found to their dismay that some wards contained no occupant capable of reading them. Undaunted they purchased a dozen copies of Leigh Richmond's didactic *Annals of the Poor* and Richard Baxter's *Call to the Unconverted* to be distributed in each of the wards.)[44] Swearing, cardplaying, drinking, and "impertinence" were typical grounds for discharge in antebellum hospitals. Managers and superintendents fought a similarly ceaseless battle against tobacco. "No smoking," the Commissioners of the Poor House in Charleston warned in their "Rules for Patients," and no "loud talking, boisterous conduct, crowding around the stove, spitting on or defacing the floors shall be allowed." Inmates "without exception" were required to attend "the religious exercises of the House, on Sundays." All lights were to be extinguished in the wards at eight in the winter and nine in the summer. Visitors were carefully regulated. As late as 1868, for example, the Pennsylvania Hospital limited visitors to the hours between twelve and one (except Sundays), while nurses and domestics were to have visitors only between the hours of two and six on Sunday. At New York's Lying-In Asylum, no male visitors at all were to be allowed without the written permission of the board's executive committee.[45] Most hospital and almshouse rules stipulated that all inmates, including, as we have seen, housestaff, nurses, and domestics, request permission for a "pass" when they wished to leave the grounds, even for a few hours. To be an "inmate" was to barter independence for security, to subject oneself to the physical and moral authority of trustees, administrators, and attending physicians.

Convalescent and ambulatory patients were expected to work in the hospital. Male patients at New York's Bellevue helped row the boats that plied between the mainland and the hospitals and prisons on Blackwell's Island. Expectant mothers at Bellevue scrubbed floors within hours of their delivery. At both Blackwell's Island and

Philadelphia's Almshouse hospital, venereal patients were expected to work for a suitable length of time after their recovery so as to repay the costs of their hospitalization. The Philadelphia hospital maintained a punishment cell in which patients could be incarcerated "for cause"—usually intemperance, "eloping," and "fighting." At this and other hospitals, the cells were supplemented by cold showers as punishment for the alcoholic and impertinent. In 1846, for example, the Hospital Committee at Philadelphia's municipal hospital approved that

Caleb Butler be put in the cells on Bread and Water for 48 hours, and soon as the Physician in Chief says his health will permit, he is to receive one shower bath per day for one week, and two shower baths per day for two weeks . . .

Even at the Quaker-dominated New York Hospital, the Board of Governors' inspecting committee found it necessary early in the century to punish intractable patients by transferring them to the lunatic asylum and limiting them to a "low diet."[46] In most hospitals, authorities withheld the patients' clothes so as to control their comings and goings. Discipline was complicated, as we have seen, by the fact that most patients were ambulatory, often egregiously so, in an institution that was as much boarding house and convalescent home as it was a site for treating the acutely ill.

As oppressive as is this picture of energetic and overbearing stewardship, conditions in these institutions seem to have been rather different from those prescribed in hospital bylaws or envisaged by hospital managers. Enforcement was often lax, and throughout the first three-quarters of the nineteenth century, physicians and trustees complained again and again of failures in discipline. Most of these were relatively minor. Patients spat where they were not supposed to, emptied bed pans with casual insouciance. Visitors presented a particularly vexing problem; the patient's friends and family embodied a latent conflict in cultures as they pressed into the ward bearing forbidden fruit and drink. Other infractions could be even more serious. At the New York Hospital, the sailors, paid for by the marine hospital fund, created disturbances when placed among other patients—and brawled and scaled walls for evenings of carousing when housed in their own building. In 1852, for example, the Hospital's Board of Governors voted to fit twenty-four windows in the North (Marine) House with bars in order to foil such escapades. Patients at Philadelphia's Almshouse hospital defied efforts to keep men and women apart, as well as using their windows for the informal disposal of bottles and other "offensive matter."[47] Prostitutes, like sailors, tended to be difficult and outspokenly "ungrateful"; they saw no need to respect the norms of lifestyle and deference assumed by their social superiors.

The persistence of punishment cells and cold showers illustrates an endemic truculence among at least some antebellum hospital patients, as do repeated thefts of food and the smuggling in of alcohol. A black market in whiskey and tobacco flourished in every hospital despite the best efforts of superintendents and governing boards to end it. In particularly egregious cases, the clothing, furniture, and bedding of the hospital itself could serve as trade goods for its more entrepreneurial inmates. There were even more direct ways of avoiding the hospital's oppressive regulations. One was to elope, or in the patronizingly whimsical words of a Cincinnati General Hospital physician, "take French leave," "move the goods," or "give leg bond." In every nineteenth-century hospital, annual statistical compilations included a special category for the eloped just as they did for the "died" and "recovered." Patients sometimes—on occasion defiantly, more often surreptitiously—rejected medicine prescribed by the attending physicians.[48] A passive but final mode of resistance was suicide, a problem that plagued large urban hospitals well into the twentieth century.

But everyday ward realities must have necessarily been more significant than direct resistance in insulating patients from the paternalistic intentions of trustees and attending physicians. Both public and private hospitals seem to have been administered on a day-to-day basis by men and women who failed in some measure to share the moralistic assumptions of those individuals who wrote the formal rules. Moreover, the structure of authority in the hospital was such that no single group defined the environment confronting the patient. There were inevitable conflicts between medical board and lay managers, between physicians and superintendent, between nurses and physicians. Order and a "decent gratitude" might be expected of the dependent patient, but they could hardly be guaranteed in so fragmented an institution.

The hospital staff was organized and recruited in a fashion that implied such diffusion of authority. Most important, nurses and attendants were not professional in the sense we have come to understand the term. In both public and private hospitals they were drawn from among recovered patients or from men and women with some nursing or housekeeping experience outside the hospital. In either case, they represented a social stratum and social experience very different from that of the lay trustees or physicians who nominally controlled the institution.

Despite informal recruitment and training, there was a certain professionalism within the antebellum hospital's workforce, and ward nurses often enjoyed long terms of employment. At the Pennsylvania Hospital, for example, Mary Falconer died in 1805 after having been "3 years a patient, near two years Matron, and about 18 years a nurse in the house." Massachusetts General Hospital wards had by the 1840s come to be called after nurses identified closely with their management; they were Becca Taylor's ward or Miss Styles's, not the first medical or second surgical. In 1871, to cite another example, the medical superintendent at MGH presented the case of Mary Sweetman to the trustees. She had worked in the hospital "for the past thirty-five years and is now broken down by age & infirmities & incapable of longer performing duty here or of doing much toward earning her living."[49] The relatively brief careers of most nurses and attendants only magnified the influence of that minority devoted for decades to the institution. Such men and women were professionals in terms of length of tenure and accumulated skills, but their conception of an appropriate role did not imply a necessarily close identification with medical men and medical ideas.

Servants, attendants, washerwomen, and coachmen all found a place for themselves within the hospital. Almost all lived in and many were paid quarterly; an unquestioning paternalism was assumed, but as in many such relationships the would-be patriarchs were ordinarily far away—either physically or emotionally. Physicians often complained of their inability to control and order servants, even the servants' refusal to sweep floors or make beds when requested. Authorities sometimes complained that a well-understood and intractable underground dominated ward life. As early as 1808, for example, a committee of Philadelphia's Board of Guardians reported that they could no longer tolerate the theft, the smuggling in of whiskey, "drunkenness, elopement and fornication, and the perfectly systematized and good understanding which exists between the persons concerned." A generation later, a spokesman for Sisters of Charity working temporarily in the same almshouse hospital complained that they could no longer work without "protection of their feelings from the rude assaults of such persons as are necessarily in . . . [the] institution, and regard it as their own."[50] Such a state of things was not limited to municipal hospitals. The house physicians at the Massachusetts General Hospital in 1857 complained formally of the seeming disorganization that they encountered in the wards. "The servants clan together," as one put it, "and are not in subjection" to the steward. "There is no system or order & no one knows precisely his duty or keeps to it." When we learn from the parallel testimony of another resident that the hospital employed "a brother & 3 sisters, a father 2 sons a daughter, & several brothers & sisters," we can only assume that there was indeed a well-defined order in the hospital, but one for which the ambitious young physician felt neither empathy nor understanding.[51] Thus, at least two subcultures coexisted within the hospital: that of the patients and attendants who cared for them, on the one hand, and that of the hospital's lay trustees, medical staff, and superintendent.

Class lines did not end at the gatekeeper's box. A revealing aspect of the voluntary hospital throughout the nineteenth and into the twentieth centuries were the distinctions between paying and free patients. In all private hospitals in the antebellum years and in some until the twentieth century, paying patients might bring their own servants (causing occasional problems with regard to hospital discipline. Would a private patient's servants obey the superintendent? Or would they be paid more than the hospital's regular attendants and thus arouse jealousy?). Paying patients were not called upon to perform the cleaning and nursing demanded of free patients, nor were they exposed to the eyes and hands of medical students as "clinical material." Private patients might supplement their diet with wines and other delicacies. Even medical treatment was to some extent shaped by class identity. Reformer Elizabeth Blackwell could, for example, write enthusiastically about her sister's growing mastery of surgery—emphasizing that Emily would soon perform her first operation on a private patient.[52] Though the limited number of private patients (exclusive of sailors and the insane) made such distinctions in some ways marginal to the experience of the great majority of nineteenth-century hospital patients, they do underline the ways in which a hospital's daily routine reflected the more general social relationships that characterized the world outside its walls.

Society reconstructed itself within the hospital, mirroring in microcosm those values and relationships that prevailed outside its small stage. Education, piety, genteel dress and diction brought appropriate respect; venereal disease, alcoholism, and low ethnic status brought a parallel disdain. Blacks probably fared worst. Wherever numbers made it possible, they were segregated and routinely placed in the hospital's least desirable location: attics and basements were favored. At the Philadelphia Almshouse in 1846, for example, when more space was needed for lunatics, the black male medical ward was appropriated and its inhabitants moved to the attic.[53] A similar disdain shaped the treatment of alcoholic and venereal patients, sufferers from conditions at once ailment and manifestation of moral incapacity. Venereal patients were, as we have seen, routinely charged more than other private patients. The New York Hospital only accepted male venereal patients, since it was assumed that female sufferers would necessarily be prostitutes. In antebellum Charleston, even the municipal almshouse demanded a guarantee of payment from brothel inmates or their employers. Attending physicians at the New York Hospital were chronically unwilling to visit certain wards, particularly the black and venereal. At the Pennsylvania Hospital, blacks and patients suffering from "a certain disease" were housed in a small structure separate from the main building.[54]

Ironic as it may seem, the gap between social classes must to some degree have protected the patient in his or her autonomy, especially in hospitals in which the ratio of middle-class emissaries to the hospital's inmates was always small. Even nurses and attendants were few in number, and, as we have seen, they occupied a marginal status somewhere between that of patient and employee. Philadelphia's Almshouse was atypically understaffed, but in the 1820s enjoyed an attendant to patient ratio of roughly one to seventy-five. At night, even the normally tenuous structure of authority disappeared. Nursing was a 5:00 A.M. to 9:00 P.M. occupation, and "watchers" were engaged to oversee only the critically ill at night. Convalescent patients normally cared for their more seriously ill brethren after dark. At the Pennsylvania Hospital, medicines were to be administered by the night watchman if required, but his duties were prudently limited to the male wards.[55]

The hospital's medical staff also played a small role in enforcing a rigid order. House physicians, young men who lived in the hospital and provided the great bulk of daily care, began their terms of residency with little clinical experience or status. On the other hand, the prestigious attending physicians who often served long terms appeared infrequently—to admit patients, oversee an occasional difficult case, or to teach during the brief medical school year. In those few hours they could exert comparatively small influence on the hospital's internal environment. Throughout the nineteenth century, moreover, attending physicians and surgeons rotated responsibilities, with three- or four-month periods of duty diluting still further the attending physician's potential influence. Resident physicians came and went, attending physicians stayed but infrequently visited; ward nurses, the Mary Falconers and Becca Taylors, endured.

Still another characteristic of the medical staff minimized their impact on the hospital's internal life. The recruitment of hospital physicians in the first three-quarters of the century guaranteed a maximum social distance between doctor and patient. Hospital staff positions were only for the ambitious and economically secure. Those young "medical gentlemen" successful in their quest for a resident physicianship tended to see hospital patients in terms of aversion or condescension. The attitude of house physicians veered between the sentimental depiction of an occasional winsome lily, sullied by the soot of the venereal ward or a genteel maiden lady or governess sunken in fortune—to a visceral revulsion at the "brutes" kenneled when healthy in the city's slums and when sick in the hospital's wards. The house physician's contacts with his ward patients might often be characterized by a casual brutality, but its casualness was as significant as the brutality. Nevertheless, American physicians often recoiled from the far greater degree of inhumanity that characterized doctor-patient interactions in old world hospitals. "For brutality I do not think his equal can be found," a young Bostonian wrote of one of Paris's leading clinicians in 1832. "If his orders are not immediately obeyed, he makes nothing of striking his patient and abusing him harshly. A favorite practice of his is to make a handle of a man's nose, seizing him by it and pulling him down on his knees."[56]

Ethnic and religious differences between physician and patient also widened the social distance that separated them. For example, the patient population at the Philadelphia Almshouse in 1807 was over 50 percent foreign-born, more than half of them Irish. At New York's Almshouse in 1796, of 622 inmates only 102 were American-born. By the early 1840s—before the height of the famine emigration from Ireland—the Irish rivaled the native-born in numbers even at the conservative and Quaker-dominated Pennsylvania Hospital.[57] With the mid–1840s and 1850s the rapidly growing number of poverty-stricken immigrants created something approaching a crisis in American hospitals. In 1840–1841, 46 percent of those admitted to the Philadelphia Almshouse were born abroad, while in 1850–1851, the percentage rose to 68; of these almost three-quarters were Irish. At New York's Ophthalmic Hospital in 1854, 686 patients had been born in Ireland and only 373 in the United States (the latter figure included the children of such immigrants). In the same year, New York City Alms-House Commissioners treated a large number of cholera victims during an epidemic; three-quarters of the patients were foreign-born, 77 percent of them in Ireland. A Brahmin trustee, alarmed at the numbers of Irish laborers treated at the MGH in 1851, suggested that it might be advisable to construct a "cheap building" or rent one in the vicinity of the hospital in which these ignorant foreigners might be treated. "They cannot appreciate," he explained, "& do not really want, some of those conveniences which would be deemed essential by most of our native citizens." In the same year, the Governors of the New York Hospital barred priests from routine visiting when, as diocesan protests emphasized, the great majority of its patients were Catholic.[58]

More general social assumptions were reaffirmed within the hospital on the administrative level as well. As the lay trustees viewed the institution, it was to be defined by a due order, and the only appropriate model for the internal life of such institutions was the family writ large. The superintendent or steward was the father of this extended family; the trustees exerted their legal authority through him. He was responsible for purchasing, for discipline, for hiring and firing within the "house" he administered. The terms "house" and "family" were thought of as only in part metaphorical. The resident physicians and apothecary ate at the superintendent's table, while his wife normally served as matron in particular charge of the women's wards and such "female departments" as cleaning and laundry. The qualities desired in an antebellum hospital superintendent were neither hospital experience nor medical training, but rather the prudence, responsibility, and piety one might hope for in a business partner or vestryman. It was expected throughout the nineteenth century that the superintendent would live, with his wife and children if any, in the hospital and eat every meal with his house staff and apothecary. When the trustees sought to fill vacant superintendentships, recommendations of wife as well as husband were solicited, for she too bore an appropriate responsibility for maintaining the institution's moral health. The superintendent and his immediate family represented virtue and prudence in an otherwise alien environment—an ambassador from an ordered world to a culture ominously different. Like a good father, the superintendent was expected to assume personal responsibility for the physical and moral condition of his charges. Ironically, of course, the more earnestly he functioned as patriarch, the more intrusive he must have seemed to patients and nurses as he made his daily way through the wards.

The Ward Perceived

Normally, of course, historians can only extrapolate the feelings of ordinary men and women in the past. We have comparatively little evidence bearing directly on the antebellum hospital patients' felt experience; they were rarely consulted during their lives and remain generally mute to the historian. We can only infer the way in which the routine of a particular ward impinged on the individuals residing in it. However, the diary of at least one such American has survived. John Duffe, a ward nurse and almost certainly one-time sailor and patient in New York Hospital's Marine House, kept a journal during 1844. It provides at least one fragment of perceived ward experience.[59]

Duffe had few illusions and less patience for the benevolent paternalism of his betters. Charles Starr, the hospital's superintendent, did indeed inspect Duffe's ward each day, but hardly endeared himself to the objects of his paternal concern. Duffe was only too pleased on those days when Starr "went off without growling."[60] The superintendent's relentless evangelicalism seemed mere hypocrisy to the Catholic nurse. When indignant at the rotten butter served up to the nurses and patients, Duffe felt it

useless to complain because if we do it may irritate the religious feelings of our superintendent and he will soon point out the way to the gate. There is one thing that we have to complain of and that is the table for if putrefied vituels be injurious to the stomac I am shure we will soon be all rotton for our butter is rotton and stinks worse than a Sconk but it must be borne with for like everything else if we complain our godly Superintendent will tell us you may consider yourself discharged for the Lord sent it and you must eat it you hireling.[61]

The ex-sailor had as little faith in the character and intentions of the visiting physicians, arrogant demigods who demanded immediate and total attention as they swept into each ward. On one occasion, for example, visiting physician John Watson flew into a rage when he entered the ward and Duffe was away

because he had no water soap nor towel to all of which house surgeons offered to help him but he declined thretening the nurse with dismissal in case he should not soil his unmentionables sooner than be absent again when the knight of the lancet was again on his rounds.[62]

At the same time, Duffe entertained few illusions in regard to patients and fellow nurses. Theft and dissimulation were everywhere. One nurse had a watch stolen from a nail at the head of his bed, while furniture and bedding were constantly disappearing. And though most of his patients were genuinely ill, others were, as Duffe called them, victims of acute "Shamaticks."

What is most striking, however, are the length and diversity of Duffe's duties. He was an experienced dresser of wounds and infections, and administered countless baths and enemas. At the same time, and with occasional help from the healthier patients, he scrubbed the floors, washed the sheets, fetched dinner for the men on the ward. And until the hospital arranged to have the city's new water supply introduced in pipes throughout the building, much of his work consisted of "carrying and luging (sic) of Slops and all kinds of filth and dirt." On those rare days when he received "liberty," Duffe had to find a patient healthy and reliable enough to substitute for him. "So ends this days work," he noted at the close of one long day, "for work we may call it without end."[63]

To visitors from the world of middle-class order, Duffe's little world seemed altogether different. To the handful of respectable laymen who entered America's antebellum hospitals as administrators or chaplains in these years it remained—as it had been for Ezra Stiles Ely at the beginning of the century—a moral desert. In addition to the chance existence and even more unlikely survival of John Duffe's diary, we have, coincidentally, a journal kept by the same hospital's chaplain seven years earlier, from 1837–1838.

John Moffett Howe was a zealous young evangelical, and 1837 marked the height of a particularly widespread and deeply felt period of revivalism. Howe was enthusiastic at the prospect of redeeming the souls of those sick and dying in the New York Hospital's wards, indeed so enthusiastic that he was warned by a representative of the Board of Governors as he received his appointment not to "be too religious—don't be bigoted—nor sectarian—have charity for all."[64]

Howe was appalled by the misery and spiritual desolation he encountered. "Like brutes they live," he confided to his diary, "like brutes they die." Much of this brutishness was exemplified in the "mummery" and superstition that enveloped the Hospital's Catholic patients. "Hardened infidels," he described them, "despisers of the Bible—of the means of grace."[65] Extreme unction epitomized the spiritual deadness of Romanist practice and the frustration facing the young clergyman; impending death provided both dramatic structure and spiritual opportunity, yet it was opportunity that Howe could seize only rarely. Few of the dying or acutely ill rejected their Catholicism; they were supported in their faith by fellow patients who, as even Howe conceded, nursed and comforted them. A German woman was brought into the hospital in a feverish delirium, for example, and was soon attended by a priest her fellow patients summoned.

. . . although as insensible as a block he administered to her the Sacrament of the Lord's supper—The other Catholic women kneeling about the bedsides—with all apparent devotion—The Priest dressed in his cassoc on ground—The cerimony was imposing—but perfectly uninteligable to the ignorant attendants & to the insane dying woman.[66]

And if many of the patients were well enough to walk about, fetch their own meals, and nurse their sicker wardmates, others like the woman near death with fever were in agony for days. Howe described another German woman in such pain that she tried to commit suicide by choking herself with a handkerchief.[67]

Yet even among the scenes of torment and spiritual disarray, the young clergyman could find a consolatory moral order. The superintendent of the hospital, he noted with satisfaction, was one of the kindest of men, "he may in fact be said to be but the father of this large family."[68] More significant was the ultimate moral logic implicit in the particular instances of sickness and death he witnessed.

"All the diseases, or Nine out of 10," he observed, "are produced by bad habits—or rum. This is the opinion of the clerk of the house—nay more . . . if *rum* was put away & men would be correct in their ways you might shut up the house & the Physicians would have nothing to do." Illness and accident were always revelatory of more fundamental realities. When a nine-year-old was crushed by an iron gate on the Sabbath, Howe reflected that it would not have happened had the child been at Sabbath School: "let children who play truant or profane the Sabbath take warning."[69]

Physicians in the 1830s might seek to redefine their conceptions of disease and arrive at an understanding of the pathological mechanisms associated with its various manifestations, but to most Americans its meaning had still to be sought in another realm. Like the assumptions of social responsibility and hierarchy that informed the actions of trustees and philanthropic supporters, these ideas long antedated the nineteenth century. They would not be easily discarded.

CHAPTER 2

Vocation and Stewardship: Inconsistent Visions

Both physicians and trustees saw the hospital in similar terms; its wards were dominated by people and behaviors alien and unsettling. But if trustees and their medical staff agreed on matters of class definition and the social styles appropriate to those definitions, they often disagreed in other areas. Most such disputes grew out of the physicians' professional needs. Autopsy and teaching privileges and the control of admission and discharge all occasioned recurrent conflict. Ordinarily, such differences remained potential, for the antebellum hospital was characterized by a sharing of authority between laymen and physicians that tended to circumvent open antagonism.

This equilibrium was not to outlast the nineteenth century. By 1900, the needs and perceptions of the medical profession had come to dominate the hospital, as the hospital was itself coming to play a gradually more prominent role in the provision of medical care. The roots of these developments were evident much earlier. America's hospitals had played a central role in the careers of ambitious urban physicians since the end of the eighteenth century. By 1850 America's larger hospitals had already created forerunners of our familiar internship and residency programs. An elite antebellum physician would have become acquainted with the hospital even before graduation from medical school. In all likelihood, he would have first been a private student of an attending or resident physician, then served as house officer, then perhaps substituted for an attending or outpatient physician. The pinnacle of medical accomplishment lay in obtaining an attending physicianship, with its prestige and prerogatives. But such positions, however, were to be enjoyed by only a comparative handful of the most accomplished and well connected. The path to professional eminence was clearly marked—yet only a few were equipped to set out upon it.

A Goodly Stewardship

Although we tend to see the hospital as an institution structured by medical priorities and defined by medical needs, this conception is inappropriate to the reality of American hospitals through most of the nineteenth century. At no time during the century was the institution dominated by one group or one point of view. It was a creature neither of physicians nor of laymen. Medical men, as we have seen, had played a key organizing role in the founding of America's first hospitals and dispensaries. And lay trustees, though they often opposed specific requests by medical staff members for teaching privileges, always conceded a general legitimacy to the claims of medical education. Yet throughout the late eighteenth and nineteenth centuries, lay authorities maintained a careful day-to-day control over hospital policy and personnel. Or at least they always sought such control; to do less would have been a denial of their responsibility as stewards of society's wealth. Through this day-to-day commitment, community values played a prominent role in shaping hospital realities. In the late twentieth century, the term "community control" has assumed a specialized political meaning—that of power to the potential users of a particular institution. The lay trustees of our early hospitals were not potential patients. Nevertheless, their attitudes toward social responsibility demanded and structured a role for community norms in the hospital. In both public and private institutions, lay managers felt no temptation to subordinate their sense of personal accountability to medical authority. Christianity and the imperatives of traditional stewardship, not the values of the medical profession, often determined particular hospital policies. When, for example, in 1846, the Massachusetts General Hospital attending physicians urged the erection of a medical college in the hospital's vicinity, the trustees stated flatly "that they cannot perceive any advantage to this institution to arise therefrom."[1] Hospital practice, as the New York Hospital Board of Governors put it in 1820, should be conducive to the promotion of medical science, but only in accordance with due economy and only insofar as consistent with their primary responsibility—promotion of their patients' comfort and cure.[2]

Perhaps the most helpful way of looking at authority within the antebellum hospital is to imagine a division of responsibility between trustees and administrators, between laymen and physicians. Occasional conflict was inevitable, given differing lay and medical notions of an appropriate division of responsibility. The resulting differences must not be seen as simply a series of trivial squabbles over power and prerogative—they were conflicts between world views. In most respects, physicians' attitudes were no different from those of laymen who served on hospital boards of trustees or those less secure members of the middle class who served as hospital stewards or superintendents (and their wives as matrons). All were drawn from a similar social background and often shared religious as well as class identity. But as members of a profession, staff physicians had assimilated peculiar values, peculiar ways of behaving, and peculiar tactics for achieving status within the profession.

One kind of conflict arose out of the very smallness of the antebellum hospital in conjunction with the paternalism of the lay trustees. No detail of hospital routine was too trivial an object for their concern. Subcommittees chosen on a rotating basis from among the board members provided the accepted mode of structuring this meticulous supervision. The New York Hospital, for example, had two such committees, a "visiting committee" entrusted with overseeing admissions and discharges and an "inspecting committee" charged with touring the hospital at least once a week and seeing that "a proper economy" was observed, that the floors were scrubbed and the walls whitewashed, that the nurses and matron treated the patients with kindness. At the Charleston Almshouse, the city's Commissioners for the Poor chose a subcommittee to visit at least twice a week and report "any disobedience, immorality or irregularity" to the full board. Trustees at the Massachusetts General Hospital voted that their rounds be made unaccompanied by medical staff so that patients and nurses could express possible grievances.[3]

Trustees took their work seriously indeed. H. I. Bowditch could, for example, boast in 1851 that as a group the Massachusetts General Hospital's attending managers had missed only twelve meetings since the opening of the hospital in 1821. Pennsylvania Hospital's Board of Managers imposed fines of fifty cents for absence or twenty-five cents for lateness. Visiting committee minute books preserved at both New York Hospital and Massachusetts General Hospital (MGH) underline the care with which trustee responsibilities were carried out; in the hospital's early years, for example, MGH visiting committee members would excuse themselves for not having called on particular patients—perhaps because they were bathing, or "abroad" on a pass; in one case because a female patient's case was of a "delicate nature."[4] At the same time, it will be recalled, the visiting committee had to approve each admission and ascertain possible means of payment or approve the extended stay of particularly worthy patients. The most frequent reason for refusing a certificate of admission was "no free bed." Other applicants were refused as incurable (and referred to the Overseers of the Poor) or simply "unfit," and some as sufferers from delirium tremens, epilepsy, or paralysis. One applicant was categorized as "unfit in consequence of leaving house against the advice of surgeon & now applying for free bed."[5]

At the New York Hospital, similarly, members of the inspecting committee were assiduous in carrying out those inspections during the institution's early years: inquiring as to the cleanliness of blankets and bedding, sampling the bread, noting leaks, urging that male and female patients have separate privies, checking as to the regular attendance of physicians and surgeons, even disciplining individual patients guilty of impertinence, profanity, and drunkenness.[6]

In exchange for this personal solicitude, the managers expected an appropriate deference. The visiting committee at New York's Asylum for Lying-in-Women could describe a Mrs. Wilson with enthusiasm. Frail and unable to leave her bed five weeks after confinement, she still retained

the same grateful patient character. In speaking of her mercies, she expresses herself thus. "I have everything earth can give to make me comfortable." Such an instance of patience under suffering, and of gratitude to all around her; connected with such abject indigence, will, I think, stimulate every member of this board to double their exertions to promote the interests of the institution.

The trustees expected, and in at least some cases received, an appropriately Christian and deferential version of suffering on the ward.

"Many a lesson of patient endurance," H. I. Bowditch wrote of his visits to the Massachusetts General, where he served for so many years as trustee, "may be learned at our visits. Many a bright version recurs to my imagination of sufferers who, by their truly Christian resignation and fortitude . . . warmly enlisted the sympathy and regard of all who saw them."[7] It was just such pious sufferers who might attract the continued patronage of individual trustees.

This sense of personal involvement was strengthened by the long terms of service that characterized board membership in the nineteenth century. Samuel Coates's forty-year tenure (1785–1825) at the Pennsylvania Hospital was an extreme example of such lengthy service, but not entirely atypical. In 1857, for example, George Newbold and Benjamin Swan retired from New York Hospital's Board of Governors: Newbold after forty-eight years on the board and having served as its president for twenty-four; Benjamin Swan after thirty years of membership. These were men who worked hard to be worthy stewards and did not easily delegate responsibility.[8]

And when they did, of course, it was to men whose ideas and social background were, insofar as possible, like their own. The antebellum hospital superintendent had not emerged from some professional training program in hospital administration; ordinarily he had had no training at all in hospital work. Prospective administrators were men of business and piety. Letters of recommendation refer to their moral and religious virtues and to the estimable qualities of their wives (and hospital matrons presumptive). "I feel assured that this lady is regarded with much esteem," a letter of endorsement for the prospective superintendent of the Massachusetts General Hospital described the applicant's wife in 1825. "She is in reputation for prudence, activity, industry and intelligence. Her disposition is amiable, her deportment conciliating, her acquirements solid and useful."[9] Such virtues were indispensable if the superintendent and his wife were to serve as father and mother to the hospital's ill-assorted family. Antebellum hospital administrators clearly owed no loyalty to a "profession" or to other men who happened to occupy similar positions; instead, their allegiance lay with the particular trustees who had appointed them and to the values they shared. Neither superintendent nor trustee would have felt morally secure in delegating administrative responsibility to medical men exclusively. They assumed, indeed, that conflict might arise between attending physicians who acted and felt as medical men and the interests of patients and lay administrators. It was only natural that many hospitals refused to allow medical men to sit on their governing boards.

Physicians, of course, had a rather different set of priorities, yet priorities clothed with a moral urgency equaling that which shaped the decisions of their lay coworkers. Thus, medical needs might not only clash with the trustees' desire for personal control, but with their sense of what constituted an appropriate stewardship. Such conflicts appeared and reappeared in a number of predictable areas: conditions of medical teaching and student access to patients, admissions procedures, control of autopsy policies, staff discipline and performance, and even disagreement over seemingly technical aspects of therapeutic practice.

The most frequent conflicts developed and reenacted themselves over medical education and its impact on patient care and patient dignity. Trustees of both private and municipal hospitals objected repeatedly to an excessive amount of student contact with patients. When the Massachusetts General Hospital sought in 1824 to attract students, it warned that they could be admitted to its wards only with the understanding that they "carefully abstain from any gesture or remark which may tend to alarm the sick." Students could examine patients only with specific authorization from the attending surgeon or physician. "It is obvious that the greatest inconvenience must arise, if such examinations are commonly made by the pupils." Philadelphia's Board of Guardians of the Poor endorsed a similar principle in 1845. "There are rights possessed even by the recipients of charity," they emphasized, "which should be guarded, and feelings which should be respected." No patient was "to be presented to the class against his or her consent." And in every hospital, contemporary mores made administrators particularly wary of young physicians or students being present when "examination of females of a private character are made."[10]

Trustees sought to shield not only individual patients within the hospital, but, equally important, that larger group of fearful patients outside it. The nineteenth-century hospital never ceased to be a source of anxiety to its prospective clients. The very youth of students and housestaff aroused suspicion in a period when lay expectations included white hair and a suitable air of gravity. "None of them 'ere assistants should ever practice on him," one truculent patient vowed. Even more alarming to ordinary working men and their wives were age-old fears of therapeutic experimentation, the conviction that charity patients would pay with their bodies for the board and care they received. Such worries had constantly to be allayed. An evil-minded physician, the trustees of the Massachusetts General Hospital soothed fellow Bostonians in 1822, would hardly plan to experiment upon patients in a hospital where he would be scrutinized by other physicians and a visiting committee that examined each patient once a week: "It is not reasonable to suppose that a public Hospital would be selected for these wicked and inhuman practices." Neither patients, nor trustees, nor the majority of practitioners were ready to accept the academic physician's view that every treatment was in some measure experimental, but a necessary experiment while medicine's therapeutic understanding remained inadequate.[11]

Yet, despite such popular qualms, all of America's antebellum hospitals tolerated clinical teaching—limited and unsatisfactory as such opportunities may have seemed to many physicians. The relationship, in other words, between lay and medical authority was complex. Lay trustees at all the hospitals felt called upon to circumscribe teaching, although they rarely challenged the need for clinical instruction in the abstract. Physicians could even less plausibly question the authority of lay trustees, but nevertheless sought ever-expanded teaching opportunities. Thus, the recurrent quibbles over the number of students to be admitted to the ward, their bearing and decorum while in the hospital, and the right of patients to refuse to serve as "clinical material."

The seemingly logical connection between medical school teaching and clinical appointments in hospitals was never accepted by nineteenth-century trustees. They were jealous of their appointment powers, and thus another conflict endemic to hospitals inevitably acted itself out. Without a hospital position, a medical school professor could not lecture in its amphitheater or demonstrate cases on its wards. Some hospitals and medical schools did have special relationships (Harvard and the Massachusetts General Hospital, the Pennsylvania Hospital and the University of Pennsylvania), but even here conflicts over appointments might arise. The fact that a man had been appointed professor in a medical school did not, trustees emphasized, create any obligation on their part to parallel that appointment with one as attending physician. And if trustees felt it inappropriate to have choices dictated to them, physicians in turn made it increasingly clear that they considered it inappropriate that laymen hold so much power over professional matters.[12]

Controlling senior attending physicians was never an easy task. Throughout the nineteenth century, for example, such medical eminences proved themselves often unreliable in attendance. It was difficult, however, for trustees to enforce punctuality on senior physicians; as if to make up for this failure of discipline, trustees sought all the more energetically to control the behavior of those fledgling practitioners who served as resident house staff. In their unquestioned view of themselves as stewards of an institution populated and staffed by moral and economic minors, lay trustees felt strongly that young physicians must submit to their authority. This meant in practice that house officers had, like patients, and orderlies, to accept the routine surveillance of a lay superintendent, ask permission to leave the hospital, and observe bylaws that forbade drinking, gambling, smoking, or socializing with female nurses. Not surprisingly, young men of twenty or twenty-one found such restraints confining and squabbled with superintendents, matrons, or ward nurses. Often they resented being forced to eat with the superintendent's "family." In other cases, conflict arose over the desires of house officers to play cards, drink, or fraternize with an occasional nurse or patient. Groups of high-spirited medical students could also irritate the trustees' paternalistic sensibilities. In 1806, the entire University of Pennsylvania medical school class protested a series of trustee reprimands implying, as they put it, "that the Managers suppose . . . blackguard and medical student synonymous terms." House pupils at the Medical College of Virginia's dispensary in 1860 were similarly indignant when new rules specified that alcohol be kept under lock and key, to be doled out only by the janitor.[13] When conflict arose between physicians and lay antagonists, moreover, the reaction of trustees was often to chastise the medical men.

Even therapeutics might serve as an occasion of disagreement between lay and medical authority. Although trustees did not ordinarily presume to judge the effectiveness of particular drugs or surgical procedures, they felt it entirely within their competence to evaluate the economic and moral aspects of the physician's accustomed practice. A particularly long-standing conflict developed, for example, around the traditional medical reliance on alcohol as a stimulant and tonic. From the 1820s until the end of the century, hospital physicians had to withstand a sometimes vigorous opposition to their routine therapeutic use of alcoholic beverages—if alcohol was so destructive to man's health, the argument followed, how could it help restore that health once impaired. The evangelicalism of the 1820s and 1830s only reinforced the urgency that impelled activist laymen to banish rum from the hospital.

Economic considerations, however, more frequently than temperance qualms led to the questioning of therapeutic practice. Outpatient physicians were routinely limited to a handful of specified drugs (and on occasion warned that they must write no more than one prescription per case). In several antebellum institutions, physicians were warned against the use of costly leeches to draw blood; the lancet had served well enough in the past. At other times, lay committees approved lists of drugs to be made available in hospital dispensary practice. "The strictest economy is to be recommended," the managers of the Boston Dispensary warned their volunteer physicians in 1812, "in the distribution of Medicines and Wine; one quart only of the latter shall be ordered at one time and that to be Lisbon or Sherry, or some other not exceeding their value. Port may sometimes be directed if thought to be peculiarly beneficial; giving preference to the cheapest will suit the case."[14] At midcentury such watchdog committees often questioned an increasingly lavish use of beef tea and other dietary supplements. For example, a subcommittee of New York Hospital's Board of Governors in 1845 deplored the use of "very expensive medicine & in quantities which have not been used—and a prodigal use of Lint & Leeches." They did not, the report concluded, "intend to cast . . . censure upon the Resident Physicians & Surgeons. Ardent young men," it seemed, "in the pursuit of Science are not likely to be very careful of expenditure."[15] New and costly drugs could alarm frugal laymen, despite the medical man's conviction that they were demanded by contemporary knowledge. "Allow me to say," a physician at the Charleston Almshouse protested when criticized for the extravagant use of such newly fashionable remedies as cod liver oil and silver nitrate,

that as chemistry progressively invents, & therapeutics determine their remedial value, so must the Phys. avail himself of them. Most of these articles, but little used in former years, possess virtues, but recently discovered, for instance chloroform.[16]

This was 1853. Such arguments were to become increasingly commonplace in the next half century as medicine's technical resources grew more varied, more expensive, and more efficacious.

Trustees were always careful to assert their ultimate authority whenever it was explicitly questioned. In 1852, for example, the "house pupils" at the Massachusetts General Hospital complained that one of their number had been charged by a trustee with the "careless and unprofessional" use of a catheter. The young medical men were indignant; it did not seem right that they should be subordinate to laymen in matters purely clinical. The board, on the other hand, was categorical in affirming its ultimate authority. "In matters purely medical or surgical," the trustees conceded, they relied on

. . . the ability and discretion of Gentlemen selected by themselves, and would not think of interfering with their prescriptions or practice. But should a specific charge be made against any Physician or Surgeon, either of a want of competency or skill, or of humanity or delicacy in the treatment of a patient, the Trustees would feel it to be not only their right but their duty to investigate the circumstances of the case and to act as in their opinion should be required by due regard to the interests of the Institution and of the Community. So likewise the Trustees will not interfere with the professional duties prescribed to medical and surgical pupils by their immediate superiors, but will, nevertheless, at all times, hold them accountable for the performance of those duties in an exact, kind and proper manner.

The board concluded by "expressing their surprise" at the original question: "an inquiry which would seem to be founded on an entire misapprehension of [the house pupils'] own true position and an unwillingness to recognize the paramount authority of this Board."[17]

Less significant in terms of the hospital's day-to-day realities, but nevertheless revealing as to its fundamental attitudes, were sporadic clashes in regard to postmortem and autopsy policies. Throughout the century physicians sought liberal autopsy privileges, ones that would allow the performance of postmortems in ambiguous or interesting cases. Trustees sought to enforce regulations that would minimize the possibility of offending the late patient's family—and thus the community generally. Their primary responsibility, as lay trustees understood it, was to provide medical care for a particular constituency. Popular fears that the hospital was a place where patients would be experimented upon while alive and dissected after death obviously interfered with the carrying out of that responsibility. As late as 1872, a trustee's committee at the Massachusetts General Hospital explained that

The trustees are to consider that their special duty is to make the Hospital useful to the greatest possible number of patients, as a curative establishment. This duty is paramount to the duty of making it subserve scientific purposes: and they must therefore remove from the popular mind all apprehensions which may deter persons from entering its wards.[18]

Physicians, on the other hand, contended that the advancement of medical knowledge justified the occasional inconvenience of a particular patient's family. Such arguments recurred periodically throughout the history of every large and important American hospital. Although circumstances might differ, the conflict itself remained essentially unchanged, for it reflected fundamental differences between lay and medical perceptions. The medical ethos dictated a vision fixed inward toward the body as mechanism and toward the ideas and collective opinion of the profession; lay attitudes looked outward toward the place that the body had occupied in a particular society. Yet physicians at the same time assumed that they spoke to an even larger community, that of the world of medicine and, through it, to all those who might ultimately benefit from improvements in medical understanding.

Significantly, the arguments of physicians who sought unfettered access to patients for teaching were strikingly similar to those justifying demands for liberal autopsy regulations. The particular patient, they emphasized, was not as important as the lessons his illness might impart to student physicians. The momentary discomfort of an individual was a small price to pay for the increased clinical competence that a whole class of students might later apply in practice (often, it was contended, in rural areas where opportunity for observing "obscure" cases was infrequent). J. C. Warren, pillar of the Massachusetts General Hospital attending staff, explained this deeply felt medical assumption in 1845:

Medical treatment at the hospital alleviates the sufferings of some one or two hundreds of persons who, from year to year, resort to its wards, but the advancement of medical science confers important benefits upon the community at large, and every individual, throughout the extent of our land, who becomes the victim of disease or accident, directly participates in them.[19]

Thus stated, the benefits of clinical teaching far outweighed any immediate discomfort it might create. Self-serving as such arguments may appear, they were nevertheless rooted in a fundamental distinction between the motivating imperatives of medicine and those of society generally. Both laymen and physicians saw their particular attitudes as morally compelling, and the very tenacity of their convictions guaranteed that neither view would entirely dominate the nineteenth-century hospital.

Advantages of Place

To most trustees the hospital was one among many concerns—a challenge to their benevolence and stewardship, but ordinarily less absorbing than business activities or legal practice. To the physicians who practiced in its wards, however, the hospital was a fundamental aspect of their "business." It was only natural that ambitious young medical men should have competed eagerly for a handful of unpaid hospital appointments. Hospitals could casually refer to the "advantages of place" as a fair substitute for salary.[20] In a period before board certification, well-endowed professorships, and research grants, a hospital attending physicianship (often with a related medical school appointment) was the profession's single most important badge of success. Hospital physicians were almost by definition an elite in the hierarchical world of urban medicine, and the recruitment of staff was never a problem for trustees. When considering an increase in the number of their attending physicians in 1842, for example, a committee of New York Hospital's Board of Governors pointed out that

. . . The practice & Experience, gained at the Hospital, are deemed so important, & so great are the advantages it offers, that the situation is sought for, and can at all times be filled by the most talented of the profession.[21]

The "advantages" were too well understood to need elaboration.

Even though historians and sociologists tend to speak of "a medical profession" or "physicians" as though they constituted a unified group, nineteenth-century American practitioners were characterized as much by diversity as similarity. Medicine was not one profession, but several, marked by a hierarchical distribution of influence, knowledge, and institutional position. Only their position in the doctor-patient relationship itself bound together all those who called themselves physicians. The relationship of the medical man to the hospital underlines this particular reality; in another sense it helped create and perpetuate an internally differentiated and stratified profession. Although the hospital ordinarily played no role in the training or practice of rural physicians and almost as little in the education and practice of most urban doctors, it was always central to the plans of an ambitious and well-connected minority, to those physicians who treated not artisans and small shopkeepers but merchants, professionals, and men of influence. The hospital was their primary locus of clinical training, of the accumulation of status, of entrée in many cases to circles from which a successful practice might be expected to develop. The values and career options of this numerically small medical elite were to play a formative role in the creation of the modern hospital and in the reshaping of medicine generally.

The very casualness of most formal medical school requirements in antebellum America, and especially the lack of clinical training, served only to intensify the hospital's importance to the medical elite. An aspiring physician with some means and seriousness of purpose would not limit his training to the perfunctory steps specified in early licensing laws. Although the particular provisions of such laws varied widely in Jeffersonian America, none had a significant impact in defining the nature of clinical preparation or limiting access to the medical marketplace. "There is an act of the Legislature," a prominent New York physician wrote in 1799, "relative to the practice of Physick and Surgery, but it is a poor stupid thing, and I believe few pay any attention to it." All one needed to begin practice was a certificate from a local doctor attesting to the candidate's having studied two years with his preceptor. Once such a certificate was filed in the county clerk's office, a young man was ready to hang up his shingle and treat the unwary sick. State laws varied widely throughout the first half of the nineteenth century, but none were rigidly enforced or intellectually demanding.[22]

These casual requirements had little relevance to the aspirations of the would-be medical elite. Such ambitious young men followed a far more demanding path. After a relatively substantial premedical education, including graduation from college in many cases, they would begin their medical training with apprenticeship to an urban, hospital-connected physician. Their first contact with the hospital would have come as they followed their teacher through its wards, possibly recording prescriptions or dressing ulcers. After graduation from medical college there was competition for a house officership; then if finances warranted, a European visit; finally, a position as dispensary or outpatient physician, or as temporary substitute for a regular visiting physician—all the while patiently lobbying for a permanent inpatient position. In the 1820s and 1830s, the older apprentice-based system of clinical training began to decline, to be replaced by one based increasingly on formal medical school attendance. Yet even the most ambitious of the nation's medical schools lacked adequate clinical facilities. Hospital work thus loomed ever more prominently in the career plans of that minority of young physicians who could realistically enter the demanding race for eminence in urban medicine.

Not surprisingly, the first generation of American hospital physicians, like their antebellum successors generally, were prominent and well trained. Of ten medical men who served the Pennsylvania Hospital as visiting physicians in the last fifteen years of the eighteenth century, nine had received at least some European training and five held degrees from Edinburgh, then Europe's most demanding medical school.[23] And this was at a time when the majority of American practitioners had never seen the inside of a medical school classroom, let alone the ward of a great general hospital. The elite in American medicine has always been cosmopolitan and urban.

The city was inevitably the elite's arena for social and intellectual achievement. And the larger the city, the more elaborate its medical institutions, the more seductive it appeared to ambitious young men. It provided the "clinical material" and the institutions in which an elusive trade might be learned and taught, a circle of similarly motivated and well-informed physicians, and the wealthy patients and lucrative consultations necessary to a successful practice. Before the Civil War, Philadelphia was the most important such American medical center and its hospitals an intellectual and social magnet for young physicians. Thus, a bright young Bostonian could write in 1809 that "Philadelphia is to be the seat of medical science before all other places in the United States. Would that my lot had fallen in so pleasant a place." A third of a century later, a Southern physician explained in similar terms that he had decided to remain in Philadelphia because it boasted the best medical schools, teachers, libraries, collections of anatomical and pathological specimens. The "atmosphere of Philad. is Medical," he enthused, and he had "determined to remain within its influence."[24] The problem of finding adequate medical care for small towns and rural areas was not as urgent in antebellum America as it was to become in the twentieth century, but many of the factors that account for the urban preferences of medical men were already present.

Such medical priorities had always been essential to American hospitals and almshouses, for these benevolent institutions were ordinarily dependent upon the willingness of physicians to serve without pay. Young doctors in search of clinical experience and older men eager for status and intellectual opportunity had always sought hospital work. In Philadelphia, for example, both the almshouse and Pennsylvania Hospital employed "medical apprentices" as early as the 1770s. It was a practice almost inevitable: indispensable to the hospital, desirable for aspiring practitioners, and consistent with the dominance of the apprentice model in other areas of eighteenth-century life.

The archives of the Pennsylvania Hospital indicate how this traditional system still functioned in the first decade of the nineteenth century. A young man would apprentice himself to the hospital for five years and provide bond in the amount of "one hundred pounds per annum for every day that he absents [himself] without leave from the Managers." If accepted, the young man had to bring his own feather bed. Beneath the quaint requirements that surrounded the award of these proto-internships lie significant realities. Perhaps most obviously, a young man without substantial financial backing could hardly consider such a lengthy period of economic dependence. One aspiring physician from North Carolina, for example, had to turn down the possibility of serving as hospital apprentice.

Altho I should disregard the Labour & confinement, I do not think it would be possible (stranger as I am) to find satisfactory security in Philadelphia. I am besides possessed of very little property, too little I am certain to enable me to find my cloaths and pocket money for five years.

It was expected, moreover, that the applicant would have at least some prior medical training before undertaking hospital work. The youthful North Carolinian who found himself financially unable to apply for an apprenticeship had already studied medicine for eighteen months and had "acquired a competent knowledge of the virtues & doses of all medicine used in modern practice" and was "acquainted with Pharmacy, with bleeding and treating of wounds."[25] Such training was necessary, for in the hospital's small world, house physicians were expected to be jacks of all medical trades, beginning with the more routine and less desirable tasks and ultimately accumulating ever-more-responsible duties.[26]

By the 1840s, America's hospitals had already discarded this traditional system of apprenticeship (as it was similarly being rejected in other areas of American society). One year was now the normal term and most house officers had completed at least one course of formal medical lectures; many held the medical degree before assuming their grueling responsibilities. Throughout the century, such young men were expected to eat and sleep in the hospital, to serve as the hands and eyes of the institution's attending physicians. Since these senior clinicians visited for only a few hours a week and rotated terms of duty, a handful of partially trained young practitioners constituted the only continuing medical presence in the antebellum hospital. House officerships remained in short supply throughout the first half of the nineteenth century, and even well-connected young men might have to be content with an almshouse or dispensary post if a staff position could not be arranged in the more prestigious private hospitals. Jonathan Mason Warren, for example, the son of Harvard and Massachusetts General Hospital surgeon John Collins Warren, could write his father from Paris, where the young man was studying surgery, asking that he submit his name for an almshouse position.[27] Physicians at whatever stage of their career were proud to add their hospital appointments to letters of application, to the title pages of books and monographs, to insert them carefully in memoirs and eulogies.

As we have seen in the case of the apprentice system at the beginning of the nineteenth century, house officerships were with few exceptions only for the ambitious and at least moderately well-to-do. At the New York Hospital, for example, house physicians throughout the first two-thirds of the century were recruited only from among those young men who had been fee-paying pupils of the institution's attending physicians and then served as "walkers" or clinical assistants in the wards. Until the end of the century, house officers at both the Massachusetts General and Pennsylvania hospitals were chosen by the institution's socially prominent board members. Men with no social standing, financial support, or contacts in the community would have had a difficult time in finding a place (or supporting themselves while they occupied it). At the Philadelphia Almshouse Hospital, the largest and to medical students most desirable of the municipal hospitals throughout the century, the house pupils had to pay a fee through most of the antebellum period, at one time as high as $250.[28] In addition, they had to have attended at least one course of medical lectures and been approved by the hospital's senior medical board. In some hospitals, fees might be paid to senior resident physicians by undergraduate students eager for clinical experience; such fees purchased access to patients on the resident's ward. This was a difficult school of medicine—for patients as well as practitioners.

A house officership was only the first step in an elite medical career, but it was a necessary step along the path that might culminate in an attending position, profitable practice, and prestigious and, in some instances, lucrative teaching posts. Attending physicianships were, in addition, long-term or permanent, even at hospitals that formally renewed appointments each year. As an attending physician approached the age of retirement or as his private practice grew to unwieldy size, he could look forward to the largely honorary post of consulting physician. Although never quite as powerful and autocratic as their English counterparts, American attending physicians were clearly an elite within the urban medical world. And if they were not paid a salary, their duties were comparatively light. The custom of rotation limited responsibilities to three- or four-month periods. In the summer months, as all familiar with hospitals understood, it was often difficult to guarantee regular attendance from the physician unfortunate enough to have been selected for that dreary stretch of duty.

As a response to such staffing problems and to steadily increasing numbers of patients, some hospitals had by midcentury created the post of salaried resident physician—less desirable than the more senior attending physicianship, yet more responsible than the role of house officer or house pupil. These full-time positions were also highly sought after. (Titles had not yet become uniform. "House pupil" corresponds most closely to our intern, while "resident physician" might be likened to a twentieth-century chief resident.) Many applied again and again in hope of receiving such posts. But even repeated failure might not discourage a would-be resident; the stakes were high enough to justify continued efforts. "The lessons to be gained from a connexion with the best Surgical Institution of our country," a tactful if unsuccessful applicant wrote to the Pennsylvania Hospital, "afford too bright a prospect to the Clinical Student to be relinquished on first disappointment."[29] The career of an elite practitioner might well be visualized in the form of a ladder; the placement of its rungs was both obvious and crucial to those young men who sought to ascend them.

The biographies of successful nineteenth-century practitioners have a repetitive quality. Let me simply outline the career of one such physician in his own terms as he applied in 1856 for an attending post at the Pennsylvania Hospital. Alfred Stillé's curriculum vitae was typical of those forged by the ambitions and institutional realities of his generation. He could point to a career nicely calculated to prepare himself for the position he sought. "My whole life," Stillé explained, "has been devoted to preparation for the dept. of medicine." He assumed that the Board of Managers sought a physician "whose knowledge of *scientific and practical* medicine is great, and whose *habit of teaching* is formed." While still in medical school, Stillé had undertaken private clinical work with a then resident of the hospital. When he graduated from medical school a year later, Stillé had applied for the resident physicianship, but lost out to a physician in residence at the city's almshouse hospital. Stillé was then chosen to fill the unexpired portion of his successful competitor's term. (A neat example, it should be noted, of the difference in prestige between the two hospitals. The municipal institution was desirable but not quite so desirable as its private counterpart.) Stillé then studied in Europe for two years and returned to compete—this time successfully—for the Pennsylvania Hospital resident physicianship he had at first failed to obtain. In 1844, he was appointed lecturer on the practice of medicine in the "Philadelphia Association for Medical Instruction," a summer school in which medical students could purchase the individualized clinical instruction not yet available in the regular medical school curriculum. While still lecturing in this informal school, Stillé was chosen in 1849 as attending physician at the newly organized St. Joseph's Hospital, then spent nearly six months "at Vienna in the Great Hospital of that city distinguished as the most perfect *clinical institution* in the world." In 1854, he was selected to fill the Chair of Theory and Practice of Medicine in the Pennsylvania Medical College, one of Philadelphia's lesser medical schools.[30] This teaching position, in conjunction with his attending post at St. Joseph's, meant that Stillé had attained a rung just below the highest in

Philadelphia medicine's ladder of eminence. He had now only two goals left to pursue: a clinical appointment at the Pennsylvania Hospital and a chair at the University of Pennsylvania. He was ultimately to attain both. Most of his competitors were, of course, not so successful.

But in order to play the game at all, one needed to be dealt the appropriate cards. And, as we have seen, these included, in addition to some intellectual capacity, the ability to take advantage of special summer and tutorial arrangements, to travel to Europe, and to serve unpaid years as house officer. No young man of humble origins could easily embark on this lengthy and ill-paid road to medical eminence, nor could he have enjoyed the social connections so helpful in seeking hospital appointments. A far less typical case, that of Patrick Nolan, a young man serving as "senior medical walker" (a position akin to extern or fourth-year medical student) in New York Hospital in 1858, is in its own way as revealing as the account of Stillé's experience.

Nolan's career was so out of the ordinary that senior attending physician John Griscom took up the young man's case with the hospital's Board of Governors, asking that Nolan be offered the privilege of living and boarding in the house. Nolan had been the "artificer of his own position as a Physician," Griscom explained. "He commenced a penniless emigrant, and by dint of hard labor and close study, without borrowing a cent, has paid his way through the College of Pharmacy, and the College of Physicians & Surgeons." Nolan had managed to work his way through both colleges as an apothecary's clerk, but now, Griscom elaborated, such outside income would cease in consequence of his hospital duties. The hard-working Irish immigrant desperately needed the board and room normally provided only for house physicians.[31] The young Irishman's struggle upward was not impossible, but it was difficult, demanding, and highly uncommon.

It was a frustrating situation for the average young medical graduate, eager to accumulate clinical experience, yet dependent on income from practice for his daily bread. Easily available internships and paid residencies were far in the future. A few medical students could compete for the scarce house positions. The still ambitious, but less able or well-to-do were more likely to content themselves with volunteer outpatient work in hospitals and dispensaries, while grimly enduring the months and years of genteel poverty that preceded the gradual establishment of a secure private practice.[32] A

few paid positions as "outdoor" physicians to hospitals and almshouses existed in the largest cities, and these might help pay a
young practitioner's bills. Such outdoor physicians treated the indigent poor in their tenement homes. Simon Wickes, for example, a
Yale graduate who had attended medical school in Philadelphia,
decided to establish a practice in this bustling city and opened an
office in April of 1833. He paid four dollars a week for board and
one hundred dollars a year for rent and was happy to be hired as
outdoor physician to the city's almshouse at one hundred dollars a
year.[33] The position paid his office rental, allowed him to add a title
to his unadorned M.D., and offered an opportunity to accumulate
clinical experience and contacts among working people who might
in better times be able to pay for his services. But there were comparatively few such positions. To most novice practitioners, a gradual path upward into their city's hospital and teaching establishment was not to be contemplated.

A Balance of Power and Function

Within each city, the ranks of hospital physicians tended to be
close and exclusive. And, although I have pointed to areas of recurrent conflict, the relationships between such medical men and the
members of lay hospital boards were ordinarily placid. They were
often social equals, possibly even acquaintances; their children
might know each other; a hospital's attending physicians might
serve as family practitioners to prominent board members. Long
terms of office on the part of both laymen and physicians helped
strengthen their natural community of interest. By midcentury,
most of our hospitals had negotiated an implicit division of labor,
and thus authority, between lay and medical spheres. Attending
physicians often nominated house officers, for example, though
formal appointive powers remained in lay hands. Admissions had
become a largely medical decision, although still influenced on occasion by trustee guidelines and arbitrary and personal intrusions on
behalf of the occasional favored patient. Therapeutics too were
ordinarily controlled by medical men, with the exception of sporadic bursts of trustee economy or moralism.
Stability depended upon a continued balance of power between

the board of attending physicians and their nominal lay superiors. Attending physicians naturally objected to any change that might disturb this stalemate and thus their power in the wards. When, for example, the Massachusetts General Hospital trustees sought to appoint a salaried resident physician to undertake a portion of the steward's administrative duties and report directly to the trustees, the proposed reform was opposed by the hospital's attending physicians. It seemed a step toward unification of authority under the hospital's lay trustees. Similar proposals at the Philadelphia Almshouse Hospital and New York's Bellevue had also been opposed by senior attending physicians.[34]

But it was difficult to oppose such administrative innovation forever. The need for an experienced resident physician had become increasingly pressing by mid-century. It was a natural response to growing numbers of patients, exacerbated by a disproportionate increase in trauma and emergency cases—which could hardly be scheduled at the convenience of a hospital's attending staff or consigned to the unfledged skills of house officers alone. As early as 1807, Benjamin Rush and other attending physicians had urged the Pennsylvania Hospital's Board of Managers to hire a salaried resident house surgeon, not to exert administrative responsibility, but to attend outpatients, treat and admit emergencies, and oversee the carrying out of attending physicians' orders. At mid-century, the Massachusetts General Hospital created the position of "admitting physician," an experienced practitioner who would be required to visit applicants for admission in their homes as well as be available to treat emergency cases at the hospital.[35] This position was a logical response to institutional necessity; it survived at Massachusetts General Hospital until the appointment of a full-time paid "resident physician" in 1858.

The office of resident physician was in fact well-accepted by mid-century and its duties almost standardized. At the hospital of the Medical College of Virginia, for example, the resident physician in 1856 was required to sleep in the building, prescribe in emergencies, and examine candidates for admission, rejecting "such as may be affected with any contagious or infectious febrile disease, or with insanity." He was to make rounds every morning and evening and oversee the hospital's "house students."[36] By the time of the Civil War, the medical staffs in America's largest hospitals had already assumed a structure recognizable to twentieth-century eyes. At Philadelphia's municipal hospital, for example, the attending staff in 1859 consisted of four physicians, four surgeons, and four obstetricians; in addition, eight residents served two-year terms (rotating through different services and accumulating increased responsibilities). These resident house officers were all holders of the medical degree and were selected by examination. The older system in which it was assumed that house officers would in many cases be undergraduate medical students and attend lectures in hours snatched from their hospital duties was no longer a viable means of providing day-to-day care in an ever expanding institution.[37] America's hospitals had evolved an increasingly elaborate organizational structure. The situation was already quite different from the one that prevailed at the beginning of the nineteenth century, when a few partially trained students and intermittently available senior physicians cared for the handful of predominately chronic patients occupying America's few hospitals and almshouse medical wards.

This new staffing system reflected a necessary functional logic; both medical education and patient care demanded an increasingly structured and intrusive medical staff. And those staff members inevitably reflected the values and specific knowledge of a rapidly changing medical community. The hospital was integrated precisely into the career patterns of the medical profession. But at the same time the staffing of nineteenth-century hospitals reflected the larger community's values and social relationships. Just as patient populations reflected prior social status, so did the decisions that determined hospital appointments. Eminence in medicine certainly implied intellect and achievement, but it reflected family connections as well, often specific ethnic or religious ties. It implied, as we have seen, opportunities available to only a small minority of would-be physicians. Publications and teaching responsibilities were as much legitimation as they were objective criteria for membership in the profession's urban elite. The hospital was very much a community institution—even as the medical men who served in it acted out their identity in another and more specialized professional community.

CHAPTER 3

The Medical Mind: Tradition and Change in Antebellum America

Older physicians in mid-nineteenth-century America recognized that they had lived through a revolution in thought. The past half-century, a prominent Albany physician explained to his state's Medical Society at its semicentennial in 1857, had seen enormous changes.

When our medical colleges or schools were limited to five, and the hospitals of this country but a little more numerous; when the whole apparatus, chemicals and chemical tests of the chemist's laboratory could be almost packed in a bushel; when the anatomical museum of a college consisted of two or three smoky skeletons, a handful of disjointed bones, and a few coarsely injected preparations—and when a pathological cabinet was not known in our country; it requires no very great stretch of the imagination to draw the contrast between the advantages of 1807 and those of 1857.[1]

The direction and desirability of change could hardly be questioned. Science was relentlessly uncovering the secrets of man's physical nature and physicians had steadily incorporated that knowledge into their practice. The era of Thomas Jefferson and Benjamin Rush was a distant and primitive time.

The hospital had played a prominent role in this half-century's accumulation of knowledge. Paris with its sprawling hospitals and innovative teachers had replaced Edinburgh as magnet for America's most ambitious young physicians. Like their counterparts from

England and the continent, these privileged Americans flocked to Paris, hoping to absorb its newly elaborated understanding of pathology and arsenal of specialized clinical skills. Many returned, committed firmly to the city and to the hospital. These were the only battlefields on which the laurels of publication and innovation could be won. Nevertheless, America's antebellum hospitals remained the professional domain of a small medical elite, irrelevant to the care of the vast majority of Americans and to the careers of those practitioners who treated them. The hospital helped both structure and justify the gap that separated the ordinary (in most cases, rural) physician from his aspiring urban counterpart.

The world of American medicine shifted more slowly in practice than it did in the publications and programmatic statements of a self-conscious minority of strivers after intellectual and institutional status. The mid-nineteenth-century world of medical practice remained in some ways closer to that of the eighteenth than to that of the twentieth century. There was little in the way of diagnostic or therapeutic technique that could not be provided as well outside as inside the hospital, little available to the physician that the patient could not sense, evaluate, and—in his or her fashion—comprehend. A flushed face and rapid pulse, a coated tongue and griping diarrhea would be apparent to laymen just as to physicians; and grandmothers as well as senior consultants could and did make reasoned prognoses. Much of hospital medicine was little different from domestic practice. Bleeding, cupping, purging, all seemed routine and comprehensible to laymen. There were, of course, no x-rays, no clinical laboratory, no thermometers, and, at the beginning of the century, not even a stethoscope. Surgery ordinarily enlisted the humble skills of the nurse and wound dresser, not those of the hospital surgeon, whose incursions were indeed dramatic, but infrequently employed. Diagnosis and therapeutics still created a bond, not a barrier, between doctor and patient.

Similarly, ideas about the nature of disease and its transmission and thus the physical organization of hospitals—the size of wards, placement of windows, drains, and fireplaces—reflected social attitudes as much as empirical findings. Even the writings of the most vehement and would-be empirical reformers of the mid-nineteenth-century hospital drew upon older moral certainties in fashioning a blueprint for reordering that flawed but necessary institution. A line between social and medical thought could hardly be drawn at the beginning of the nineteenth century; at mid-century these ancient patterns of assumption had only begun to change. It was inevitable that America's antebellum hospitals would continue to be shaped as much by dependence and traditional notions of class, deference, and social responsibility as they were by the categories and capacities of medicine.

A Body Distressed

It is difficult to recapture the medical world of 1800; it was a world of thought structured about assumptions so fundamental that they were only occasionally articulated as such—yet assumptions alien to a twentieth-century medical understanding. The key to making sense of therapeutics and pathology at the beginning of the nineteenth century lies in seeing it as a system of belief and behavior participated in by laymen and physicians alike.[2] Since the human body was only intermittently accessible to the physician, it was all the more necessary that he believe in and practice a medicine that used his limited understanding of that body, its products, and its responses to the drugs that made up his pharmacopoeia. It was equally necessary that this medicine be intelligible to patients and family members who also could observe a rapid pulse, a coated tongue, the effects of a disordered colon.

Central to the logic of traditional medical practice was a particular way of looking at the body. It was seen metaphorically as a system of ever-changing interactions with its environment. Health or disease resulted from cumulative interactions between constitutional endowment and environmental circumstances. One could not well live without food and air and water; one had to exist in a particular climate, subject one's body to a particular style of life and work. Each of these factors implied a necessary and continuing physiological adjustment. The body was always in a state of becoming—and thus always in jeopardy.

Two subsidiary assumptions organized the shape of this lifelong interaction. First, every part of the body was related inevitably and inextricably to every other. A distracted mind could curdle the stomach; a dyspeptic stomach could agitate the mind. Local lesions might reflect imbalances of nutrients in the blood; systemic ills might be caused by fulminating local lesions. Medical theory found numerous ways to explain this relationship—but all served the same function relative to pathology and therapeutics. All related local to systemic ills; they described all aspects of the body as interrelated and tended to present health or disease as general states of the total organism. Second, the body was seen as a system of intake and outgo—a system that had to remain in balance if the individual were to remain healthy. Thus, the traditional emphasis on diet and excretion, perspiration and ventilation. Equilibrium was synonymous with health, disequilibrium with illness. Traditional bleeding and purging as modes of adjusting the body to seasonal changes—ancient practices still very much alive in the nineteenth century—were understood within the same framework. Similar attitudes explain the routine domestic use of cathartics, often to anticipate and avert ill health as much as to cure. Physicians warned that such lay practice could easily be carried to excess. "I was well," a medical epigram explained, "wished to be better, took Medicine & died."[3]

The idea of specific disease entities played a relatively small role in this system of ideas and behavior. Neither learned physicians nor educated laymen saw most ills as having a discrete cause and characteristic course. Not surprisingly, early nineteenth-century hospital case records often fail to record a diagnosis, for disease was seen as a general state of the organism in relation to its environment—as a disordered individual adjustment, not as a patterned and predictable response to a particular cause. Within this traditional world of patients, and not of diseases, the medical man could easily maintain his customary explanatory and therapeutic role. The physician's most effective weapon was his ability to "regulate the secretions"—to extract blood, to promote the perspiration, the urination, or defecation that attested to his having helped the body regain its customary equilibrium. Even when a disease seemed not only to have a characteristic course but (as in the case of smallpox) a specific causative "virus," the hypothetical pathology and indicated therapeutics were placed within the same explanatory framework. When mid-eighteenth-century physicians inoculated or early nineteenth-century physicians vaccinated to protect against smallpox, they always accompanied the procedure with an elaborate regimen of cathartics, diet, and rest; the body had to be helped to contend with this antagonistic substance. Physicians could not easily accept the idea that a specific substance could prevent or cure a specific ailment. It undercut the elaborate physiological framework that justified their customary ministrations and at the same time reminded them all too forcefully of their profession's quackish competitors who had for centuries hawked specific remedies.[4]

The pedigree of these ideas can be traced to the speculations of classical antiquity. They could hardly be superseded, for no information more accurate or schema more socially useful existed to call them into question. Most important, the system provided a framework in which the physician could at once reassure the patient and justify his prescriptions. The physician's own self-image as well as his social plausibility depended on the creation of a shared faith—a conspiracy to believe—in his ability to understand the cause and course of the ills that afflicted his patients. This system of ideas provided a place for his diagnostic as well as his therapeutic skills: Prognosis, diagnosis, and therapeutics all had to find a consistent mode of explanation.

The American physician in 1800 had no diagnostic tools beyond his senses, and it is hardly surprising that he would find congenial a framework of explanation that emphasized the importance of intake and outgo, the significance of perspiration, of pulse, of urination and menstruation, of defecation, and of the surface eruptions that might accompany fevers or other internal ills. When the physician entered the hospital ward, he could ask patients how they felt, examine their tongues, inquire into the regularity of their "evacuations." A doctor would feel the patient's pulse, but describe it in qualitative—as full or shallow, for example—not quantitative terms.[5] When Patrick Flinn, a forty-nine-year-old Irish laborer, was admitted to the New York Hospital in 1809 complaining of a fever, his examination was easily summarized by the house physician: "Pulse full and somewhat tense, moderately frequent, skin cool, tongue clean; belly regular, appetite impaired; sleep not much disturbed; nightly perspiration considerable." A resident physician at the Philadelphia Almshouse Hospital in January of 1826 could similarly report the condition of Anthony McGill, forty-seven, a laborer suffering with an eye infection. "The temperature of the surface was considerably above the natural standard—pulse frequent and moderately full but very compressible & tongue very foul—respiration not materially affected—thirst urgent."[6] There was no clinical laboratory or thermometer to help the antebellum physician in evaluating his patient's symptoms.

These biological and social realities had several implications for the doctor-patient relationship. Drugs had to be seen as adjusting the body's internal equilibrium. In addition, the drug's action had to alter, if possible, those visible products of the body's otherwise inscrutable internal state. Thus, the popularity of drugs that promoted sweating or urination or defecation. Logically enough, drugs were not ordinarily viewed as specifics for particular disease entities; materia medica texts were often arranged not by drug or disease, but in categories reflecting the drug's physiological effects: diuretics, cathartics, narcotics, emetics. Quinine, for example, was ordinarily categorized as a tonic and prescribed for numerous conditions other than malaria. Medical men found it easier to generalize from its effectiveness in malaria and prescribe it for a variety of ills rather than to see it as a remedy with a specific and limited efficacy.[7]

The effectiveness of the system hinged to a significant extent on the fact that all the weapons in the physician's normal therapeutic repertoire "worked," worked that is by providing visible and predictable physiological actions: purges purged, emetics caused vomiting, opium soothed pain and moderated diarrhea. Bleeding seemed to alter the body's internal balance, as evidenced both by a changed pulse and the very quantity of blood drawn. Not only did a drug's activity indicate to both physician and patient the nature of its efficacy (and the physician's competence), but it provided a prognostic tool as well, for the patient's response to a drug could indicate much about his condition, while examination of the product elicited—urine, feces, blood, perspiration—could shed light on the body's internal state. The body seemed, moreover, to rid itself of disease in ways parallel to those encouraged or elicited by drug action. The profuse sweat, diarrhea, or skin lesions often accompanying fevers, for example, all seemed stages in a necessary course of natural recovery. The remedies he employed, the physician could assure his patients, only acted in imitation of nature:

Blood-letting and blisters find their archetypes in spontaneous hemorrhage and those . . . exudations that occur in some stage of almost every acute inflammation; emetics, cathartics, diuretics, diaphoretics, etc. etc. have each and all of them effects in every way similar to those arising spontaneously in disease.[8]

Medicine could provoke or facilitate, but not alter, the fundamental patterns of recovery built into the human organism.

Physicians and laymen shared a similar, although of course not identical, view of the manner in which the body functioned, and the nature of available therapeutic options reinforced that view. The secretions could be regulated, a "plethoric" or overly full state of the blood abated through blood-letting or leeches, the stomach emptied of a contents potentially dangerous. Recovery must, of course, have often coincided with the administration of a particular drug and provided an endorsement of its effectiveness. Thus, experience seemed to "prove" that fevers were often healed by the purging effects of mercury or antimony. Similarly, a physician could describe a case of pleurisy as having been "suddenly relieved by profuse perspiration" elicited by the camphor he had prescribed.[9] When Catherine Wayland, for example, arrived at the Cincinnati General Hospital on March 17, 1838, she had been exposed to the cold and damp on the deck of a steamboat for three nights and complained of severe diarrhea and pain in her back and legs. The resident physician prescribed opium and calomel (a mercury compound used widely as a cathartic) and then castor oil the next day when the calomel failed to "operate." On the twentieth, the resident was able to report that "the oil of the 18 operated and she is now convalescent."[10] Drugs reassured insofar as they acted, and their efficacy was underwritten by the natural tendency toward recovery that characterized most ills.

Therapeutics thus played a central role within a highly structured doctor-patient relationship. On the intellectual level, therapeutics confirmed the physician's ability to understand and intervene in the physiological processes that defined health and disease; on the emotional level, the very severity of drug action assured the patient and his family that something was being done. In the hospital, even more than in the private home, physicians depended on the administration of physiologically active drugs, for the attending or resident physician's care was rushed and episodic. He could not call upon the confidence and familiarity that developed naturally in a more conventional family practice; and the advice on diet, exercise, sleep, stress, and work that figured prominently in private practice was hardly applicable to the hospital's ordinarily poverty-stricken inmates. The physician's art, in the hospital perhaps even more than in private practice, centered on his ability to employ an appropriate drug, or combination of drugs and bleeding, to produce a particular physiological effect. This explains the apparent anomaly of physicians employing different drugs to treat the same condition; each drug, the argument followed, was equally legitimate, so long as it produced the desired physiological effect. The selection of a proper drug or drugs was no mean skill, for each patient possessed a unique physiological identity, and the experienced physician had to evaluate a bewildering variety of factors, ranging from climatic conditions to age and sex, in the compounding of any particular prescription. The same speculative mechanisms that explained recovery explained failure as well. One could not hope for a cure in every case; even the most competent physician could only do that which the limited resources of medicine allowed—and the natural course of some ills was toward death. The treatment indicated for tuberculosis, as an ancient adage put it, was opium and lies. Cancer too was normally incurable; some states of disequilibrium could not be put aright.

Individuals from almost every level of society accepted, in one fashion or another, the basic outlines of this conceptual framework. Evidence of these beliefs among the less educated is not abundant, but does exist. Surviving hospital records, for example, indicate the widespread dissemination of such ideas. One broadly shared assumption was the interconnectedness of the body's various organs and functions. Thus, a Cincinnati carpenter could explain in 1837 "that his eyes sympathize with his stomach and bowells [sic]" and became infected "when much nausea of stomach obtains."[11] Hospital patients also understood that a sudden interruption of perspiration might cause cold or even pneumonia, that such critical periods of developmental instability as teething, puberty, or menopause were similarly dangerous. The metabolic gyroscope that controlled the balance of forces within the body was finely tuned and might easily be thrown off balance. It was natural for servants and laborers reporting the symptoms of their fevers to an almshouse physician to ascribe their illnesses to a sudden chill; the interruption of any natural evacuation would presumably jeopardize the end implicit in that function; if the body did not need to perspire in certain circumstances, or discharge menstrual blood at intervals, it would not be doing so. These were mechanisms through which the body maintained its health-defining equilibrium and could thus be interrupted only at great peril.

A widespread faith in emetics, cathartics, diuretics, and bleeding is evidenced as well by their prominent place in folk and patent medicines. Domestic and irregular practice, like regular medicine, depended on eliciting predictable physiological responses; home remedies mirrored the heroic therapeutics practiced by regular physicians. In the fall of 1826, for example, when a Philadelphia tallow chandler fell ill, he complained of chills, pains in the head and back, weakness in the joints, and nausea. Then, before seeing a regular physician, he

was bled till symptoms of fainting came on. Took an emetic, which operated well. For several days after, kept his bowels moved with Sulph. Soda, Senna tea, etc. He then employed a Physician who prescribed another Emetic, which operated violently and whose action was kept up by drinking bitter tea.[12]

Only after two more days did he appear at the almshouse hospital. Those physicians skeptical of extremes in therapeutics complained repeatedly of lay expectations that worked against a suitable moderation; medical men, for example, might be subject to criticism if they should fail to bleed in the early stages of pneumonia. Parents often demanded that physicians incise the inflamed gums of their teething infants so as to provoke a "resolution" of this developmental crisis. The indications for bleeding, to cite another example, were carefully demarcated in formal medical thought, yet laymen often demanded this procedure even when the state of the pulse and general condition of the patient contraindicated loss of blood. Laymen frequently bled themselves and friends, sometimes with such enthusiasm that they found themselves in a hospital bed. Some patients demanded, as well as expected, the administration of severe cathartics and emetics; they feared danger in too indecisive a therapy.

We cannot know how particular nineteenth-century patients experienced their hospital stay, for those Americans who found themselves in an antebellum hospital bed were hardly the sort who kept diaries or published memoirs. But we can at least try to understand something of their feelings about the remedies to which they were subjected. Hospital medicine duplicated in modified form practices that would have been employed in the home or a physician's office. Patients knew and "understood" the familiar action of purges, emetics, and diuretics. Even most surgery, as we have noted, bore little resemblance to twentieth-century procedures, but consisted of the dressing and tedious redressing of wounds and ulcers. These lesions were on the body's surface and accessible to the eyes and hands of ordinary men. Similarly, fractures, breaks and dislocations—less frequent than such lesions but still a routine staple of hospital admissions—required little in the way of conceptual sophistication. Bones could crack or break, joints pull apart; such injuries were serious but not mysterious. And, even in trauma, much of the treatment rested on adjustment of the patient's diet and secretions and not on surgical intervention.[13]

The hospital was no temple to the mysteries of an esoteric body of medical knowledge. The ordinary man or woman might not comprehend the physician's ministrations within quite the same framework as the physician, but there was a significant overlap of experience and understanding. Medicine itself, as well as traditional social attitudes, determined that the antebellum hospital would be an institution defined more by need and deference than by the categories of medical diagnosis and the tools and techniques of medical therapeutics. Theories of disease causation also were suitable to an unspecialized society in which medical knowledge was intricately related to social thought generally. The body could not be seen apart from the society in which it worked, ate, and breathed. The ideas I have described concerning the body and health were all-inclusive and antireductionist, capable of incorporating every aspect of a person's physical and emotional life in explaining his or her state of health. Just as the body interacted continuously with the environment, so did the mind with the body, moral with physical health. The realm of causation in medicine was not distinguishable from the realm of meaning in society generally—just as the antebellum hospital could not be removed from society's values and accustomed roles.

But this traditional way of understanding disease and its remedies was not to remain undisturbed. By 1800, the first signs of change had already manifested themselves and by mid-century the system was no longer intact. The very nature of disease was being redefined, and in an increasingly professional and self-consciously scientific medical world, the hospital was to play a central role: first in the careers of a small elite of professors and practitioners, then gradually in the treatment of ever larger numbers of the sick.

Sources of Change

Scholarship helped define the successful urban practitioner. Without social connections or extraordinary good fortune, of course, scholarship could not guarantee a medical school chair or hospital attending physicianship, but neither could social connections without the appearance of scholarship. This generalization holds true for the entire nineteenth century. In the course of that century, however, the definition of scholarship was to change fundamentally. Until 1850, research in the twentieth-century sense—even systematic clinical observation—was no necessary part of medical learning. Scholarship meant wide experience and ripe judgment allied with a mastery of the available clinical literature. Innovation was honored, but not required for the would-be teacher of medicine. A learned physician spent his leisure hours in the library, not the laboratory.

Most antebellum American practitioners were unlettered by European standards, but even in 1800, America's handful of educated urban physicians were well integrated into the international world of medical learning and aspiration. An influential minority of America's late eighteenth-century physicians had studied in Edinburgh (and often in London hospitals and on the continent as well); the acquisition of advanced training had always brought with it high prestige. Although few in number, such men of cosmopolitan learning claimed a disproportionate share of available teaching and hospital positions.[14] They were to be the instructors of a new generation of ambitious practitioners. And despite an overwhelming orientation toward the day-to-day necessities of patient care, at least some early nineteenth-century American physicians sought opportunities to perform postmortems and improve their anatomical skills. Much of such dissection was casual and crude, partially because of a lack of training, partially because of a lingering cultural antipathy toward desecration of the body; opportunities for autopsy were relatively few and the motivation of those performing them necessarily high. In retrospect, however, the desire of at least some physicians to perform postmortems, often in difficult if not actually dangerous circumstances, is more significant than the technical limitations of their work.

Similarly, the casual experiments that often figured in early nineteenth-century doctoral dissertations and journal articles are hardly impressive by twentieth-century standards, but their existence indicated how closely the interests and aspirations of world medicine figured in the shaping of American medical careers. Edinburgh's professors had encouraged an interest in pathology and anatomy as well as a cautious experimentalism.[15] The world of European thought and practice was never far from the consciousness of that minority of American physicians who waited eagerly for each ship that brought a fresh stock of medical journals and monographs: the intellectual world of Boston and Philadelphia was no farther from London than the six weeks it took a sailing ship to cross the Atlantic. When Edward Jenner's new mode of vaccination first became known at the end of the eighteenth century, for example, Americans were among the first outside of England to experiment with it. When digitalis was first introduced into the world of academic medicine as a treatment for "dropsy," it was rapidly adopted by American physicians eager to find a remedy for the incapacitating and ultimately lethal edema and weakness that often tormented their patients.[16] The attraction of novelty allied with the inescapable demands of clinical practice guaranteed an eager constituency for promising new ideas and therapies.

Hospitals were inevitably the stage for many of these explorations. It was the only place where one could normally hope to undertake postmortems (except for an occasional instance in which forensic evidence might be required). It was the only place where surgery could be carried on in a systematic and even innovative fashion. As early as 1819, for example, surgeon Valentine Mott had performed a pioneering operation in the New York Hospital for an arterial aneurism. The patient died, he reported to the Board of Governors, but the hospital's attending surgeons had learned new and important facts. It was their professional duty, Mott contended, to experiment so that lives might ultimately be saved.[17] A greater future good could justify clinical experimentation just as we have seen it legitimate the use of patients in teaching. Ever since its eighteenth-century origins, the American hospital had been regarded by its medical staff as a kind of postgraduate school and clinical laboratory—thus, the repetitive demands by antebellum attending physicians for better instruments, for convenient postmortem facilities, for books with "more accurate and *recent* knowledge."[18] Medical men similarly urged that they be allowed the extra manpower needed to keep accurate clinical histories. "Hospital practice is the best school of medicine," as one group of physicians put it in 1827, "and offers the most certain source of improvement by the accumulated experience it derives from the numerous cases." But without adequate records, this knowledge would die with the men who had accumulated it.[19]

Although such values could encourage the uncritical publication of new and unproven remedies, they also promised enduring rewards for the successful innovator. Despite a necessary practicality of orientation among most physicians, knowledge as such was always respected among the profession's leaders and their educated and economically secure patient constituency. In addition to the value placed upon intellect, a sense of vocational seriousness and high moral purpose was often present in elite motivations. Inevitably, indeed, one of the key elements encouraging change in the nineteenth-century profession was an alliance between this seriousness of purpose and the respect accorded intellect; it made the struggle for reputation and advancement that shaped every young physician's career morally acceptable. To many such young men, a career devoted simply to the accumulation of dollars would have been intolerable. Some aspiring physicians would, indeed, have chosen between medicine and the ministry; both would have been pursued with appropriate gravity. George Shattuck, for example, a founder of Boston's dynasty of medical Shattucks, was quite explicit in explaining his choice of medicine over the pulpit. "Not the employment, but the faithful & honorable discharge of the duties of the employment, is most acceptable to him, to whom we must hold ourselves responsible. These things being impartially weighed, it appeared evident to me that I could acquit myself with more honor to myself and my God, in physick, than divinity." Shattuck was by no means unique. The same cultural values that guided and sanctioned his vocational choice flourished widely in the antebellum years. "If God had given me any ability," a mid-century aspirant to medical eminence warned himself, "it becomes me not to despise the talent and bury it in the earth." If he would be a successful practitioner, he must improve the means God had provided and avoid diffidence and overconfidence alike.[20]

Not only did one pursue a professional career with wholehearted zeal, but, in theory at least, the physician, like the clergyman, pursued a vocation whose rewards transcended those accruing to the mere buyer and seller of goods. Of course, physicians throughout nineteenth-century America were inevitably participants in a highly competitive marketplace (for there were no clinical chairs, few well-paid professorships, and only a handful of physicians with private income sufficient to allow systematic attention to clinical or laboratory investigation). Doctors, even professors and hospital staff members, supported themselves through patient fees, and only the most successful could attract enough of such fees to live in comfort.[21] Many of those physicians most assiduous in their efforts to write articles and monographs and most faithful in fulfilling their unpaid hospital duties saw such activities as at least in part a means of establishing a reputation and thus "accumulating business." In the world of antebellum medicine, intellectual laurels were inevitably advertisements for clinical services. But the prospect of material rewards did not preclude such achievement having a personal meaning transcending that of economic advantage. Meaningful distinctions between material and nonmaterial benefits could hardly be made. The very interdependence of these two kinds of reward allowed men of principle to seek a "flattering business" as well as "honorable reputation." This configuration of ideals and mundane benefits was a central factor in the encouragement of change in nineteenth-century medicine.

The Lure of Paris

To understand that change, we must turn from those values that encouraged the assimilation of new ideas to the source of such ideas outside American society. Much of the inspiration for change in antebellum American medicine grew out of developments in contemporary France, the world's acknowledged leader in the first half of the nineteenth century. Paris added new concepts and a new vocational intensity to the traditional structure of knowledge and vocation.[22] The Paris Clinical School—as it has come to be called by historians—crystallized a new way of looking at disease and of investigating it. This point of view (novel in impact even if some of its elements had been anticipated earlier and elsewhere) undercut in several ways the ancient mode of visualizing the body that we have seen as fundamental to traditional therapeutics and thus to the doctor-patient relationship. Older pathological views tended to see sickness as a general physiological state and to deemphasize the specificity of particular ailments. The French Clinical School on the other hand tended to see diseases as specific entities with predictable courses and related clusters of symptoms. These symptoms, moreover, could often be associated with underlying lesions identifiable at autopsy. It was the investigator's task to correlate these symptoms and lesions. At least some intellectually ambitious young physicians began to seek out the autopsy room and not the library as the principal theater in which to earn their intellectual laurels. Although only a handful of physicians did systematic autopsy work themselves, well-educated physicians at mid-century were coming to assume that most ailments had a distinct natural history (even if many felt that man would never unravel their ultimate cause). A disease such as smallpox, with its characteristic manifestations and origin in a discrete transmissible substance, became an increasingly plausible model for other infectious ills, and not simply the atypical and in some ways anomalous case it had been at the beginning of the nineteenth century.

This point of view had practical as well as conceptual implications. It implied the possibility of turning each ailment and each organ into a subject of ordered and systematic investigation. It encouraged specialty practice and endorsed an increasingly intimate relationship between medicine and surgery. The hospital was central in all of these developments. The second quarter of the nineteenth century was, in the words of a prominent medical historian, an era of hospital medicine.[23] The challenge of German laboratory medicine did not become a reality for most ambitious American physicians until the twentieth century. The careers of their nineteenth-century predecessors would necessarily be centered in the hospital, for it could alone provide the "clinical material" necessary for the following of a group of cases from admission to death and then postmortem.

Central to this complex of ideas and aspirations was a point of view that denigrated rationalistic theorizing and urged instead an almost exclusive emphasis on the data of the senses—aided by the scalpel and stethoscope—in defining and treating disease. This position reflected a particular philosophical stance, but, equally important, implied a program for medical investigation and shaped an academic style of clinical activity oriented not toward the care of particular patients, but toward the accumulation of knowledge based on the treatment (and possibly autopsy) of numerous patients with similar ills. With an immediate progenitor in eighteenth-century empiricist philosophy, the French emphasis on "medical observation" also invoked a more remote pedigree which saw its legitimate ancestors in a tradition of precise and sophisticated clinical description that ran from classical antiquity to Thomas Sydenham in the seventeenth century. No a priori assumptions could be admitted to a serious place in medical science.

Consistently enough, a number of prominent leaders in French medicine remained skeptical of, or uninterested in, the findings of the microscope or the chemical laboratory. Both pursuits seemed in their different ways to encourage speculation and come between man's senses and the biological phenomena those senses sought to comprehend. To the most dedicated among American acolytes of the French clinical school, a truly systematic investigation of disease implied the use of quantitative procedures to order and present the data gathered in bedside and postmortem observation. This "numerical method" was associated most prominently with P. C. A. Louis, a Paris clinician and teacher particularly influential among American students. Just as a chemist would specify the conditions and substances with which he worked, so Louis would specify the case he studied, list its chief symptoms, and subject each patient during life to physical diagnosis and at death to autopsy.[24] Instead of such accustomed terms as "often," "characteristically," or "usually," he could cite specific percentages of the incidence of a particular symptom or lesion and thus build up a seemingly objective picture of a disease.

Paralleling these developments were changes in the techniques of diagnosis that made the correlation between symptom and lesion even more plausible and the hospital increasingly central to the teaching of clinical medicine as well as pursuit of clinical learning. I refer, of course, to the introduction of physical diagnosis, to the use of auscultation and percussion as well as the stethoscope.[25] All increased the physician's ability to penetrate beyond his ancient dependence on the patient's subjective account of his symptoms, his appearance, and that of his bodily products. Thus, for example, in the case of tuberculosis (the most important single cause of adult death in nineteenth-century Europe), physicians could for the first time correlate general appearance and raised temperature with particular localized sounds during life and particular kinds of lesions after death. Or to cite another example, that of chronic kidney disease and the work of Richard Bright (1789–1858). As a young physician with little private practice, Bright worked long hours in the wards and autopsy room at Guy's Hospital in London. He was able to associate dropsy with albuminous urine during life and abnormal kidney appearances at death—and thus suggest that clinical entity, chronic nephritis, which as Bright's disease would provide him an enduring and eponymous fame. Such studies became a model for the professional aspirations of ambitious young physicians not only in Paris, but in Vienna, Dublin, London—and in Philadelphia, New York, and Boston.

By gradually reducing older holistic and general theories of disease to localized problems in pathology and physical diagnosis, this new way of understanding illness necessarily underlined the hospital's importance not simply as a center for the accumulation of status and teaching privileges, but as an indispensable basis for control of the medical profession's intellectual capital. Without access to the hospital's wards, a young man could not easily find time and facilities to evaluate and accumulate clinical data and publish the results of that experience. Only a small minority of physicians felt such aspirations, of course, while even those who did seek a reputation in antebellum America ordinarily limited their professional writing to accounts of atypical cases, experience with a new drug or technique, or rambling "philosophical" reflections on the nature and cure of disease. But whatever the quality of most antebellum medical journals and monographs, the incentive to write and publish remained central to the careers of that minority of physicians who hoped to attain professional eminence. Although only a comparative handful of American physicians were exposed to the personal influence of men such as P.C.A. Louis and the enormously varied clinical opportunities of the Paris hospitals, they played a disproportionately large role in medical education and in the shaping of medical ideas. Within the small elite who occupied medical school chairs and hospital positions, the number of Paris-trained men was by no means small. In the years before the Civil War, almost seven hundred Americans studied medicine in Paris; one out of ten were to teach in American medical schools.[26] Few young medical men of ambition and some means would not have contemplated a trip to France, though practical considerations implied a more modest commitment from most: learning French perhaps or, more commonly, the mastery of a growing body of clinical and pathological literature in translation.

The Americans who studied in France during these antebellum years were impressed not only with the clarity and rigor of French clinical standards, but with the enormous number of cases that filled the wards of Parisian hospitals. They were envious as well of the freedom enjoyed by Parisian attending physicians in treating and then autopsying their indigent patients. Perhaps most significantly, they were impressed by a dedication and professionalism that manifested itself in twelve-hour workdays, limited private practice, and the production of clearly argued monographs on particular ills or organs. The most ambitious sought in their necessarily limited way to duplicate this pattern of dedicated professionalism. "I continue my observations at our own little hospital," a Philadelphian reported after a Paris sojourn, "although I regret much the slender materials I possess and the difficulties wh[ich] seem inseparable from observation in this country."[27] Nevertheless, youthful Doctor William W. Gerhard managed to use the Philadelphia Almshouse Hospital "materials" to such good effect that he was able to make a significant clinical distinction between typhoid and typhus fevers. Gerhard's commitment to clinical investigation was emulated by scores of other ambitious if less discerning physicians. A youthful house officer at Bellevue, for example, sought in 1851 to test the diagnostic value of a red line along the gums that had been urged as a characteristic symptom of tuberculosis. Of forty-four cases admitted with that diagnosis, the line appeared in twenty-nine and was lacking in fifteen. Of thirty-five miscellaneous cases—a kind of control group—only two exhibited this symptom.[28] Although most physicians continued to be immersed in the everyday necessities of treating patients and earning their daily bread, a new style of medical achievement was being forged, paralleling a new way of looking at disease.

Although study in Paris or even the enjoyment of an American hospital or teaching position were options for only the privileged and ambitious, even ordinary practitioners had begun to feel the impact of intellectual change by midcentury. Most pervasive was a gradual redefinition of acceptable therapeutics. For the questioning of traditional conceptions of disease and sources of knowledge that marked the Paris School inevitably cast doubt upon the traditional modes of therapeutics we have already described; and treatment was an aspect of medicine which no practitioner could avoid. By the 1830s, skepticism toward traditional therapeutics had become a cliché in sophisticated medical circles; an influential cadre of prominent physicians spoke of self-limited diseases, of the physician's comparative impotence in changing the course of most ills. The healing power of nature, though an ancient concept to be sure, was invoked with increasing frequency as an explanation for therapeutic humility. This point of view emphasized that the great majority of ailments cured themselves; the physician's duty was simply to aid the process of natural recovery through appropriate and minimally heroic means. Routine prescription of harsh drugs might well impede the body's efforts to restore itself to health. "It would be better," as Oliver Wendell Holmes put it in his characteristically acerbic fashion, "if the patient were allowed a certain discount from his bill for every dose he took, just as children are compensated by their parents for swallowing hideous medicinal mixtures."[29] Rest, a strengthening diet, or a mild cathartic were all the aid nature required in most ills. In those ailments whose natural tendency was toward death, the physician had to acknowledge his powerlessness and try simply to minimize pain and anxiety. This noninterventionist ideal was paralleled by that emphasis on the specificity of disease we have just described—the view that most diseases could be seen as distinct clinical entities, each with a characteristic cause, course, and symptoms. If this were the case, minor ailments need not be regarded as incipiently mortal—and thus therapeutic intervention as necessarily critical. To some extent, of course, it implied that the physician was treating a disease and not simply a patient; medical emphasis on disease as specific entity implied a gradual diminution of the role of environment and emotions, of diet and rest, ultimately of the particular doctor-patient relationship itself as significant variables in defining sickness and health.

Such ideas were central in shaping debate over therapeutics in the middle third of the nineteenth century. But we must not forget how diverse and inconsistent actual practices might be: medicine is practiced at a good many levels and in a diversity of social and geographical contexts. Even in large urban hospitals, the admonitions of Paris-trained physicians did not always determine the treatment of patients, while ordinary clinicians—the majority of them rural and many trained decades earlier—remained, far into the nineteenth century, wedded to traditional modes of practice. American physicians were tied to the everyday requirements of the doctor-patient relationship and thus, even among the teaching elite, no mid-century American practitioner rejected traditional therapeutics with a ruthless consistency. The self-confident empiricism that could deny the efficacy—and eschew the use—of any measure not proven effective in numerically ordered clinical trials seemed an ideological excess, suited perhaps to professors in Vienna or Paris, but hardly appropriate to American realities. There were enduring virtues in the old ways. "There is," as one leader in the profession explained, "a vantage ground between the two extremes, neither verging toward meddlesome interference on the one hand, nor imbecile neglect on the other." The physician had to contend, moreover, with patient expectations: "The public," as another prominent clinician put it, "expect something more of physicians than the power of distinguishing diseases and predicting their issue. They look to them to the relief of their sufferings, and the cure or removal of their complaints."[30]

Antebellum patients did have some confidence in medicine: even hospital patients expected ordinarily to be helped by the drugs they swallowed and the salves applied to their skin. Such expectations dictated the continued administration of drugs capable of eliciting a perceptible physiological response. Hospital records indicate, for example, that even elite physicians maintained a more than lingering faith in the routine use of cathartics, even into the twentieth century. To do less would have been to disappoint their patients' expectations, to replace certainty with ideology.

Physicians shaped a number of intellectual compromises in order to maintain a comforting continuity with older ideas. They still emphasized their ability to modify symptoms—in appropriate cases even to deter a mild illness from drifting imperceptibly into a more severe one. Disease specificity was too subversive of traditional views to be accepted categorically. The older assumption that drugs acted in a way consistent with the body's innate pattern of recovery was easily shifted toward new emphases; the physician's responsibility now centered on recognizing the natural course of the patient's ailment and supporting the body in its progress to renewed health with an appropriate combination of drugs and regimen. Even the course of a self-limited disease might be shortened and painful symptoms mitigated. In ills whose natural course ended in death, the physician might still avail himself of therapeutic means to ease that grim journey. No one doubted, moreover, that there were ailments in which the physician's intervention could make the difference between life and death; scurvy, for example, was often cited as a disease "that taints the whole system, [yet] yields to a mere change in diet."[31] The surgeon, finally, had still to set bones, remove foreign bodies, drain abscesses. Although the great majority of mid-nineteenth-century hospital patients may have entered their ward in a spirit of fear and resignation, they shared their culture's therapeutic assumptions and at least some of its faith in the capacities of contemporary medicine.

Another theme that was to become increasingly prominent in the relationship among doctor, patient, and hospital was a conflict between the demands of clinical practice and those of clinical investigation—or in more dramatic terms between humanity and science. The beginnings of such conflict could already be discerned in American reactions to the thoroughgoing empiricism of French clinical medicine as well as to the often brutal treatment of patients in the great Paris hospitals. "The French have departed too much from the method of Sydenham and Hippocrates to make themselves good practitioners," an unconvinced New York doctor explained in 1836. "They are tearing down the temple of medicine to lay its foundations anew. . . . They lose more in therapeutics than they gain by morbid anatomy. They are explaining how men die but not how to cure them."[32] To some American medical teachers, the newly critical demands of the Paris Clinical School seemed almost antisocial, a rejection of the physician's duty to heal the individual patient in favor of an abstract commitment to methodological purity. Echoes of such controversies were to resonate through the later history of American hospitals, helping shape interactions between lay and medical authorities, between physician and patient, and among physicians with differing values and orientations.

Therapeutics was not the only area in which such change was gradually reshaping antebellum medicine. Another, as we have already suggested, lay in the area of diagnosis. Between the early 1830s and midnineteenth century, the use of the stethoscope and of auscultation and percussion became gradually more a part of the physician's normal clinical attainments, though still far from routine—even in hospital practice. But even if the average practitioner often could not or did not practice these new techniques, student demands for the teaching of physical diagnosis underlined a far older insistence upon the integration of bedside teaching into medical education—which, of course, implied the integration of medical school curriculum with hospital practice. Such clinical arrangements were consistent with the intellectual thrust of French clinical medicine and its advocacy of close observation as the only legitimate basis for teaching and practice. In a famous admonition attributed to Cabanis, a leading ideological founder of the Paris school, diseases themselves must now serve as texts. And just as one could only learn to read with book in hand, so the physician could only learn to read the language of pathology from the living body.[33]

Such justifications for clinical instruction were well defined before the stethoscope and auscultation came into general use, and by the 1860s these techniques for interrogating the body were to be joined by the ophthalmoscope, otoscope, and laryngoscope. The use of these new tools could only be taught individually or in small groups, and the hospital and dispensary were the only convenient places for such instruction. With the lingering demise of the apprentice system in antebellum America and the unwillingness of private patients to allow themselves to be used as teaching aids, the hospital and its passive charity patients loomed ever more prominently in the pleas and plans of would-be reformers of medical education.

The experience of Paris underlined the cosmopolitanism of medicine as much as it helped define its new clinical orientation. To be intellectually respectable was to strive for success and acceptance within the community of world medicine. The moral stature, social connections, and manual dexterity that had figured so prominently in the requirements for an attending physician's or surgeon's post or medical school chair in the first third of the century began to seem increasingly incomplete. When Elisha Bartlett published his forcefully argued *Essay on the Philosophy of Medical Science* in 1844 (an American restatement of the French clinical school's leading principles), he was careful to arrange for its distribution to leading French and English medical journals. He sent two copies to Pierre Louis and four to other prominent French physicians (and, of course, copies to a half-dozen American friends scattered from New Haven to Charleston).[34] At least some antebellum American physicians aspired to a world larger than that of their local peers and patients and rewards other than those of a thriving practice. Even if most nineteenth-century American clinical publications were of a quality that might inspire little confidence today, they did represent a commitment to the forms of advanced medical learning. As the century progressed, at least a minority of Americans grew ever more able to approximate the content as well.

The Balance of Tradition

This chapter has thus far emphasized change and the values that promoted and rewarded it. But the world of midnineteenth-century medical practice was still in reality, if not in programmatic statement, much the same as it had been in the century's first decades.

Ancient modes of diagnosis and therapeutics could not be easily discarded—especially when so little of proven therapeutic worth existed to replace them.

Much of diagnosis and prognosis still rested on the patient's own report of his symptoms, his appearance, and that of his bodily products. The stethoscope remained largely a tool of the elite consultant until after the Civil War; in the 1830s a cautious physician could still write that it was an impractical fad that only the most sophisticated of practitioners could ever hope to master. Only time could tell, as one such physician cautioned in 1831, whether the stethoscope would prove a blessing or a curse.[35] Traditional modes of diagnosis and prognosis at mid-century still emphasized individual idiosyncrasy and the emotional centrality of the doctor-patient relationship itself. Students were still warned that anxiety might affect pulse rates, that the pulse should not be taken immediately after the physician entered the sickroom, but rather postponed until the patient had been put at his or her ease.[36] It was still assumed that anxiety or psychic stress as well as family circumstances could interact to shape the course of a particular disease. "When the close connection which exists between the mind and body is considered," a Boston editorialist explained, "it is not strange that practitioners in every period and country should have regarded a due deference to the former as an important means of producing a salutary effect on the latter."[37] Hospital medicine must to some extent have mirrored these traditional assumptions, although altered by the social distance that normally separated doctor and patient and the brusque and episodic quality of most hospital care.

Therapeutics too was modified in practice, but hardly in ruthless consistency with the programmatic demands of those who would purge all unproven or traditional elements from the physician's therapeutic arsenal. Older modes of practice did not die, but, as we have suggested, were prescribed less routinely, and often in smaller doses. Bleeding especially sank into disuse. The resident physician at the Philadelphia Dispensary could, for example, report in 1862, that of a total of 9,502 patients treated that year, "general blood-letting has been resorted to in one instance only . . . cupping twelve times, and leeching thrice." Residents at Bellevue in New York and at Boston's Massachusetts General Hospital had reported the previous year that bloodletting was "almost obsolete."[38] Bleeding still lingered, however, though increasingly in the practice of older men and in less cosmopolitan areas. Mercury, on the other hand, still figured omnipresently in the practice of most physicians; even infants and small children endured the symptoms of mercury poisoning until well after the Civil War. Purges were still routinely administered in spring and fall to facilitate physiological adjustment to the changing seasons. The purposely induced blisters and excoriated running sores so familiar to physicians and patients at the beginning of the century were gradually replaced by mustard plasters or turpentine applications, but the ancient concept of counter-irritation still rationalized their use. In hospitals, the individual patient suffering from an acute ailment probably did benefit from a somewhat more liberal and "strengthening" regimen; he or she was more likely to receive tonics and a fortifying diet than to be bled and purged, or at least bled and purged to the extent likely in the first third of the century.

Change did not only come about through moderation of doses and an increasing faith in nature's healing power, but through the availability of entirely new therapeutic options. By midcentury, hospital patients were being exposed to a number of new and, in retrospect, significant additions to the materia medica. French pharmaceutical chemistry had purified such drugs as morphine, strychnine, and quinine: dosage levels could be more systematically controlled and the quality of the drugs themselves grew increasingly reliable. Even more dramatic was the introduction of surgical anesthesia in the late 1840s. First demonstrated in a public operation in the Massachusetts General Hospital in 1846, ether was internationally known and almost as widely accepted within a few years. There were, of course, some skeptics, and even enthusiasts used anethesia in far fewer procedures than we would consider appropriate; yet it and its English rival, chloroform, were quickly adopted into surgical practice.[39] By the 1860s, there was more controversy over the relative merits of ether and chloroform than there was over the usefulness of either.

But the dramatic introduction of surgical anesthesia did little to reshape the more fundamental realities we have already outlined. Surgeons had for millennia sought ways of avoiding pain—alcohol, opium, and hypnotism, for example, had all been employed with varying degrees of success in the years before the introduction of ether. In itself, surgical anesthesia could neither revolutionize surgery nor reshape the hospital's public image. The frequency of surgery almost certainly did increase in the generation after 1846, but without a knowledge of antisepsis and the gradual solution of a host of less dramatic technical dilemmas, the possibilities for the growth of surgery were limited. Until late in the century, surgery remained largely an affair of setting bones and, more frequently, dressing wounds and infections. Operative procedures remained the exception rather than the rule, even in hospital cases admitted to surgical wards.

Fundamental notions of pathology changed more deliberately still. Older ideas about the nature of disease remained indispensable. To most physicians at mid-century, one disease could still shade into another; illness was still in many ways a place along a spectrum of physiological possibilities—not some categorical entity capable of afflicting almost anyone with the same patterned symptoms as the more devoted advocates of French medicine contended. Holistic definitions of sickness as a general state of the organism were consistent with social attitudes toward need and dependence, in that both included moral as well as material elements. In both, the interplay of individual and environment could bring about health or disease, prosperity or poverty.

At mid-century, every aspect of the relationship between medical knowledge and the hospital was uncertain and subject to future negotiation. And it was a period when a newly critical spirit of reform aggressively questioned every aspect of the traditional hospital—from architecture to therapeutics. No student of the institution as it existed in the English-speaking world could remain content with the crowding, the casual nursing, the seemingly unavoidable incidence of hospital-connected illness that at once characterized and indicted mid-century hospitals. And no would-be advocate of the building of new, or the reform of old, hospitals could avoid this debate and its increasingly insistent demands for improvements in architecture, in cleanliness and order, in nursing and plumbing, and in ventilation. Thinking about the mid-century hospital became an exercise in self-conscious social engineering.

But before much could be done to reshape America's hospitals, they were engulfed by a far more general conflict. The flowering of hospital reform would have to wait until Appomattox and the restoration of civil order.

PART II

A New Healing Order,

1850–1920

CHAPTER 4:

Expanding a Traditional Institution: Social Sources of Hospital Growth, 1850–1875

In many ways the Civil War marked a turning point in the consciousness of Americans. The war seemed—even to contemporaries—to constitute a new kind of experience, one demonstrating that technological change, economic growth, and immigration had made America a very different sort of country from that which had fought for and gained its independence in the eighteenth century.

At the beginning of the conflict, medical facilities were entirely inadequate: a handful of career surgeons, a few men from the ranks serving as they always had as nurses and orderlies, no ambulance service, and, of course, no proper hospitals to treat the flood of sick and wounded.[1] By the end of the War, however, American military hospitals (and, significantly, both Union and Confederacy adopted many of the same policies) had become models for European observers to praise and for their armies to emulate—enormous, well organized, and with surprisingly low death-rates. American ingenuity had assimilated and articulated in institutional form lessons of hospital construction and administration learned during a century of European military campaigns. By the time of Lee's surrender in 1865, the Union alone had more than two hundred hospitals with almost 137,000 beds.[2] But the Civil War medical man's therapeutic resources had changed far less than the technology that had produced the railroads, the telegraph, and the breechloading rifles so important in shaping a new style of warfare. With the exception of anesthesia, the everyday therapeutics employed by a physician in Ulysses Grant's army would have been recognizable by his counterpart in George Washington's. Diet, warmth, cleanliness, and venti-

lation were at least as important as any particular therapeutic intervention in ensuring recovery. Surgery, of course, loomed more
prominently in military than civilian hospitals, but the great majority of actual operations were unavoidable responses to battlefield
necessity—and, in any case, failed to impugn the assumption that
rest, diet, and adequate ventilation were as important to the healing
process as the surgical procedure itself.

Nevertheless, as contemporaries saw it, the Civil War hospital
represented a triumph of scientific rationality. Not therapeutics or
diagnostics, but the physical and administrative structure of the
hospital had been transformed. Cleanliness, order, and ventilation
were the requirements for a modern hospital and, as Florence Nightingale had dramatically contended in the 1850s, these requirements
could be guaranteed by proper design and a newly professional
internal order.

More than a million men were treated in Union hospitals alone.
They experienced a death rate of less than 10 percent, a remarkable
record given both previous military experience and the conditions
prevalent at the outbreak of hostilities. For the first time a broad
cross section of the male American population experienced the reality of institutional care. Not only the urban poor, but farmers,
miners, small town clerks, and carpenters might have been
wounded in battle or, more likely, found themselves hospitalized
with dysentery or fever. And the quality of hospital care improved
steadily throughout the war. Contemporaries were particularly impressed with the way in which the enormous rear hospitals were
managed—laundry and meals and nursing provided, the wards
maintained in scrupulous order. Most important, physicians and
administrators had managed to hold in check the dangers of hospi-
tal-originated fever and infection previously regarded as an almost
inevitable consequence of bringing together large numbers of the
sick and wounded. There seemed to be a lesson here, a lesson that
at least some American physicians and philanthropists were to take
to heart.

The moral was simple enough. The hospital was a viable as well
as necessary institution, certainly for treatment of the dependent
and the urban working poor. And it was an institution that could
be made as safe as it was indispensable, as safe in fact as a middle-
class home. The Civil War experience helped crystallize an activist
consensus around the specific elements that constituted a good hospital and in doing so contributed to the motivation of those who

sought to make that new-model hospital a reality. If it could be made to work effectively during the stress of war, it could certainly be made even more efficacious in peacetime. Many of the most prominent advocates of hospital reform were men and women who had experienced the war and been changed by it. Some were physicians, but others active in the medical and philanthropic aspects of the war were clergymen, lawyers, lady teachers—even a landscape architect in the energetic person of Frederick Law Olmstead.[3] For a brief time at least, the hospital experience had become a public experience, not isolated in the ranks of the poor and inarticulate or a comparative handful of physicians.

Then the war ended. The enormous administrative and logistical apparatus evaporated even more rapidly than it had been assembled. Foot soldiers returned to their homes where ordinarily the chances of being treated in a hospital, often of ever seeing a hospital, were minimal. Only for the freedman, the merchant seaman, and a tiny cadre of professional soldiers did medical care continue to be a federal responsibility. The Civil War exerted a substantial but elusive influence on the development of hospitals in America.

The movement to expand and improve hospital facilities had, in fact, already begun in the late 1840s and 1850s and been marked by the same reformist agenda that would be instrumental in upgrading military hospitals during the war. The hospital movement was to gain impressive impetus well before medical ideas and medical men had done much to change the institution's technical capacities or to reshape lay expectations. For this generation of reformers, the hospital would remain a refuge for the less fortunate, for men and women very different from themselves. The years between midcentury and the early 1870s were marked by the founding of new hospitals and by an intensified spirit of activism motivating this institutional growth. But it was an activism informed by traditional views of social welfare and individual responsibility; medicine occupied a necessary but still clearly subordinate place. Growth did not bring immediate change in the mission or internal order of America's hospitals.

Commonwealth and Commonhealth

The new nation that came into being in Philadelphia in 1787 had almost four million citizens; when the Civil War broke out in 1861, its population had increased eight times to almost thirty-two million.[4] America had moved westward from the Atlantic Coast and extended itself across the continent. The population had not only grown steadily but, perhaps more relevantly for our discussion, America's cities had expanded with particular speed and visibility, a visibility enhanced by the fact that foreign immigration as well as natural increase had played a prominent role in that urban growth.

By mid-century, the city was not only growing alarmingly but was filled with a seemingly alien population. Six percent of Americans lived in towns of more than twenty-five hundred in 1800; in 1860 their proportion had increased more than three-fold to almost 20 percent, in actual numbers over six million.[5] Between 1790 and 1819, only a comparative handful of immigrants had settled in the United States. In the 1860 census, over four million Americans recorded themselves as foreign-born.[6] America was becoming larger, more disparate, increasingly different from what seemed in retrospect to have been a simple, self-reliant—and healthy—society. In this generation, the connections between physical and moral well-being were still unquestioned; those conditions that made for infant mortality made also for intemperance and corrupt politics, all those brutal realities that blighted such English cities as Manchester, London, and Birmingham.

In a generation newly attracted to the power of statistical truth, there seemed increasing evidence to support this view.[7] Statistics showed that Americans, like Frenchmen and Englishmen, lived longer in the country than in the city, and rural areas seemed better able to contend with their limited problems of deviance and dependence. In a society that presumed inevitable moral and material progress, in which growth and technological development were seen by the vast majority of Americans as unambiguously good, the nation's ever more visibly deteriorating urban health conditions seemed both alarming and inexcusable. Cholera epidemics in 1832–1834 and 1849–1854 underlined the dangers of large cities as well as the unpleasant realization that America could no longer be spared the debasing circumstances of English and European industrial life.[8] The provision of medical care for the city's indigent population was at once a pious reflex and a pragmatic response to felt necessities.

More than alliteration bound poverty and progress together. In the words of an Episcopalian layman appealing for funds to care for Philadelphia's sick in 1851, every steamboat and locomotive, every increase in commerce and urban population meant a disproportionate increase in sickness and injury. "The young men employed in our workshops and factories," he pointed out, "or engaged in the various laborious pursuits which furnish the means of living, are boarded, at low rates, in small rooms crowded to repletion; very generally sleeping in double beds. . . ." They suffered discomfort in even the most trivial ailment; when beset by serious ills, their poverty might constitute the difference between recovery and death or permanent disability. Attentive nursing, an appropriately nourishing diet, quiet, and rest were a necessary part of medical care—but were amenities often unavailable to the poor and working classes. Many Philadelphians, moreover, who employed servants or apprentices could not even "with the best wishes" find the time or space to care for such dependents at home as tradition enjoined.[9] Added to these victims of sickness who found themselves in mid-century hospital beds were an ever-increasing number of unfortunates injured in accidents at work or while traveling to it.

Twenty-five years ago, the same advocate argued, the fracture ward at the Pennsylvania Hospital was often empty for weeks at a time; in 1827 the hospital had admitted only 140 cases of accidental injury, of which 45 were fractures. In 1837, the number of trauma admissions had risen to 292, of which 119 were fractures; by 1847 the number of accident admissions had risen to 400. The trend was only to intensify. In 1846, there had been an average of twenty-nine beds filled by accident cases; in 1855–1856, this average had increased to fifty-six.[10]

In previous decades America had been able to exist with only a handful of hospitals. Most citizens had the means to employ a private physician and be treated in their own rural or village homes. It was not simply that there were no adequate accommodations for the growing number of sick and injured among the urban working classes, but that the lack of hospital beds meant in practice the consigning of worthy and hard-working citizens to the almshouse. Every thoughtful philanthropist agreed as to the injustice of such a fate. Forty years ago, a New Haven Hospital committee reported in 1871, their city had been much smaller and of a "different charac-

ter"; few demanded hospital accommodations. "It would be a re-
proach to the city to allow the present state of things to continue":
the almshouse must not be the working man or woman's only
refuge when ill.[11]

America's handful of voluntary general hospitals simply could
not handle the burden of sickness. At midcentury, for example,
Boston's one voluntary hospital, Massachusetts General, provided
beds for only 110 patients, and 23 of these paid all or some of their
"board."[12] Any others among Boston's working population who fell
ill or were injured had recourse only to the almshouse when their
resources and those of their families proved inadequate. The perception of a crisis in benevolence was underlined by the prominence
of new immigrants among prospective hospital patients. Single
working men appeared disproportionately in hospital populations—and the new immigrants of the 1840s and 1850s were over-
represented in this dependent group. In 1866, when Bellevue Hospital treated 7,111 new cases, only 2,143 had been born in the United
States—3,705 were Irish and 602 were German. Jersey City's Charity Hospital reported that between 1869 and 1875, of a total of 4,225
patients admitted, 1,185 had been born in the United States and
1,959 in Ireland, 400 in Germany, and 412 in England or Scotland.
The Quaker managers of Philadelphia's Pennsylvania Hospital reported in 1867 that during the previous decade only 7,312 of 19,478
admissions were native-born; over 7,000 were from Ireland. Even in
the less industrialized city of New Haven, roughly two-thirds of the
community hospital's admissions were foreign-born.[13] Recent immigrants had always filled a disproportionate number of beds in
American hospitals, but the scale and visibility of the problem had
increased alarmingly. Like the increase in trauma that it paralleled
in time, the growing number of indigent foreign-born applicants for
medical aid made clear how much America's cities had changed
since the beginning of the century.

Even though such need might increase the costs of public and
private philanthropy, there was no other option. Fellow creatures
could not be allowed to die in streets, doorways, or tenement cubicles. "If it shall ever become our theory that society ought to get rid
of its useless members," as one steward of that society's wealth
contended,

instead of taking care of them, the moral effect upon the useful members
will totally change the aspect of modern life, if it does not speedily re-

verse that process of development by which beasts are said to become men.[14]

Although critical thinkers warned again and again of the dangers indiscriminate relief posed to the recipients themselves—the demoralization contemporaries referred to as pauperism—most of the benevolent conceded that inpatient hospital care would not easily be abused, as payments in cash, food, or even fuel might be.[15]

If poverty is an evil, or disease a misfortune, then certainly, where they coexist, the miseries of each are intensified by the presence of the other, and the sum total is multiplied an hundred fold. And as the political economists have not yet succeeded in finding any means for preventing pauperism,—nor the physicians, in discovering any method of wholly annihilating disease,—it follows that society must still continue to provide for those of its members who are, by either or both of these calamities, incapacitated from taking care of themselves.

And anyone familiar with urban realities knew that it was not simply the lowest orders of society who might find themselves in need of care; many respectable and otherwise deserving Americans were locked into the grinding interstices of city life. Prospective hospital patients included not only "the humbler classes, but . . . clerks, etc., and small salaried men; the corresponding class of females, working for low wages, and lodging in cheap, comfortless unhealthy boarding houses."[16]

No matter how hard they worked in ordinary times and how moral their behavior, a respectable family might not be able to provide for themselves during sickness. Many families in fact required the income of more than one member to survive even in periods of good health and regular employment. Hospital fundraisers often referred to such grim realities; they sought to help the worthy, not the unworthy poor. They had had no intention of raising money for the care of those whose proper receptacle was the almshouse.

Society's benefits would transcend the mere provision of episodic medical care. In a period when the connections between sickness and health, moral obliquity and prudent self-control, psychic and physical environment were simply assumed, the hospital played an important and only partially technical role. Advocates of hospital care were well aware that drugs and surgery could often do little.

On the other hand, rest, warmth, nourishing food, and adequate nursing might make the difference between life and death. Many among the sick, as a group of women philanthropists urged in 1866, remain "without any effectual remedy, solely because the sufferers cannot command rest, suitable food, and the soothing surrounding indispensable to the full success of medical appliances."[17] Curing an illness brought more than transient benefits, for it might produce individuals better able to withstand sickness in the future. This was particularly the case with children. "It is well known," as one group of children's hospital advocates put it, "that the combined evils of poverty tend to cause a chronic condition of all the complaints of childhood, inducing symptoms and conditions which yield reluctantly to medical treatment." The means employed in curing a child from one ailment might help to ". . . establish a strengthening and confirming of the whole bodily condition, which should give the child, through life, a firm and vigorous constitution."[18]

Related to this holistic orientation were two other sentiments. Perhaps most important to the founding of mid-century hospitals was a sense of pious activism. The second quarter of the century had been a period of religious awakening, and the hospital was, to at least some philanthropists, a place in which they could act out the grace that energized them and in which the objects of their benevolence would benefit spiritually as well as medically. "How many aching, suffering hearts have been encouraged and strengthened by the unexpected kindness and sympathy they have met in this elegant home for the sick, and how sweetly from Sabbath to Sabbath, the voice of prayer has been heard in these halls, and the songs of Christian praise have pervaded these wards of suffering! How Christ-like the work!"[19] A cynical and secularly oriented observer might choose to emphasize that this particular exhortation to piety was written in praise of a hospital that treated Pittsburgh's industrial workers and was supported in good part by the dollars of families whose wealth had been won in the city's new industries.[20]

This coincidence suggests a second theme in the movement for extension of hospital care. This was an appeal to the interest of employers. In retrospect, one might well attribute a kind of economic rationality to the nineteenth-century hospital; it both restored working men to their labors and at the same time assuaged the lingering pangs of traditional conscience. And advocates were on occasion willing to see the hospital in these instrumental terms. One such argued in 1874 that society could not "afford to lose the pecuniary value of the life or health of any citizen, and that it finds in every possessor of a sound mind in a sound body, a positive addition to its social forces."[21] Interest no less than humanity demanded public support for hospitals. Such appeals were, for example, invoked routinely by advocates of free ophthalmological treatment. One could hold out to possible contributors (and legislators) the prospect of timely intervention to save the eyesight of workers and their families who would otherwise become public charges. There was no chance that such funds would be used to foster "idleness and dishonesty"—the ever-present specter of pauperism—among the poor. Economy allied itself with humanity in urging the support of such institutions.[22] Occasionally, moreover, factory owners were appealed to as a class, as potential beneficiaries of a hospital's therapeutics. The growth of industry implied new forms of benevolence. The hospital's benefits to the working man would aid not only him but his employer and, ultimately, society generally. "Order and efficiency will thereby be secured; and the operative quickly restored to his family and factory."[23] But such mundane appeals were far less common than arguments based on traditional stewardship. And when they were made, these pragmatic contentions were used to supplement, not contradict, the more pious and paternalistic appeals that tended to characterize hospital publications. The hospital was assumed to be a class-structured institution and the motives of its mid-century lay supporters were predicated on traditional notions of Christian responsibility and the obligations of class. Certainly this is how they saw themselves.

The hospital was, in fact, an accepted and understood part of an enlarged concept of stewardship organized around a vision of the common good—one in which a potential conflict between interest and Christianity could not exist. The stewards of society's worldly goods were necessarily the proper stewards for the interests of their community's less fortunate members. In this sense, there was no such thing as a truly private hospital in America during the first three quarters of the nineteenth century.[24] The trustees of voluntary hospitals thought of themselves as serving the community, not as running a private enterprise. It was no narrow legal authority they exerted, but a more general stewardship, justified by the responsibilities appropriate to their class and demanded by the common good. Thus it was only natural for the legislatures of many states to have provided for nominally private hospitals in one way or another, through lotteries, or cash grants, or auction fees, or even the proceeds of an insurance company chartered by the state. And once this practice was begun, emulation between the states served as a powerful argument for the further outpouring of legislative subsidies.

It was an entirely appropriate object of Commonwealth support, as an advocate of the Massachusetts General Hospital contended in 1819. Any costs to the state would be repaid within a few years by savings in welfare. But such actuarial benefits were only a subsidiary issue, for the fact was that communities, like individuals, were subject to the will of the Most High. Neither could escape their moral obligation to care for those unable to care for themselves. (And then the argument naturally, if rather more mundanely, followed that Massachusetts should not be outdone by Pennsylvania and New York who had in their different ways already chosen to support voluntary hospitals.)[25] The result of such assumptions was the growth of a tradition of casually mixed public and private support—though under private control. As early as the 1750s, the provincial legislature of Pennsylvania had provided "matching funds" to establish North America's first general hospital in Philadelphia. Later, New York State provided regular subventions for the operating expenses of the New York Hospital (though significantly neither state supported its chief city's municipal welfare facilities).[26] Louisiana's Charity Hospital routinely received funds from the state, though in a variety of forms including taxes on gambling houses (1823) and theaters (1838). Ophthalmic hospitals in Boston, New York, and Chicago all received state funds at mid-century; the Massachusetts Charitable Eye and Ear Infirmary was in fact to enjoy a state grant every year between 1837 and 1919.[27]

This discussion of motives has thus far been synthetic, drawing upon examples from a number of different institutions to illustrate the social circumstances and values that shaped the hospital movement at mid-century. Let me turn to a specific instance, that of the Hartford Hospital in Connecticut. America's earliest hospitals had all been in port cities, and Hartford represented the trend toward establishment of hospitals in a second tier of middle-sized but steadily growing communities such as Albany, Troy, New Haven, and Louisville. In conjunction with a few "benevolent gentlemen," a group of Hartford physicians at mid-century had organized a "Society for Providing a Home for the Sick," but had attracted little support until a boiler explosion at a local factory left numbers of dead and injured workmen—and the realization that the city had already become industrial but had failed to develop means for dealing with the injury and sickness inevitably the lot of factory and construction workers.[28]

A large public meeting presided over by the mayor and attended by many of the city's physicians and clergymen crystallized hospital sentiment. During the winter of 1854–1855, over one hundred local citizens became members of the projected hospital association for a year, pledging ten dollars each, while "several liberal gentlemen had already made subscriptions, some of one thousand and others of five hundred dollars."[29] The city's economic elite had clearly chosen to support this new charity. The General Assembly of Connecticut had granted a charter (May, 1854) and the legislature also appropriated ten thousand dollars the next year on the condition that an additional twenty thousand be raised from private sources. Within a short time, over thirty thousand dollars had been pledged, and the Hartford Hospital opened in a temporary rented home. Soon the first few patients were admitted with board set at three dollars a week. By 1859, citizens of Hartford were able to congratulate themselves on the dedication of a permanent hospital building; they had given $39,556 in addition to the ten thousand provided by the state. A year later the legislature voted two thousand dollars toward the institution's annual operating costs and in 1861 this was made an annual grant.[30]

From the very first, the hospital's experience seemed to bear out the contention that an enormous need existed among the community's working poor. Rural and village workers as well as the foreign-born had begun to converge on the state's growing cities. "These people are crowded together in large boarding-houses, or accommodated in private rooms." Adequate care was impossible in such surroundings. The situation could only be expected to worsen. "Manufacturing interests are increasing in most of the towns in the vicinity of Hartford. Thousands of people," hospital spokesmen argued, "are employed in these manufactories, whose daily subsistence is entirely dependent on their daily labor." How were they to be cared for in the event of sickness or injury? The experience of other communities had demonstrated that "well regulated hospitals, properly ventilated, are the only true modes of providing for this class."[31]

These persons are human, and must not be left to suffer uncared for in a Christian land. . . . It is a burden that is placed on community and there is no escape from its responsibility. The intelligent sick, fallen from respectable positions by the cruel hand of misfortune, without any fault of their own, cannot be passed by in a Christian community and left to die.[32]

The "intelligent"—that is the middle class in lifestyle—sick deserved a place where they could be cared for and spared the humiliating associations and permanent stigma of the almshouse. Their hospital, the Hartford trustees reported in 1866, was free to

. . . persons of temperate and industrious habits, who, from sickness or accident required care or attention, for which they are unable to pay; . . . We would not have this Hospital a receptacle for persons degraded with vice or intemperance, or a home for the hopeless pauper. It is a home for the honest mechanic and laborer, who by temporary disease or accident, is unable to support himself or family. . . . It is a home for respectable domestics who cannot be made comfortable in their attic chambers or receive necessary attention however well disposed the family in which they reside.[33]

From its inception, donors to the Hartford Hospital had been assured that their alms would not be misapplied. A hospital could guard against fraud as the individual philanthropist could not. Only the genuinely sick would be admitted, and these could hardly be demoralized by the care that restored them to health.

Given the harsh realities of urban life, advocates claimed, Hartford would ultimately save money by supporting its new hospital. The provision of care to one family member might in the long run preserve the health of all. The scenario was not hard to imagine. "One member of a family becomes sick. The watching, nursing, and increased expense impoverish them, in consequence of which they must all be provided for at the alms-house. If the sick person could be provided with a free bed at the Hospital," the argument followed, "the family could be stimulated to effort, and would be able to sustain themselves without assistance from the town."[34]

By 1870, the Hartford Hospital had grown increasingly like its institutional peers in the older port cities, its clients largely foreign-born and working-class. In 1870, the hospital admitted 284 new cases, 131 "Americans" and 153 "foreigners." Private donations helped by state and city subventions eked out a frugal budget. (Hartford pegged its support at a rate of $2.00 per patient week, at a time when the institution contended that its true costs were $5.58—a shortfall prefiguring what was to become, and has continued to be, a chronic problem for urban hospitals.) Like most of its counterparts, Hartford admitted a highly disproportionate number of males, 201 of 284 patients; a ratio of almost exactly three to one. Of these male patients 82 were classified as laborers, 67 as mechanics, and 13 as seamen.[35] This was no cross section of the Hartford community as a whole. Just as the size, number, and industrial infrastructure of cities expanded, so did the hospital. It was a natural community response to perceived social need—a response in which medical men often played a crystallizing, but rarely a dominant, role.

Patterns of Hospital Growth

In 1848, Philadelphia, still America's medical capital, boasted only one general hospital aside from the city's almshouse medical wards. New York also had one private general hospital, and both these institutions, the Pennsylvania and New York hospitals, were already old and well established by 1848. Yet this period saw the beginning of aggressive hospital growth in New York and Philadelphia.

New York's Catholics founded St. Vincent's Hospital in 1849 and the Episcopal St. Luke's opened its doors a year later. The city's Jewish population followed suit and established Mt. Sinai Hospital in 1852, while Catholics opened a second hospital, St. Francis, in 1865. The well-endowed Presbyterian Hospital received its first patients in 1868. These were explicitly religious institutions. Other motives led to the founding of Roosevelt in 1871, German (now Lenox Hill) in 1869, the Woman's Hospital in 1857, the New York Medical College and Hospital for Women in 1863, as well as an assortment of specialty hospitals: Manhattan Eye and Ear (1869), Metropolitan Throat Hospital (1874), New York Ophthalmic Hospital (1865), and New York Orthopedic Hospital (1867).[36] And this enumeration does not include several homes for foundlings; a Society of the Lying-In Hospital, which provided obstetric care for poor women in their homes; and several refuges for the chronically ill and consumptive. Nor, most important in terms of numbers, does it reflect the steady expansion of the city's own facilities for the sick and infirm poor.

At the close of the Civil War, New York's Commissioners of Public Charities and Correction were responsible not only for the sprawling, thousand-bed Bellevue Hospital, but also for a chronic disease hospital (Charity), smallpox hospital, fever hospital, infant or foundling hospital, and units for incurables and epileptics, paralytics and lunatics, all on Blackwell's Island, as well as a Children's Hospital and Idiot Asylum on Randall's Island. Bellevue alone treated 7,725 inpatients in 1866 and Charity, 7,574.[37] And these figures were insignificant compared to the amount of outpatient care provided the city's working people during the same year by New York's freestanding dispensaries, hospital outpatient departments, and the city's own "outdoor" physicians. Other large cities had experienced a similar growth of hospitals and dispensaries, though perhaps none so luxuriant as that supported by New York's booming economy. Institutional treatment, both inpatient and outpatient, had become central to the health care of the urban working classes just as it had already become indispensable to the career aspirations and teaching plans of the city's medical elite.

Newer cities followed the lead of their East Coast peers. Chicago, still a village in the 1830s, could also by the early 1870s boast an assortment of hospitals pleasing to any civic-minded citizen. Largest was Chicago's own Cook County Hospital founded in 1865; almost as large was Mercy Hospital founded in 1850. Like Mercy, St. Joseph's, St. Luke's, and the Alexian Brothers Hospital had all been established by religious men and women. But the striving new metropolis also boasted the Illinois Charitable Eye and Ear Hospital (1866), Chicago Hospital for Women and Children (1865), and the Woman's Hospital of the State of Illinois (1871).[38]

Although New York and Chicago might well be seen as atypical in the scale of want created by their explosive growth, motives for the expansion of hospital facilities were similar in smaller cities. One, as I have suggested, was a secular manifestation of a pious activism—evident even in the assumptions of an overtly secular hospital like Hartford but more explicitly central in the establishment of a group of midcentury hospitals by enthusiasts in the Episcopal Church: St. Luke's in New York, Episcopal in Philadelphia, for example, or the Church Home and Hospital in Baltimore and St. Luke's in Chicago. "No one," a Philadelphia Episcopal philanthropist contended in 1851, "who believes that sickness is one of the means appointed by Divine Wisdom to prepare the heart for the reception of divine truth, can hesitate to admit the importance of introducing religious instruction and ministrations, prudently and affectionately, into every chamber of sickness, . . ." It was humiliating, moreover, to contemplate the possibility that members of the Episcopal confession might enter an almshouse to be supported by public taxation and not the sympathy of fellow Christians.[39]

The growth of Catholic hospitals has to be seen in a rather different light—a consequence not simply of the specific history and commitment of the church and its religious orders, but of the isolated and defensive character of the Catholic immigrant population in American cities. Similar motivations help explain the contemporary movement for Jewish hospitals. In both cases, advocates emphasized that existing hospitals, no matter what their formal auspices, were in reality Protestant and all-too-often proselytizing institutions. An unmarried Jewish peddler, just like an Irish longshoreman, might find himself sick and alone in one of America's new cities. In neither case did their coreligionists feel it morally appropriate that they be at the mercy of almshouse administrators—or of the trustees and physicians of a Protestant-dominated voluntary hospital. By 1885, the Catholic community had opened 154 hospitals throughout the United States, more than had existed in the United States *in toto* in the late 1860s.[40]

The Catholic hospitals especially could not only offer a sense of ethnic identity, but also the dignity of being treated as a paying patient. For the great majority of early Catholic hospitals did charge, although at rates not much different from those prevalent at working-class boarding houses. With such payment, a mechanic or domestic could avoid the stigma of receiving charity in an alien institution. In 1858, a physician at New York Hospital complained, for example, that they could not compete with St. Vincent's for the patronage of industrious members of the working class.

Other things equal, most of our domestic servants prefer that institution, and find there watchful and attentive nurses, whose social rank is superior to their own. The patients of that institution all pay; and the charge, I believe, is three dollars a week for each person.[41]

The attending physician's reference to "our" servants made very clear the class identity of both those providing care and those who would be its natural recipients. Episcopal Hospital in Philadelphia faced a similar problem in the early 1850s; it could hardly hope to compete with the modest rates charged by St. Joseph's Hospital (founded only a few years before) or the spiritual comforts provided by the nursing sisters who staffed it.

Both German and Jewish hospitals appealed to a language-centered identity as well and, in both cases, to a network of existing benevolent societies and activities. Philadelphia's German Hospital, for example, was founded (1860–1861) with the aid of a number of societies and firms that purchased hundred dollar life memberships in the hospital. Such sponsors included the Cabinetmaker's Beneficial Society, the German Society of Pennsylvania, the Canstatter Volksfest-Verein, and the J. & P. Baltz Brewing Company.[42] In all these cases, an ethnic or religious community's honor was in some sense at stake in providing for its own. Thus, Philadelphia's Jewish Hospital could appeal for funds in 1867 on the grounds that it was a visibly Jewish institution: "It is a credit and a pride to its projectors and supporters; therefore the *honor* of the Jewish people is involved in maintaining it properly."[43] Emulation too could serve as an argument for institution building. In 1864, for example, when Philadelphia's B'nai Brith Lodge No. 3 issued an appeal (in German and English) for the founding of a Jewish hospital, they urged that if New York and Cincinnati as well as so many European cities had been able to found such institutions:

It reflects the greatest discredit on so large a Jewish population as that of Philadelphia, to force friendless brothers to seek, in sickness and the prospect of death, the shelter of un-jewish hospitals, to eat forbidden food, to be dissected after death and sometimes even to be buried with the stranger.[44]

Not the peculiar technology of medical diagnosis and therapeutics, but rather the need for good and familiar food, for warmth, cleanliness, and dignity justified the founding of such ethnic and religious hospitals. Home remained the ideal place to treat the sick—but if that home proved inadequate, the hospital was a necessary recourse. And like a good home, the hospital must provide for the souls and dignity as well as for the bodies of those it nurtured.

Such assumptions guaranteed that the new ethnic hospitals would expand the categories of those treated; many, for example, made a point of admitting chronic, and often aged, patients, a group generally excluded by the older private hospitals. In 1869, for example, when the Roman Catholic Carney Hospital opened in Boston, it welcomed aged patients. The sisters reserved one of its five floors for "old people who may not be sick but come here for a home."[45] The hospitals founded by Episcopal benevolence in this period rejected the traditionally rigid rules excluding chronic patients. In New York, St. Luke's admitted some chronic patients, and in addition, Episcopal laymen also saw to it that a Home for Incurables was established just outside the city. Nowhere else but at the "forbidding almshouse," Chicago's St. Luke's reported in 1866, would the aged and feeble be cared for; thus, the hospital found a place in its wards for some "aged men who are there simply because nowhere else could they have the decencies and comforts of life to which none who knew them would deny they are entitled."[46] Some of the religious hospitals also admitted tubercular cases, normally avoided by voluntary hospitals which regarded them as difficult and unpleasant as well as generally incurable. Cancer, too, ordinarily disqualified a patient from voluntary hospital care. But such admission criteria were antithetical to the assumptions and motives of many midcentury philanthropists. "Next to promoting a restoration to health and strength," the trustees of one Episcopal Hospital explained

there is perhaps no greater charity than that of giving a hopelessly ill man or woman a comfortable bed to die in; and in very many intermediate cases, while recovery cannot be hoped for, much may be done by medical skill and kind care, to prolong life and alleviate suffering.[47]

This was a sentiment entirely understandable in the middle third of the century, yet one that was to find less and less assent as the nineteenth century drew to a close, and the power of medicine to intervene in acute illness seemed to increase dramatically.

Different and perhaps less pious motives led to the organization of other sorts of hospitals in this period. One direct consequence of economic growth was the founding of the first industrial hospitals, organized to care for workers in areas where dispensary or hospital care (and often families) were unavailable. An early example was the institution created by the Lowell textile corporations in 1839 when they agreed to sponsor a hospital "for the convenience and comfort of the persons, employed by them respectively when sick or needing medical or surgical treatment."[48] After the Civil War, railroads and coal towns began to concern themselves with the provision of hospital facilities for workers in industries with extraordinarily high accident rates. In 1869, for example, the Central Pacific railroad built a hospital exclusively for its men—financed by employee contributions of fifty cents a month. (Retired railroad men were also eligible for treatment, an aspect of the plan aimed presumably at encouraging worker loyalty in a notoriously unstable industry.)[49] In Pennsylvania, a complaisant legislature encouraged local coal mining communities to apply for subventions in aid of their particular hospitals.[50] But the vast majority of nonurban industrial, mining, and agricultural workers remained without practical access to hospital care. Despite sporadic (largely physician initiated) attempts to establish hospitals in smaller towns, few such community hospitals actually came into being before the late 1880s.

Specialty hospitals developed out of the energy of ambitious clinicians acting symbiotically with lay perceptions of a growing need among the city's poor—and in the case of women's hospitals with a proto-feminism. Female philanthropists were also interested in the health of children and were prominent in the work of establishing children's as well as women's hospitals. America's first children's hospitals date from this period as do a number of important ophthalmic and orthopedic hospitals. Specialists in these fields were anxious to control their own clinical facilities, for they enjoyed little success in fighting their way into the attending staffs of older hospitals dominated by physicians and general surgeons. America's established hospitals were often resistant to the ambitions of youthful specialists. A minority of socially conscious physicians was also acutely aware of the need for improved facilities for abandoned and orphaned infants (foundlings, as they were termed by contemporaries)—in place of the traditional almshouse provisions in which death rates routinely approached 100 percent.[51]

As we shall see, medical men and medical ambitions were to play an ever-increasing role in the creation of new and redefinition of old American hospitals. But in these postbellum years at least, their therapeutic resources were limited; at least in retrospect, it seems apparent that there was little physicians could do in 1875 that they could not have done in 1830 or 1845. Anesthesia constituted the most visible single novelty. But even this dramatic innovation initially had a limited impact. Until the adoption of antiseptic surgery much later in the century, the surgeon's realm remained extremely circumscribed. More surgery was performed in 1875 than was undertaken before the introduction of anesthesia thirty years before, but results in individual procedures were not always more favorable. (And, as we have suggested, a certain amount of the increase in surgery was a consequence of the increase in trauma, not simply a response to the availability of anesthesia.) It is true that the style of the surgeon had changed—the emphasis on speed, for example— but the place of operations in the hospital was still relatively small. Most surgical admissions were still for the treatment of lacerations, ulcers, and simple fractures.

Diagnosis was beginning to change by the 1870s, especially in hospitals where use of the stethoscope and of auscultation and percussion had become almost routine in diseases of the chest, lungs, and abdomen. The thermometer was gradually, and for the first time, becoming more than a curiosity; the first temperature charts began to appear in hospital case books in the mid–1860s. And where symptoms hinted at a kidney ailment, physicians would routinely test urine for the presence of albumin. But, of course, an experienced practitioner still learned much from his patient's appearance alone, and, as conservatives emphasized, new diagnostic tools added little to such skilled—if impressionistic—judgments.

Not only were medicine's therapeutic resources small, they remained limited almost exclusively to measures as easily applicable outside as inside the hospital. Drugs remained fundamental to medical care, but they were used more cautiously and in smaller doses than they had been in the century's first quarter. Bleeding too was employed with decreasing energy and frequency. Most important, as the majority of midcentury clinicians would have conceded, there was no substitute for rest, a nourishing diet, warmth, cleanliness, and good nursing.

The increasingly conservative therapeutics of this generation only underlined the peculiar relevance of the hospital to the poor. For the beef broths and sherry, the rest and adequate ventilation, the tonics that a wealthy patient could provide for him- or herself could only be made available to the poor in a hospital. In this sense it was difficult indeed to disentangle need from diagnosis as criteria for hospital admission. A limited technical capacity as well as prevailing social values and relationships defined the hospital's patient population.

Inside the Walls: The Persistent Institution

The hospital was a reality that the urban poor had to accept, if at best with resignation. No one wanted to enter a hospital in the mid-1870s, except for that small minority of the least enterprising and lacking in self-respect. It was an object of fear and an "asylum" for the dependent and socially isolate; even a "wretched and filthy hovel" seemed often preferable. Or so it seemed, for example, to a young Philadelphia woman facing childbirth. As soon as her friends heard she might enter one ". . . they strenuously endeavored to dissuade her, by saying that they had heard of cases of ill treatment in *'Hospitals'* and that she would be far better off at home."[52]

It was easy enough for contemporary critics of the medical profession to appeal to such sentiments. "The poor," one such hostile commentator argued, "are peculiarly objects of commiseration, for they are considered fair game for experimenters. Young physicians, . . . are much more apt to try experiments on patients, than those who have gained experience by practice; and hospitals are the place where they exercise their ingenuity in killing, or curing, with impunity."[53] Stories of the desecration of bodies after death and cruel treatments during life continued to color popular images of the hospital. Such fears were intensified by the humiliation implicit in the taking of alms for any purpose. It is not true, however, that the mid-nineteenth-century hospital was no more than a place where the poor went to die; the worst hospitals at the worst times rarely had death rates of more than 10 percent, and these were municipal institutions burdened with large proportions of chronic and incurable cases.

Even those who had little realistic prospect of ever becoming patients in hospitals found them disquieting. Perhaps it was a necessary institution, but one best contemplated from a distance. Even advocates of hospital expansion conceded that they could be genuinely distasteful. "The prejudice which prevails against hospitals," a supporter of Boston City Hospital argued in 1860, "in the immediate vicinity of dwellings, is due, in great measure, to the unsightly and repulsive objects often seen about such institutions." Among those repulsive, and perhaps dangerous, sights were the patients themselves. This particular hospital planner suggested that the proposed institution be erected around a center court, ". . . which is thus effectively cut off from the view of neighbors and passers-by."[54]

The siting of hospitals could be a political minefield, unless they were built in remote and unpopulated areas or placed among the poor who had far less capacity to make their objections felt. Quarantine hospitals were particularly unpopular—and on occasion destroyed by irate neighbors—but lay fears of contagion shaped attitudes toward all hospitals.

Not surprisingly, the hospital remained in this period of midcentury expansion as it had begun in the late eighteenth and early nineteenth centuries in theory, a deferential, and in practice, a class-structured institution. Disciplinary codes remained unbending. Every aspect of the patient's life was subject to the institution's paternal oversight. St. Luke's "Rules for Patients," for example, specified that patients were expected to help about the wards insofar as their health permitted. Profane or indecent language, "infidel or immoral" sentiments, or irreverent behavior at religious services could be grounds for a patient's summary discharge. No reading matter or packages were allowed in the wards without permission and no spirits, wine, or tobacco except by prescription.[55] Most hospitals sought to control the movement of patients and employees through a rigid system of passes.[56]

The superintendent and matron remained, in their sex-segregated spheres, the parents of an extended family. And in that family the roles of authority and deference were to be carefully acted out; house staff were expected to be "kind and forbearing" and the patients "grateful, and appreciate what is done for them."[57] If anything, the middle third of the century with its widespread and relentlessly activist evangelicalism only increased the social pressure placed upon hospital patients. The women's committee, for example, became a regular feature of hospital life in this period and, with its commitment to personal visiting, brought a new and intrusive presence to the ward, impinging on the world of house physicians and nurses as well as of patients.

The social and experiential gap between the ambitious young physicians who filled house staff positions and their working-class patients remained enormous. Only rarely did Americans of diverse social-class origin interact with such intimacy—except in such stylized relationships as that of master and servant or client and prostitute. Contemporaries were well aware of the social distance between physician and hospital patient and of the problems such contacts might create. Perhaps most important, hospital brusqueness could breed a dangerous insensitivity; the habits of the ward would bring disaster in private practice—and especially among women.[58]

Criteria for discharge as well as admission reflected the primacy of social variables in shaping the mid-century hospital's clientele. It can be illustrated, for example, in the simple matter of clothing. Soon after they opened, the managers of Philadelphia's Jewish Hospital Association appealed for clothing because that removed on admission from the "poorer class of patients" proved often unfit for use. A patient pronounced cured by the attending physician might still remain on the ward because he or she lacked clothing. The lady managers of Philadelphia's Woman's Hospital discovered the same thing a few years earlier and set about making and collecting clothing for their patients.[59] In municipal hospitals, the arbitrariness of distinctions between the sick and the simply dependent was always apparent. An individual patient might be shifted along a spectrum of labels ranging from sick to aged to unemployed—each describing the same person at different points in time.[60] Any woman who was willing to give birth in a public hospital, to cite another kind of example, was either desperately poor or a prostitute. Neither condition could be understood in purely medical terms, nor in either instance did a warm hearth or familial security await the new mother and her child. The Philadelphia Board of Guardians' hospital committee resolved in 1861, for example, that women who had been in the hospital's obstetric wards for three months or more since the birth of their children should be discharged unless they provided a good reason for their continued stay.[61] In all these examples, the issue, of course, turned on the patients' economic status; their hospital admission was only one symptom of a more fundamental social ailment.

The image of genteel ladies sitting in their parlors and sewing garments for indigent patients is a useful one to keep in mind. For with the exception of the large municipal hospitals—Bellevue, for example, or Philadelphia General—midcentury hospitals remained relatively small and self-consciously personal in their sense of moral oversight. Most voluntary hospitals, with the atypical exception of a well-endowed Roosevelt or Presbyterian in New York or Johns Hopkins in Baltimore, started with small rented buildings no different from many other private residences. There seemed to be no reason that a building which could house a healthy family could not house men and women in sickness. When, for example, the Episcopal Church sought to open a hospital in mid-century Philadelphia, their plans were modest indeed.

Patients who are *able to go about,* should wash out the wards, and take meals at the Refectory. Each *Nurse* should be held accountable for the furniture &c of her own ward. *By* obtaining from . . . merchants *donations* of Muslin, Blue check, Blankets and bed ticking, the cost of the above may be materially diminished. The *cost* of *bedding* will also be less if hair &c is obtained from the wholesale stores and made up at the Hospital or by the upholsterers. . . . To furnish a *Ward for 12 patients,* which is sufficient for the commencement, would *cost* about $310. *One Nurse* would be sufficient for 12 Surgical and 15 medical patients, allowing for the performance of other house duties.[62]

Opening a mid-century hospital was not terribly different from opening a well-run boarding house. The motives that impelled hospital growth were dependent neither on the promise of an elaborate technology nor on an intimidating accumulation of initial capital.

Staff physicians and lay managers were not always content with such informal arrangements. Some physicians and laymen were already seeking ways to reshape the hospital into a more bureaucratic form, to transcend both the traditional style of working-class life and the deferential paternalism, whose negotiated interaction defined ward life. One simple measure often advocated was the use of clothing to symbolize status and responsibility. "The servants of hospitals," one young medical man contended in 1859,

should be compelled to dress in clean garments, and not be allowed to wander over the building looking like the off-scouring of the city. . . . I think that, if the nurses and servants should have some particular badge or mark, by which their station and position could be determined at sight, it would do much for the discipline of the charity.[63]

Numbers provided another tool for subduing the unruly institution. In the mid–1870s hospitals began routinely to compute costs in terms of patient days; thus the still new Roosevelt Hospital could for the first time in 1877 provide its supporters with a figure for the cost to the hospital per patient day: 97½¢. Even more effectively, it allowed them to make subcalculations, as for example that 22.1 of the total went for food.[64] Calculations were also provided for average census and total number of patient days; these figures were to become routine in the administrative procedures of all hospitals as boards sought to control steadily rising costs.

Medicine provided still another tool for ordering an institution's "inmates." This was diagnosis itself. Mirroring the shift in medical thought toward a more specific view of disease entities, hospital records began to reflect this shift; the inmate was gradually becoming a case. In the Pennsylvania Hospital rules of 1848, for example, the resident physician was required to fill in each patient's name and date of admission on a piece of paper to be inserted in a tin frame at the head of his or her bed. Eleven years later, the hospital rules were amended so as to require that a diagnosis be added to the admission card.[65] Such procedures were only part of a more general effort to keep careful clinical records.

But these efforts to enforce a more impersonal order could not abruptly reshape a traditional institution. They could not banish older notions of social responsibility, of the nature of sickness and dependency that still informed the social roles acted out within its walls. Mid-century America, like the hospitals that necessarily reconstituted it in microcosm, was a society with its ideological structures perhaps less changed than its social structure. Disease was still no random event; poverty was still both stigmatizing and often unavoidable; the hospital was still a refuge for the unfortunate and the inadequate. Although medicine could make claims for autonomy within the hospital and in society generally, it too was still very much part of a traditional world. Disease could never be divorced from its social and moral meaning (while medicine could do little to intervene in its course). This could be seen most obviously in the way lifestyle seemed to predispose to disease—as for example, in the precision with which venereal disease scourged the transgressor. "The specific diseases of these organs consequent on promiscuous indulgence," as one midcentury medical man explained

will almost warrant the belief in the direct interposition of Providence for the punishment of the violators of the seventh commandment. . . . It is an admitted fact, that nearly all the chronic diseases to which the system is liable, are the consequences of some violated laws that Infinite Wisdom has imposed upon the animal economy.[66]

Moral causes and pathological consequences still fit together. Let me cite a parallel example, drawn more directly from the hospital. The

vaginal speculum had recently been introduced into clinical practice—to the accompaniment of charges that it was inappropriate to
the treatment of private patients. It had emerged from specialist
practice in the syphilitic wards of Parisian hospitals, and critics
contended that it should remain confined to such moral plague
spots. It was only natural for a defender of this new diagnostic tool
to concede that although it might indeed have developed in the
venereal wards of Parisian hospitals,

—does not Providence often bring good out of evil? And on whom could
it be more justifiable to make investigations and experiments, that might
redound to the benefit of the good and virtuous, than on the vicious and
profligate of the same sex?[67]

This was still a world of moral certainty in which the connections
between sickness of body and soul seemed both appropriate and
inextricable.

But such views could elicit change as well as guard against its
impact. For in just this period of growth, existing hospitals were
under attack by reformers inspired both by a humanitarian activism
and a specific vision of the shape an ideal hospital should assume.
The hospital movement of the 1850s, 1860s, and 1870s was in good
measure a response to demographic and economic reality, but it was
a response shaped by the motivating alliance of would-be scientific
rationalism, pious commitment, and traditional stewardship. Such
motives and assumptions inspired a vigorous expansion of hospital
facilities well before the arrival of those technical capacities that
have come in retrospect to seem indistinguishable from the hospital
itself.

CHAPTER 5

Ventilation, Contagion, and Germs

The hospital has become so central to medical care that it is difficult to reconstruct a world in which it played only a marginal role. It is more difficult to imagine circumstances in which even this limited role seemed questionable. Yet this was the case in the 1850s and 1860s. Critics in England, in France, and in America invoked the alarming results of statistical studies that pointed to increasing rates of something called "hospitalism"—the incidence of hospital-origi-nated fevers and infections that made care in even the best-known urban institutions more perilous than treatment in a cotter's simple hut or the tents of a well-disciplined army encampment. In the words of James Y. Simpson, a Scottish surgeon and perhaps the most influential of such medical critics, a patient "laid on an operat-ing-table in one of our surgical hospitals is exposed to more chances of death than the English soldier on the field of Waterloo."[1] In a much-quoted study, Simpson presented data indicating that English surgical mortality rates increased in proportion to a hospital's size—ranging from one in 2.4 in general hospitals with three hundred beds to one in seven in hospitals with fewer than thirty-six beds.[2] Paral-lel American statistics documented similarly dismaying realities. At Philadelphia's Pennsylvania Hospital, for example, during the dec-ade 1850–1860, death rates in amputations were 241.23 in a thou-sand—and an even more alarming 266.89 in the next ten-year period.[3]

Progress seemed in this instance at least to be marching backward not forward. Lying-in statistics from both England and France pointed toward similar conclusions. A poor woman was safer with a midwife or private practitioner in her own home, no matter how deprived, than in the best staffed and endowed of hospitals.[4] The direct relationship between the scale of a hospital's size and prestige and its mortality rates seemed particularly unsettling, for the larger metropolitan hospitals enjoyed the services of the most eminent surgeons on their attending staffs. It was difficult to understand why their results compared so poorly with those obtained by unpretentious country practitioners. The explanation had to be sought in the character of the hospitals themselves and the patients they treated, not in the qualities of the men who staffed them. The increase in mortality was, as J.Y. Simpson put it, a result of "our system of huge and colossal hospital edifices, and to the hygienic evils which that system has been made to involve."[5] The mid-century movement for hospital reform was emotionally and intellectually predicated upon a conviction that large urban hospitals were fundamentally disordered, a necessary yet paradoxically improper institution that endangered the physical and moral health of all those who sought help in its wards. A minority of critics even called for their abolition.

It is clear that English and American hospitals were in no danger of extinction. Both humanitarianism and an inexorably growing urban population implied—in fact demanded—continued hospital expansion, while the requirements of clinical teaching only reinforced society's need for hospitals. The arguments of Simpson and like-thinking critics were in effect not attacks on the hospital as an institution but arguments for its rationalization and continued growth.

This reform program drew a good deal of its strength and legitimacy from a particular view of disease causation, a view that both explained high levels of mortality and morbidity and pointed to ways of reducing them. The causes of fever and infection seemed both obvious and remediable to most midcentury students of hospital conditions. And that culpable gap between grim reality and attainable improvement constituted a powerful motivation for reform.

Infection, Medical Thought, and the Antebellum Hospital

We tend to think of the mid-nineteenth century and particularly the work of Florence Nightingale as beginning the identifiably modern hospital. The trained nurse, the hospital building's self-consciously hygienic design, its orderly and efficient administration all seem to originate with that extraordinary Englishwoman and her work in the Crimea. Even those little concerned with the history of medicine are familiar with the powerful symbol of the lady with the lamp, helping somehow to guide us into the path of a beneficent modernity.

But the roots of her ideas were far older than her century, and much of their power lay not in novelty but in their familiarity—allied with a zealous activism that would not tolerate the imperfections of existing hospitals. Her ostensibly medical rationale for institutional reform cannot be understood apart from its relationship to contemporary social ideas and values, on the one hand, and, on the other, to centuries-old explanations of infection.

For as long as the benevolent—and the military—had provided hospitals for the dependent, these institutions had presented seemingly linked problems of discipline and infection. Military medicine had even elaborated its own hospital orthodoxy by the end of the eighteenth century, a set of teachings that emphasized cleanliness, good ventilation, isolation of septic cases, and the avoidance of crowding in individual wards, buildings, and interconnected rooms. Even hospitals in tents or temporary barracks could, as a result of their modest scale and excellent ventilation, prove more healthful than the largest, best staffed, and most sturdily-built institutions.[6] "Hospitals," as Benjamin Rush expressed his Revolutionary War experiences with characteristic hyperbole, "are the sinks of human life in an army. They robbed the United States of more citizens than the sword. Humanity, economy, and phylosphy, (sic) all concur in giving preference to the convenience and wholesome air of private houses."[7]

The reasons seemed obvious enough. The central mode of infection was the atmosphere and the more crowded and ill ventilated a building, the greater the danger to its inhabitants. Few physicians in the first half of the nineteenth century questioned the critical role of the atmosphere in promoting infection in confined spaces. Although there was much mid-century debate as to the precise mode

of transmission of certain epidemic ills, especially cholera and yellow fever, there was far less debate about the "ordinary" fevers that
appeared each year among the urban poor—or the fevers and
wound infections that seemed inevitably to haunt the wards of city
hospitals. Much of the disputatious yet poorly defined discussion
of contagion in cholera and yellow fever that cluttered English and
American medical journals in this period was never regarded as
relevant to the hospital's peculiar conditions.[8]

The very distinction between contagious and noncontagious had
little validity for contemporary hospital critics as they surveyed its
crowded and filthy wards and the seemingly interrelated occurrence
of wound infection, dysentery, erysipelas, childbed fever, and typhus. The distinction between causation and transmission was no
more meaningful than that between contagion and noncontagion;
all disease could become infectious if conditions were sufficiently
congested and ventilation inadequate. The larger the number of
patients crowded into a common space, the greater the contamination of the atmosphere they breathed. This understanding of hospital infection fit neatly into those ancient ideas of the body and
sickness that we have already discussed in chapter 3. How could the
body maintain its health-defining equilibrium if every breath of air
was vitiated, unnatural, "loaded" with the products of abnormal
metabolism? "Think," one physician warned in 1876,

of the changes continually taking place in the atmosphere by healthy
persons breathing it. How much more readily then must these changes be
produced by those who are sick, the exhalations from whom are highly
morbid and dangerous, inasmuch as they are one of nature's methods of
eliminating noxious matter from the body, in order that it may recover
health.[9]

Given such assumptions it was hardly surprising that wound infections seemed often to induce typhus or dysentery, or that erysipelas
in one ward should induce childbed fever in another.[10] Local conditions allied themselves with the physiological idiosyncrasy of patients to dictate the form and incidence of hospital ills. Few contemporaries regarded them as the predictable effects of specific
disease-producing agents.

The most discussed and feared of antebellum hospital ills were,
in fact, childbed fever, wound infection, and erysipelas—the first
particularly frightening because it killed young and otherwise

healthy women in the course of a normal physiological process.[11] In surgery, lingering illness from postoperative infection was so widespread that it ordinarily caused no special alarm; such infections were assumed to be an aspect of the normal recuperative process. Thus, generations of surgeons could blandly interpret the appearance of "laudable pus" as a sign that recovery was underway. Success in the healing process was to be hoped for, not expected; postoperative death rates as high as 25 percent were anticipated in major procedures.

Hospitals had always found these intractable problems. Private institutions, as we have seen, refused to admit fever and erysipelas cases as well as such unquestionably contagious (in the sense of person-to-person contact) ills as smallpox.[12] Some were hesitant about providing lying-in facilities, partially because of the fear of childbed fever, partially because so large a proportion of women willing to give birth in a hospital were unmarried, and no hospital trustee wished to subsidize immorality. Where lying-in cases were admitted, conventional wisdom suggested that they be carefully separated from general, and especially septic, wards.

The hospital's difficulty lay not so much in excluding the obviously ill, but in dealing with cases that broke out among patients once they had been admitted. Smaller hospitals might simply close when an epidemic erupted, dismissing patients to their homes and allowing a prudent—and presumably cleansing—interval to pass before admitting new patients. Once hospitals increased in scale, however, the option of simply closing was no longer plausible. By the 1840s, administrators had developed a well-understood set of procedures for combating hospital infection. Normal practice following an outbreak of erysipelas or childbed fever involved the removal of patients to isolated wards or rooms. The contaminated ward was then fumigated, scoured, and whitewashed, and bedding burnt or otherwise discarded. The room was then to be thoroughly "aired" so as to remove or at least substantially dilute any disease-inducing materials that might have remained in the atmosphere. Antebellum hospitals were sometimes unwilling or unable to implement these exacting measures, but no one doubted their wisdom.

A competently administered hospital sought to pursue equally well-understood policies in an effort to prevent epidemics of hospital infection and to minimize the number of sporadic cases. One was to avoid crowding, another to enforce cleanliness, a third to promote ventilation. Servants were directed to dust and clean thoroughly, change linen and empty bedpans frequently, and never allow food to remain on wards, for any decaying organic matter, not only the patients' bodily excretions, could contribute to the aggregate contamination of an institution's atmosphere. Increasing effort was devoted to designing the hospital building so that dirt could not easily accumulate. Smooth, hard-surfaced floors, metal instead of wooden bedsteads, the systematic removal of garbage, all helped minimize the accumulation of disease-inducing organic matter. Sewers and drains were also important concerns for midcentury hospital planners—the unintended escape of "effluvia" from chamber pots too long unemptied, filthy linens, or poorly designed and constructed sewers and drains could all poison an institution's atmosphere (just as they induced fevers in a city's filthy and crowded tenements).[13] Effective placement of windows, doors, fireplaces, and the siting of the building itself so as to maximize the circulation of fresh air were all established principles of hospital architecture by midcentury, even before the Crimean War and their widely publicized advocacy by Florence Nightingale.

Thus, a well-planned hospital would be carefully located in a healthful site and then designed so as to maximize the circulation of air between the building's interior (wards, corridors, and service areas) and the exterior, while minimizing the internal movement of air among wards, corridors, and service areas. The goal, as one contemporary put it, was "perfect isolation of every ward from every other ward."[14] Kitchens, laundries, autopsy rooms were all acknowledged to be sources of potentially dangerous organic emanations. Our wards, the newly completed Hartford Hospital reported in 1857

are separate and distinct from each other, and are so arranged that the contaminated atmosphere will not pass from one ward to another. The apartments for the sick have no direct connection with those apartments which are occupied by the steward and family. The kitchen is so arranged that its fumes do not pass into any other part of the building.[15]

Thus, "any number of wards," they boasted at the hospital's dedication, "can be built to accommodate any number of patients, without any fear of contamination by accumulated disease."[16]

When the benevolent and well-informed contemplated a new hospital they always sought a lot far from the city's most congested areas near open fields or, ideally, a river or body of open water from which cleansing breezes might be expected to refresh even the best-ordered hospital's inevitably tainted air. The Pennsylvania Hospital, for example, was located in the mid-eighteenth century at Eighth and Spruce streets, far from the city's busy and crowded waterfront; New York Hospital and the same city's almshouse were located on what seemed healthful riverfront sites. As late as 1849, a New York Hospital staff member could warn against the danger of erecting a new building on the hospital's still ample lot; it might impede the wind currents that did so much to sustain the hospital's increasingly tenuous salubrity.[17]

By the mid-1850s, moreover, this emphasis on maximizing the circulation of air had found appropriate architectural form in the pavilion hospital. It was, in the words of one historian, "a sanitary code embodied in a building."[18] The pavilion plan specified wards ventilated by a generous number of windows on both long sides and doors at each end; any number of such pavilion wards could be joined by connecting corridors. Since the goal was to maximize ventilation and limit density, pavilion design also implied low, one or at most two-story, sprawling hospitals and the avoidance of high-rise buildings on small lots in congested urban areas.

This body of medical and planning doctrine was not so much examined as intoned. It represented a way of organizing medical thought so deeply internalized that its constituent assumptions were rarely if ever questioned or systematically articulated; they had become the common-sense wisdom of a generation.[19] And in 1859, they were embodied in a sacred text, Florence Nightingale's *Notes on Hospitals.* [20]

Florence Nightingale: The Hospital as Moral Artifact

All of these medical, administrative, and architectural arguments were incorporated in Florence Nightingale's energetic program for hospital reform. Most of her teachings were no more than applications of these well-worn speculations—underwritten by the new-style plausibility of statistical analysis. But Nightingale made emotionally effective and politically astute use of these truisms, while adding a more novel emphasis on the need for formal nurse training coupled with a vision of administrative order inseparable from that of the hospital as physical artifact.[21]

It is always hard to contend that a particular individual has played a unique historical role. Few men or women do. But Florence Nightingale was certainly one of those influential few. Both in England and the United States her ideas and example served to focus and motivate not only the organization of nurse training schools—for which she is best known—but, as her contemporaries understood, to reform and reconstitute the hospital more generally.

Yet, as we have suggested, her ideas were hardly original. Perhaps if they had been, she could not have exerted the social influence she in fact did. And like many of her generational peers, Nightingale found it extremely difficult to accept the new ideas of disease causation that were transforming medical theory in the 1870s.[22] Her ideas of pathology and therapeutics were rooted in a more fundamental vision of society, a way of organizing and controlling the world that transcended the specifically medical form in which that vision was projected.

Beneath her invocation of statistics and experience lay ideas much older and more traditional. Like those assumptions that I have already discussed in terms of early nineteenth-century pathology and therapeutics, these ideas reflected a vision of the world in which volition and disease, environment and regimen, body and mind were woven together so as to create a meaningful structure into which health, healing, and disease could be placed.

Although mid-century opinions varied enormously in detail, there remained a fundamental area of agreement in the understanding of infectious disease. Since the 1840s explicitly—and far earlier implicitly—students of epidemic ailments had, following the influential example of William Farr, England's leading authority on vital statistics, categorized epidemic and infectious ills as "zymotic," or fermentlike. The familiar processes of fermentation and putrefaction provided plausible models for ways in which a small amount of infectious material could induce potentially pathogenic changes in a far larger quantity of material. In the case of hospital infection, the atmosphere served as an analogue to the dough of the baker or the grape juice of the vintner.[23] (It was consistent as well with the powerful example of smallpox: since the mid-eighteenth century and the introduction of inoculation it had been impossible to deny that, at least in the case of this disease, a minute quantity of a specific material substance could provoke enormous and predictable changes in the body.)

The seeming logic of this analogy was difficult to escape. The scientific debate surrounding the nature and possible specificity of fermentation was still fresh in the minds of Nightingale's contemporaries, educated laymen as well as physicians. Scientists had for decades disputed the nature of fermentation. Was it "chemical" or "vital"? Was it the consequence of some living organism's physiological processes? Or was it a progressive chemical change induced by some inorganic catalyst? But to most clinicians, this was a distinction without a practical difference, for the essential elements of the model seemed fundamentally similar whether the ferment should prove ultimately chemical or vital.

It was too useful an explanation. The ferment model seemed clothed in the garb of currently plausible science, while that science could for the moment neither test nor validate its truth. Most important for this generation, it explained how the atmosphere served as a medium for the transmission of disease. Ubiquitous and necessary to man's existence, the very indispensability of the atmosphere helped explain how it served as both cause of disease and vehicle for its transmission. Contaminated by a minute quantity of putrefying matter, it could spread cholera or yellow fever throughout a city; within the confined walls of a hospital or tenement house, it might cause any one of a score of ills as the exhalations from too crowded human bodies acted as a kind of yeast in this culture. Given such beliefs, it was only natural that ventilation and cleanliness should have seemed a necessary prerequisite to hospital health, that crowding and slovenly housekeeping would exact an inevitable toll in the form of infection, fever, and death.

Florence Nightingale shared this belief in the primary role of the atmosphere in causing disease. And it was far more than a plausible speculation, far more than one among a number of intellectual options certified as respectable by the medical community—it was a social and, in her case, emotional necessity. Nightingale's views of disease causation didactically underlined the connection between behavior, environment, and health—and thus constituted a systematic program for hospital reform. It was a program that necessarily integrated architecture, engineering, and administrative order. An institution's environment was a result of the interaction of all these factors; employee and patient discipline was as much a determinant of hospital atmosphere as the placement of windows and fireplaces or the frequency with which walls and floors were scrubbed. It was a model closely paralleling the holistic understanding of individual sickness that, as we have seen, justified traditional views of pathology and therapeutics.

Perhaps most fundamentally, Nightingale's understanding of hospital-generated infection emphasized the role of volition and behavior. And it was applicable not only to the hospital's microcosm, but to the macrocosm of society more generally. If local authorities, she suggested, would only monitor carefully the atmosphere of schoolrooms, Englishmen would hear no more of scarlet fever or other supposedly "unavoidable" childhood ills. They would hear no more of "Mysterious Dispensations"—of disease being in the hands of God—when the responsibility lay squarely in man's own hands and brain. We must, she reiterated, look first to our own habits in seeking to explain disease. God laid down the laws governing man's body; health lay not in prayer, not in hoping for miracles, but in obeying the dictates implicit in those unyielding laws. God would hardly ". . . break His own laws expressly to relieve us of responsibility."[24]

The meaning for hospital hygiene was clear enough. Only hard work and careful planning could avert fevers and infection. And when these scourges did appear on a hospital's wards, it was a consequence of institutional sloth and incompetence. As a compelling rationale for the activism demanded by her personality and her generation's social circumstances, the image of zymotic disease could hardly have been more effective. It provided both blueprint and justification for social intervention. "If infection exists," she summarized her hospital experience, "it is preventible. If it exists, it is the result of carelessness, or of ignorance."[25]

Nightingale's use of statistical arguments related closely, if seemingly paradoxically, to her use of the fermentation concept. No student of her work and that of her contemporaries in mid-century reform can doubt the centrality of their appeals to the "objectivity" of quantitative data. But Nightingale's use of statistical description and analysis was as much rhetorical as instrumental; it was a seemingly modern tool employed in ironic defense of a far older way of conceptualizing the world. Despite her well-deserved reputation for tactical skill (if not ruthlessness) in the service of pragmatic reform, Nightingale's mind ultimately saw things in morally resonant polarities: filth as opposed to purity, order versus disorder, health in contradistinction to disease. Hospital infection was thus a consequence of disorder in a potentially ordered pattern. Statistics defined the place of a particular ward or institution along the continuum shaped by these polarities. Given her unwillingness to accept the specificity of disease and her tendency to correlate incidence of fever and surgical infection with levels of atmospheric contamination, it was only natural for her to point with indignation to correlations between particularly untoward hospital conditions and atypically high levels of hospital infection. The incidence of such infection served as a seemingly objective index to culpable human failure.

The central image that at once communicated and legitimated her reform program was a view of the hospital itself. Nightingale's vision was far more than simply metaphorical, for it incorporated a careful analysis of existing realities and a blueprint for consequent change. On the other hand, it was hardly a value-free rendering of these realities. Inasmuch as it mirrored and created public attitudes, it must be seen as a powerful factor in the mid-nineteenth-century hospital movement. The institution seemed to her quite literally a microcosm of society, every part interrelated and all reflecting a particular moral order. Just as order in the body and an appropriate physical and psychological equilibrium constituted health for the individual, so an appropriately constructed and managed hospital would experience a low incidence of fever and wound infection. Similarly, in society at large, ill-health, poverty, and depravity all sprang from a sequence of remediable human acts. The hospital was a component of that society, a microcosm of the social and moral relationships that determined the health of society generally and of the individuals who made up that society. Within this framework, one could hardly distinguish between the moral and material, the individual and the community as aggregated individuals. Social health and individual health were bound together by a set of intertwined moral relationships and responsibilities; life and death on the ward illustrated these truths with didactic clarity. If man failed to obey God's physiological laws, he could only expect disease; if a hospital was badly designed, then contaminated by filth, administrative negligence, and immorality, the consequent fevers and infections were equally inevitable.

For Florence Nightingale and her American followers, the mid-nineteenth-century hospital was indeed a place of disorder. No woman of her class and education could well have encountered that would-be healing institution without finding it menacing and alien.

It is no accident that her new-model trained nurses were responsible as much for discipline as for overseeing proper diets or dressing ulcers. Indeed, the emphasis in Nightingale's etiological and pathological thought on the interaction of the patient with every aspect of his or her environment implied that the distinction between moral and physical well-being, between mind and body, was hardly meaningful. It only obscured those factors that caused disease generally and was particularly irrelevant to the understanding of hospital infection.

The mid-nineteenth-century hospital was a lower-class institution in many ways, organized in theory according to the moral assumptions of its lay trustees and administrators, but dominated in reality by values and behaviors antithetical to those Nightingale regarded as the only appropriate basis for a moral society. It was a period too when in both England and America the new industrial cities seemed to be alive with a threatening and potentially chaotic working class—a class that produced a disproportionate number of victims of epidemic disease and provided virtually all the occupants of urban hospital beds. Zymotic images were ideal for describing both the city's and the hospital's fermenting and disorderly life—a below stairs without an above stairs to control it. We need not be surprised to learn that Nightingale's widely praised and adopted ward arrangements placed the nurse's room so that she might observe all its inmates from a single vantage point.[26] It was equally logical that closets and stairwells where "skulking" might occur or where convalescents might "play tricks" must be avoided.[27] These were to be eliminated by the enlightened hospital architect, just as he avoided corners in which dust might accumulate or sewers that allowed the escape of dangerous fumes.

Within this world of nonspecific and overwhelmingly environmental causes of disease, Nightingale inevitably saw the nurses' role as both multifaceted and indispensable. At the same time it was fundamentally moral. Nightingale contended that a trained nurse's capacities must be ultimately spiritual; the technical skills she might acquire were, if not precisely subordinate to her moral endowments, at least subsequent to and dependent upon them. The same holistic pathology and hygiene that explained the incidence of health and disease also explained the numerous ways in which the nurse could help bring about the patient's recovery. Like many of her self-consciously forward-looking medical peers, Nightingale placed little faith in drugs and bleeding, or in therapeutics generally. There was relatively little the physician could do to alter the course of a disease. Medicine, she explained, was no part of the fundamental recuperative process. "It is often thought," she explained, "that medicine is the curative process." But this was far from the truth. Surgery, Nightingale explained, could remove a bullet from a wound, "which is an obstruction to cure, but nature heals the wound." Neither medicine nor surgery could ". . . do anything but remove obstructions; neither can cure; nature alone cures."[28]

All nursing could accomplish—and it was no small achievement—was to help the patient attain the best possible condition for nature to proceed with its innate pattern of recovery. In this sense a hospital could not *cure,* but it seemed self-evident to Nightingale that the institution could and must avert the spread of infection and more generally promote the body's internally generated efforts to regain health. At least a well-run hospital could prevent a patient from being inadvertently poisoned by the emanations arising from his or her own excretions and those of ward-mates. Drugs and bleeding were to play at best a minor role in her ideal hospital— nursing, cleanliness, and diet were to occupy center stage.[29]

The possibility of effective hospital administration implied its necessity. Translated into behavior, Nightingale's point of view emphasized the certainty of improvement through carefully directed activity. It is not surprising that Florence Nightingale was so resolutely hostile to the idea of contagion at mid-century or to the germ theory in later decades. The germ theory seemed, in fact, no more than a mechanism justifying a contagionism she had already staked her reputation and intellect on rejecting. In her formulation, hospital infection reduced itself to the consequence of untoward behavior. Poor planning of windows, slovenly nursing, cold and ill-prepared foods, drains and sinks placed where they might contaminate the atmosphere, inadequate ventilation, chamber vessels unemptied for hours were all remediable, all consequences of incompetence and irresponsibility.

In this interrelated world of volition and pathology, contagion seemed arbitrary, random, and thus asocial in its moral implications. If chance alone determined whether an individual should intersect with a disease-causing microscopic particle, then sickness was bereft of meaning; it could play no monitory role in a world of moral order. It was not simply an inability to comprehend the germ theory that made Nightingale hesitate to accept it, but its irrelevance—if not, indeed, its destructiveness—to her complex way of visualizing the nature of disease and its relationship to behavior. And, of course, it would undermine as well the program of environmental reform she had done so much to create.

Language is obviously affective as well as denotative, and Florence Nightingale in her analysis of midcentury hospital infection was more rhetorician than scientist. Her understanding of bodily function and the nature of infection bound together perceptions of particular realities—the sickness, the filth, the disorder of mid-nineteenth-century hospitals and cities, the everyday realities of yeast rising or beer brewing—within an explanatory language that incorporated both the contemporary prestige of science and moral certainties of a more traditional sort. Her language also communicated the perceptions of a particular class and time. In such diversity of reference lies the key to Nightingale's extraordinary appeal (and the more general tenacity of the medical ideas she and many contemporary physicians espoused).

Perhaps it was this ability to communicate as much as her social position and extraordinary energy that made Florence Nightingale the most influential and widely quoted of Anglo-American hospital reformers. Her work in Britain's military hospitals during the Crimean War (1854–1856) was widely and enthusiastically reported on both sides of the Atlantic. By the end of the 1850s, she was already being cited as an authority and inspiration by would-be hospital reformers in the United States as well as in the United Kingdom. She was able to dramatize far older calls for cleanliness, for ventilation, for skilled nursing, and for administrative order. Equally important, she placed them in a form that seemed both novel and attainable. Her advocacy of nurse training schools and the pavilion hospital provided a concrete and seemingly innovative blueprint for hospital reform. At least some American philanthropists and an influential minority of concerned physicians were ready to set out on a crusade against hospital filth and disorder.

But before America's urban hospitals could be transformed, social activists were engulfed in the Civil War. Hospital reform in American cities waited until the restoration of peace. And, as we have seen, the war's cumulative experience, in both North and South, seemed only to underline the truth of Nightingale's doctrines while helping shape an activist cadre of reform-minded men and women.

Medical Doctrine and Social Change: Germs and Ventilation

There was little difference of opinion about the requirements for a new model hospital. The pavilion plan seemed the best way to avoid the dangers of congregating too many patients in the same interconnected and inadequately ventilated space. "There will be no great single structure," as an advocate of a new city hospital for Boston explained in 1860,

towering above the private houses, and filled for its many stories with the congregated calamities of all the various subjects of its care, . . . but instead there will be presented to the eye a cluster of moderate sized, tasteful, and pleasantly grouped pavilions, such as are to be found in some of the pleasure grounds and parks abroad.[30]

Philadelphia's Episcopal Hospital had been designed in self-conscious conformity to these views before the outbreak of hostilities in 1861.[31] And during the war, thousands of men had been successfully treated in sprawling shedlike pavilions. Adequate ventilation, efficient logistics, cleanliness, and increasingly skilled nursing had allowed even the largest Civil War institutions to boast relatively low mortality rates—in hospitals containing as many as three thousand sick and wounded.[32] After the experience of the Civil War, the building of multistory hospitals in densely settled urban areas seemed no longer defensible; their cumulative opportunities for atmospheric contamination seemed to guarantee an unacceptable level of fever and infection. "Shall we profit by the lessons so dearly bought" in the Crimean and Civil Wars, a St. Louis physician asked rhetorically in 1874? Shall we ignore the "valuable lessons of reform fastened upon the public attention by the heroic efforts of Florence Nightingale . . . ?"

Shall we give heed to the teachings of science confirmed and enforced by thousands of experiments? or continue to sacrifice human life at the shrine of architectural beauty and elegance by the construction of . . . magnificent edifices closely connected, four or five stories high, and call them hospitals, and point to them with pride as monuments of public charity?[33]

What St. Louis, and by implication every forward-looking city, needed was a system of "rational pavilion hospitals" scattered around the city, rather than one large and ostentatious building. "There is no branch of sanitary science," as a New Yorker exhorted in 1864, "which, during the past few years, has been more strikingly and more rapidly developed and improved, than the construction of hospital edifices . . ." Modern architecture allied with "competent professional science" could produce results "beyond the most sanguine medical calculations" of previous generations.[34] Hospital design seemed at last to have become a practical hybrid of science and architecture. This was a program that inspired confidence as it promised results, a program that deployed reassuringly traditional medical ideas in a form that offered the appeal of efficacy and concreteness.

In the wave of hospital building that marked the late 1860s and 1870s, these architectural goals became dogma and, to a lesser extent, actual guidelines for construction. New York's Presbyterian and Roosevelt hospitals, Boston City and Cincinnati General, Philadelphia's University Hospital, Baltimore's projected Johns Hopkins all reflected these doctrines to some degree or another— and insofar as they did not, were subject to the indignant criticism of hospital reformers.[35] Older hospitals sought ways to avoid the worst aspects of hospitalism by removing lying-in services, for example, or physically separating surgical and septic cases.

There was certainly room for technical debate concerning means, especially in regard to the best modes of heating and ventilation, but not in regard to ends. The view that circulation of fresh air was the primary requirement for institutional health was unchallenged. "The condition essential to success," as one authority summarized accepted wisdom, "is the greatest attainable purity of the atmosphere, and to it all other questions should be but secondary."[36] Hospital planners, like Nightingale herself, were quick to invoke arbitrary but seductively precise formulae for the numbers of cubic feet each hospital patient (or schoolchild or tenement dweller) required to avoid infection. The maintenance of health reduced itself to the placement of beds and windows, the arrangement of flues and ventilators, the proper design of heating systems.

It was into this reform consensus that the germ theory appeared, at first in the shape of Joseph Lister's doctrine of antiseptic surgery. A prominent teacher and surgical practitioner in Glasgow, Lister (1827–1912) had been much impressed by Louis Pasteur's work, especially that on spontaneous generation. Pasteur had demonstrated in the early 1860s that the growth of microorganisms in a nutrient broth and consequent putrefaction of the broth could be prevented by avoiding atmospheric contamination. The analogy with wound infection seemed obvious to Lister, and he soon elaborated a system of treating wounds and surgical incisions aimed at "disinfecting" bits of organic life in the atmosphere. His name became permanently associated with the carbolic acid he used to suffuse surgical dressings and the atmosphere in operating theaters.

The implications of this new way of understanding and preventing infection were so inconsistent with generally prevailing assumptions that they were not so much dismissed as misperceived. So powerful and unexamined, in fact, was contemporary emphasis on the atmosphere as the medium for hospital infection that even Lister's original procedures stressed atmospheric "decontamination" or "disinfection." It seemed improbable that a minute bit of living matter could cause wound infection or puerperal fever (even more improbable that infectious ills generally might be caused by microscopic organisms).

It was more than simple inertia that guaranteed the germ theory would have a hard time making itself understood—let alone implemented. First it appeared to be inconsistent with the acknowledged importance of predisposition in explaining disease incidence. It seemed obvious that the poor, the malnourished, the imprudent would be less resistant to endemic or epidemic ills. (Defenders of large metropolitan hospitals at mid-century sometimes excused their dismaying surgical mortality rates by pointing to the poverty, chronic ill-health, and immorality of their patient population. Could one expect a drunken Whitechapel prostitute to have the same vitality as a vigorous East Anglian farmer?)[37] Second, atmospheric notions of infection were additive and nonspecific; the greater the aggregate amount of contaminants the greater the danger. Statistical evidence of mortality rates and their relationship to the size of institutions or local population densities, for example, seemed only to document this style of explaining disease, to express and legitimate it in another form. The notion that disease could be caused by discrete minute particles seemed meaninglessly random—the denial of a collective wisdom distilled from centuries of medical experience (and forcefully underlined by the conditions of mid-nineteenth-century urban life).

Only a small minority of American physicians in the early 1870s were quick to assimilate these new ideas. John Shaw Billings, probably America's most prominent late nineteenth-century authority on public medicine in general and on hospital design in particular, provides a particularly enlightening example of such intellectual flexibility. Between 1870 and 1875, Billings fundamentally reoriented his understanding of hospital infection. In the former year, Billings had been commissioned by the Surgeon General to inspect the Army's barracks and hospitals. His conclusions were predictable and conventional.[38]

The most important necessity in maintaining health, Billings concluded, was a supply of fresh air, "such that no occupant shall be compelled to breathe air which has recently passed from the lungs, or which is vitiated by the products of combustion." Part of the danger lay in the fact that such air was physiologically unfit for respiration—impregnated with moisture, lacking in oxygen, and oversupplied with carbon dioxide. Anyone unfortunate enough to breathe it would have difficulty in maintaining normal vitality. Even worse, a hospital's atmosphere was ". . . contaminated with organic matter which has a strong tendency to putrescence, and has been well described as a sort of 'aerial filth' or . . . 'a physiological miasm.' " Sometimes, as in the case of smallpox, this might be a specific poison. More frequently the danger lay in the ". . . organic emanations from a case of pneumonia or typhoid fever, in which rapid retrograde metamorphosis is going on."[39] Men in neighboring beds could hardly hope to escape these products of an abnormal metabolism, and with sufficient crowding and inadequate ventilation occupants of even distant wards would be at risk. These were views that would have been immediately understandable and acceptable to any Anglo-American physician during the hundred years preceding Billings's tour of inspection.

Only five years later, in 1875, Billings produced another report on military hygiene as well as a model plan for the projected Johns Hopkins Hospital; both expressed a very different view of hospital infection.[40] The early 1870s were years when the views of Pasteur and Lister were being widely reported in medical journals and discussed by knowledgeable English and American physicians. Billings had clearly been won over to these new ideas. He emphasized in 1875 that existing ventilation systems worked on the principle of diluting hospital air and replacing it with fresh. This was all very well for gases that might have minor deleterious effects, Billings contended: "but the real danger of hospitalism arises, from solid particles, probably living."[41] It was "these particles, known as disease germs, contagia, microzymes, micrococci, bioplasm, germinal matter, etc." that caused the great majority, if not all, of those diseases "referred to in the term 'Hospitalism.' "[42] Wound infection could arise even in well-ventilated six- or twelve-bed hospitals, most likely transmitted on surgical dressings, beds, or linen and not through the atmosphere. Attempting to dilute such particles might decrease the chance of infection, but could not avoid it. The numbers of such particles could be reduced, but the individual entities would remain intact.

We may by diluting the air remove a certain number of the germs, with the effect that in a cubic foot of air there shall be but ten instead of one hundred, and that therefore the probabilities of coming in contact with one are correspondingly diminished; but if it chances that one particle falls on the wound, the results will be nearly the same as if no dilution had been made.

   If you are standing on a plain across which a file of men are firing your chances of escape are of course better if there are but ten men shooting instead of one hundred; but if one of the ten does chance to hit you, the practical difference will probably not be appreciable.[43]

It was a striking metaphor, particularly resonant to a Civil War veteran like Billings, and it was a metaphor that communicated a very different meaning from the one conveyed in the traditional and still powerful image of a cumulatively contaminated atmosphere selectively affecting the physiologically predisposed.

   Individual volition and social circumstance threatened to have less and less to do with the explanation of sickness. Billings's metaphor emphasized the randomness of sickness as well as its mechanism—it was not who but where one was that determined vulnerability. The energetic Christian as well as the drinker and whoremonger might charge into the bullet's path. The grimly democratic message of Civil War battlefields had repeatedly demonstrated this unsettling truth. Billings's military image captured the declining plausibility of traditional holistic disease models and the symmetrically increasing centrality of a specific, reductionist, and mechanism-oriented understanding of disease.

   Of course, change was not to come quickly or categorically. Billings himself still found a place for older ideas of predisposition, both moral and environmental, and remained a worshipper of the pavilion system and the sacredness of ventilation. Neither was he convinced of the specificity of hospital infection. And most of his contemporaries were far less aware of the germ theory's ultimate implications. The majority sought to eat their cake and have it too—simply adding disease germs as one more element to an eclectic array of substances cumulatively contaminating the atmosphere of a hospital or tenement.[44]

Billings's battlefield metaphor was prophetically appropriate to an increasingly impersonal, bureaucratic, and technologically oriented society—and medical system. But let me emphasize finally that the battle between the cumulative, nonspecific atmospheric model and the germ theory was not simply one of contending metaphors (though on one level it was that), nor of simple technical correctness. The germ theory seems to us correct, not because its various versions in the 1860s and 1870s were accurate, provable, or immediately efficacious, but because they did provide a closer approximation of the natural history of infectious disease—and because the germ theory was to be built into a changing structure of technical qualification, laboratory findings, and professional status. This was a world of credentials and experts increasingly uncongenial to the holistic, individual, and moral understanding of health and illness that had for millennia helped men deal with the incursions of disease. The germ theory had immediate and practical dimensions; it was no intellectual abstraction. In the next half century it would not only reshape the hospital but help transform every aspect of medicine.

CHAPTER 6

The Promise of Healing:
Science in the Hospital

In 1866, the New York Hospital closed: its building on Chambers Street was old, operating revenues were inadequate—and its land was too valuable. For a decade the hospital's trustees and medical staff debated the institution's future. Where should the Board of Governors build a new hospital to fulfill its historical obligation to provide medical care, and what kind of building should they approve? It was not simply an esthetic or economic debate, nor simply a conflict between medical staff and laymen—though it was in some measure all these things. Ideas about germs and fevers were to play a key role in these deliberations, along with the schedules of clinical teachers and attending staff. Differences over the cause of hospital infection were not the abstract concern of scholars, but structured into matters as practical as the disposal and acquisition of real estate, the design of windows and heating ducts, the dressing of a wound.

No question was more important than that of choosing a proper site. Well-informed laymen as well as medical men unconnected with the New York Hospital felt their new building should be removed from the city's crowded center to a more salubrious—and cheaper—site where the expansive principles of pavilion design could be applied. "Ease of access to patients for physicians and students," as a Bostonian had expressed the reform consensus as early as 1861, "has hitherto determined the site of most of our large hospitals; and a central location has been too often secured at the enormous sacrifice of pure air and good drainage."[1] The New York

Hospital's prestigious consulting staff was not entirely comfortable with the practical implications of such teachings. Hours spent in unpaid ward rounds were prestigious, but necessarily marginal to an established practitioner's busy schedule. Most of the attending staff wanted to remain close to their teaching, their private practice, and, they argued, to the working-class districts served by the hospital.

When the New York Hospital finally opened its new building in 1877, the ceremony was an occasion of controversy as well as celebration. Its leaders and their architect had ignored the central axioms of contemporary hospital architecture, building a "seven-story building . . . on a space of ground only seventy feet by one hundred and seventy-five in extent," in a crowded part of the city.[2] Critics charged that the hospital's Board of Governors had scorned the most fundamental teachings of sanitary reform and allowed the demeaning logic of real estate costs and the convenience of attending physicians to outweigh the safety of patients.

Staff members were prepared to defend their design. Their architect argued that he had sacrificed esthetic considerations in order to maximize ventilation. Consulting surgeon William H. Van Buren, a spokesman for the hospital's staff, defended their design choice in more novel terms. If the findings of Pasteur and the procedures Joseph Lister had based on them proved correct, Van Buren argued at the new hospital's inauguration, then the absolute number of patients and the structure's interior design need not be crucial. "It has been shown how we can keep wounds sweet and healthy, and conduct them to a favorable ending by a shorter and surer route than that heretofore followed, and thus prevent hospital patients from poisoning each other."[3] Antiseptic procedures could prevent wound infection in any sort of building, no matter how tall or how constricted its grounds.[4] These new insights justified a high-rise structure in a site convenient to the city's business and residential center.

To many contemporaries, of course, Van Buren's words seemed no more than the strained defense of a short-sighted and economically biased decision. Lister was still an extremist, an enthusiast who, as the editor of New York's leading medical journal put it, ". . . has a grasshopper in his head."[5] It was to be another decade before antiseptic surgery and the germ theory upon which it was based won general acceptance in the medical world.

But despite such contemporary misgivings, it is clear that scientific knowledge and, equally important, the image of science had already become deeply embedded in the social process of delivering medical care. Subsequent social change in the hospital was in good measure to turn on the assimilation of intellectual change—on the reshaping of a welfare institution into a seeming laboratory of healing. General structural factors such as urbanization and industrialization were, of course, fundamental, while nineteenth-century medical science offered as much rhetorical promise as clinical efficacy. But without that promise the scale and substance of subsequent hospital development could hardly have been imagined.[6]

The actual place of science in American clinical medicine has always been ambiguous and conflicted—yet that ambiguity has never significantly undermined the faith of most educated Americans in the promise of that science. It was a faith shared by the most influential and ambitious in the medical profession. Both physicians and their hospitals were to cloak themselves in the mantle of an ever-improving, increasingly effective, and necessarily unselfish medical science. By the beginning of the present century, the hospital and the American medical profession would never look back; scientific medicine was to provide a new plausibility for physicians and their institutions. No single aspect of this new knowledge was more important in reshaping the hospital than the germ theory and antiseptic surgery.

Banishing Infection: The Measured Triumph of Antisepsis

In retrospect, the relationship between antiseptic surgery and the modern hospital's development seems neat and logical. For Lister's medical contemporaries the perceived reality was rather more complicated. Few were immediate converts to this radically new way of understanding infection.[7] Few anticipated the fundamental nature of the changes that were to overcome medical practice. As we have seen, surgery was a minor aspect of the mid-century hospital's clinical routine. Even with the stimulus of anesthesia, operative procedures, aside from the treatment of ever-increasing incidents of trauma, were still a minor part of the hospital's therapeutic work in the 1860s and 1870s. Most surgical admissions were still minor wounds and lacerations, fractures, hernias, or persistent skin lesions. "Important operations," as contemporaries termed anything more severe, loomed far larger in terms of drama and an individual surgeon's status than they did in an institution's day-to-day routine.

The quarter century after the introduction of anesthesia witnessed no revolution in surgical efficacy. Ether and chloroform facilitated longer and more elaborate procedures, but in so doing may have increased the likelihood of surgical infection.[8] Well-merited fear of such infection allied with a limited understanding of shock and related physiological problems made surgeons cautious in expanding their traditional repertoire. Intrusive voluntary procedures remained infrequent and limited to a comparative handful of operations. Hospital rules still routinely called for a formal consultation before any life-threatening procedure could be undertaken.[9] When operating on a strangulated hernia, a prominent clinician recalled, it was considered impolite not to invite every bystander to examine the wound; "my surgical colleague," he added, "amputated the limb of a corpse and a limb of the living in the same forenoon, on the same table, in the same purple gown."[10] It was not surprising that even minor operations could develop fatal complications or that hospitals could be recognized by their stench, "predominant among which was that of stale pus. It was something which could be recognized hundreds of yards away from the institution."[11]

Wound infection was seen by mid-nineteenth-century surgeons as an intractable difficulty, to be minimized though perhaps never entirely overcome.[12] In the 1860s and 1870s, dozens of prominent surgeons in England and on the Continent as well as in the United States experimented with wound-dressing procedures that would—they hoped—minimize infection. "Cleanliness" was universally if imprecisely endorsed, while individual surgeons fixed on pet systems of dressings and drainage to achieve that cleanliness and support the body's recuperative powers. Traditional holistic assumptions also dictated that rest, diet, and "evacuations" be carefully monitored both before and after an operation. It seemed obvious that a well-nourished and rested patient had the best chance of resisting infection.

There was also much interest in the possible utility of "antiseptics" in discouraging infection. As we have seen, most mid-century physicians believed that some "zymotic" or ferment-inducing substance in the atmosphere, often originating in accumulated organic matter or the exhalations of the sick, was somehow responsible for hospital infections and fevers. Antiseptics were chemicals that held the promise of neutralizing such substances, of somehow combating sepsis. Since at least the second half of the eighteenth century, physicians had experimented with such agents for use in hospitals, ships, and other crowded, enclosed, and potentially dangerous places.[13] Since the 1830s, for example, chlorine compounds had been widely advocated for their disinfectant properties, and American surgeons had used bromine and chlorine solutions for similar hospital purposes during the Civil War.

In this context, Lister's system seemed in some ways little distinguishable from its numerous competitors in the late 1860s. Even his choice of carbolic acid as disinfectant was not entirely novel, although the consistency and energy with which he applied it seemed peculiar to many skeptical contemporaries. Mid-nineteenth-century surgeons thought in terms of procedures, not pathological mechanisms: what sort of dressings should be used, how frequently should they be changed, how should drainage be managed. Few understood and accepted Lister's theoretical rationale for his idiosyncratic technique. It was hardly surprising that to many clinicians in the early 1870s, Lister's "system" reduced itself to an obsessive and arbitrary reliance on a particular chemical. It was also complex and expensive in a generation accustomed to casual procedures and meager budgets, when surgical costs were traditionally limited to the initial expense of purchasing a case of instruments.[14] The toxicity of carbolic acid seemed only to underline the arbitrariness of the Glasgow surgeon's program with its novel emphasis on operating in a spray of carbolic acid vapor. Lister's prior conversion to Pasteur's views was ignored by some and rejected as sectarian by others. Even if one believed that carbolic acid was effective in fighting wound infection, its precise mechanism remained obscure. Did it simply impede putrefaction in the exposed tissue? Or did it somehow destroy the microorganisms responsible for that putrefaction? Critics had argued for years that the finding of "parasitic forms" in an infected wound did not prove a causative relationship; the microorganisms might well be "a consequence of it, which furnished a nidus for their rise and development."[15]

The editorialists who criticized the New York Hospital's reliance on Listerian antisepsis in 1878 expressed no more than the prudent common sense of the matter. In the mid-1870s, Lister's views were still controversial—not lacking in merit, but not necessarily different in kind from numerous competitors. Prudent surgical staffs adopted many of his suggestions in the 1870s, but saw them as part of a multidimensional attack on infection. A study of surgery in the Pennsylvania Hospital, for example, boasted proudly in 1880 that only 17 of 108 amputation patients had died between 1875 and 1879. The authors attributed these good results and an unaccustomed freedom from "pyemia," or blood poisoning, to better ventilation, the "free use of carbolic acid," scrupulous cleanliness, and the dressing of wounds with flowing water.[16]

The Transformation of Hospital Surgery

It was hardly surprising that it took a generation for surgeons to incorporate this new understanding of wound infection and build it into a standard set of operating room procedures. As we have seen, it demanded a radical change in fundamental views of the nature of disease and its origins, in particular a rejection of the older, aggregate model of infection. And it implied as well a gradual decline in a centuries-old faith in the primacy of the atmosphere in promoting infection, a faith so strong that it had guided even Lister's own early work. One need only recall the carbolic acid spray that suffused operating theaters in the first decade of antiseptic surgery.

The two decades after Lister's original publications in the mid-1860s brought a gradual modification of his original procedures: the evolution of antiseptic into what came to be called aseptic surgery. By the mid–1880s, Lister's stature had been generally accepted, even as his techniques were being recast. "Lister's method has been curtailed," as one enthusiast explained in 1884,

modified, indeed in some ways every limb, so to speak, has suffered high amputation; but the grand trunk, the vital principle, still lives, still is acknowledged, that in some way, some how, by some means, it matters not what, wounds must be kept from first to last surgically clean.[17]

This shift from Lister's original antisepsis to asepsis was more process than event, for it presupposed the elaboration of an integrated assortment of techniques, tools, and procedures aimed at keeping bacteria from coming in contact with exposed tissue.

Even surgeons who considered themselves convinced advocates

of antisepsis were at first dismayingly imprecise in their application of these new teachings. Surgeons in the 1880s might drop instruments on the floor, pick them up, and after wiping them on a sleeve continue their procedure. Bandages and sutures were used without being sterilized, and natural sponges were used, washed, and used again. One jacket might serve as operating room garb for as long as a year. In a few prominent institutions, staffs were split, with some attending surgeons following what they assumed to be antiseptic procedures, while others forbade them on their services.[18] Hardly an autobiography of a physician trained during these years is without such anecdotes.[19] But the trend toward the elaboration and adoption of aseptic surgery was inexorable. By the 1890s, the introduction of autoclaves, sterilized dressings, and the rubber glove had made surgeons more inventive and confident. Most important, rapid progress in bacteriology clarified the mechanisms underlying Lister's empirical suggestions. "The principles upon which aseptic surgery is established are firm," an authority explained in the mid-1890s, "since the theories which have led the technique to its present state of perfection are confirmed by bacteriological tests."

This change, however, cannot disturb the glorious foundation laid by Joseph Lister. To Lister we owe the mother, *Antisepsis,* who, though she died in parturition, brought forth her idealization, ASEPSIS.[20]

The world of surgical possibilities had changed dramatically.

The body cavities were no longer forbidding obstacles, for example, but enticing opportunities. As early as 1886, the Massachusetts General Hospital's staff urged the institution's trustees to establish a special ward for abdominal surgery, one with an adjoining operating room in which rigid antiseptic measures could be enforced. Dangers that had seemed overwhelming only a few years before had, they argued, "been reduced to a minimum. In our Wards Erysipelas is rare, Pyaemia & Saepticemia seldom seen & Hospital gangrene has been stamped out."[21] The stakes were high for ambitious young clinicians. "Abdominal surgery is now the field where the most brilliant successes are to be attained," as one such surgeon argued two years later. "No branch of surgery can compare with it for a moment. . . . It is from the work we are now doing & hope to do in abdominal surgery (& . . . cerebral surgery as well) that the Hospital must gain its position among the hospitals of the world at the end of the next ten years. We have the choice," he warned and enticed, "now to take the lead."[22] Technical virtuosity was being inextricably related to status—for institutions as well as individuals.

By the turn of the century, the increasing complexity and effectiveness of aseptic surgery, the advantages of the x-ray and clinical laboratory, the convenience of twenty-four-hour nursing and house staff attendance were making a hospital operating room the most plausible and convenient place to perform surgery. To many surgeons, in fact, it was beginning to seem the only ethical place to practice an increasingly demanding art.

Though the prestige of surgery constituted an ever more powerful inducement, middle-class patients remained hesitant to enter hospitals. Until the 1920s surgery was often performed in private homes, and babies were in many cases still delivered in the mother's bedroom, whether attended by a family physician or midwife.[23]

But despite the slow and grudging growth of public acceptance, a trend toward hospital surgery had become increasingly clear. By the turn of the century in fact, critics of surgical euphoria were already warning against excessive and unnecessary resort to the scalpel. Appendicitis was the most obvious example; " 'Belly-ache' is now a surgical disease," one prominent clinician complained.[24] And the extraordinary number of appendectomies performed at the very end of the nineteenth and beginning of the twentieth centuries indicates that the procedure was almost certainly being abused.[25] But such reservations had little effect in moderating the trend toward increased surgery. In hospital after hospital, the proportion of surgical to medical admissions increased, as did the percentage of voluntary procedures among those surgical admissions. At the Pennsylvania Hospital, for example, over eight hundred and fifty operations were performed in the year between May, 1899 and May, 1900, more than the total number of operations performed at the same hospital between 1800 and 1845.[26]

Surgery meant an activist, intrusive style of practice and a decreasing emphasis on the conservative or expectant management of many syndromes. New York's Hospital for the Ruptured and Crippled provides an exemplary case.[27] James Knight, the leading spirit in its founding and its surgeon-in-chief from 1863 to 1887, was a physician who assumed a holistic—and paternalistic—attitude toward his patients and the hospital's work generally.[28] He placed little emphasis on operative procedures and a great deal on diet, exercise, fresh air, bandages, and appliances. Knight saw local lesions as aspects of more general conditions, just as he saw the child as potential citizen of a larger society and concerned himself with his little patients' moral education and future job prospects. Knight lived in the hospital and served as father of an extended family. By 1887, Knight had become an anachronism. He was succeeded by Virgil Gibney, a youthful and energetic orthopedist. Numbers of operations increased rapidly and lengths of stay decreased; Gibney himself lived outside the hospital. The surgeon was no longer content to guide and monitor, to negotiate a multidimensional path to physical and social health. Aseptic surgery had far more to offer many patients than the bandages, regimen, and braces of mid-century, but the new-model surgery construed its responsibilities in increasingly narrow and procedure-oriented terms.[29]

By the 1920s surgical admissions outnumbered medical.[30] Ordinary Americans had not only begun to accept the hospital, they had come to associate it with the surgeon. Hospital planners could assume that private surgical beds would always outnumber their medical counterparts.[31] Prospective patients were influenced not only by the hope of healing, but by the image of a new kind of medicine—precise, scientific, and effective. For the first time, patients came to their physician with the hope—and increasingly the assumption—that he might impose and not merely facilitate healing. The new surgery helped change physicians' expectations as much it did those of laymen. Most practitioners were as impressed as their patients with the achievements of modern surgery. It was no wonder that the specialty attracted so many bright and ambitious young men. Surgery had always played a disproportionately dramatic role in the world of medicine and medical education, and now it could claim a potential for healing that overshadowed the more humble and inconclusive efforts of internal medicine. It seemed to represent the innovative spirit of science made clinical reality. Not everyone agreed as to what that science actually was or should be—or how it might best be related to the clinician's mundane tasks. But such imprecision did little to moderate the impact of appeals to the laboratory or undercut the role of science in the forging of a new style of medical identity. Quite the contrary, a lack of precise meaning has rarely interfered with the efficacy of appeals to science and the promise of its application.

New Definitions of Disease

In retrospect it is clear that the expanding clinical role of surgery was consistent with other trends in medical thought.[32] One was toward a belief in the specificity of disease, toward seeing particular ailments as predictable sequences of symptoms growing out of localized lesions or well-defined malfunctions in some physiological process. Diseases were, in other words, entities that could now be conceived of apart from their manifestation in particular individuals.[33] As we have seen, this novel understanding of disease grew out of developments in clinical medicine and pathology, culminating in the work of the Paris clinical school during the first half of the nineteenth century. To these scholars and their followers in Paris, Vienna, and the British Isles, there seemed no necessary connection between the reality of these newly agreed-upon disease entities and a parallel agreement as to their precipitating cause. It seemed possible, if not likely, that the cause of disease would never be understood; for the moment it was enough that medicine delineate the natural history of particular syndromes in life and death.[34]

In demonstrating a connection between particular infectious ills and particular microorganisms, the germ theory underlined and explained the unity of disease patterns already demonstrated by three generations of clinicians and pathologists. But this new knowledge did more than that. It changed public attitudes toward the medical profession and raised expectations, even before laboratories could do much to transform the shape of everyday practice.

If therapeutics was at first little altered, the same could not be said of public health. By the first decade of the present century, the laboratory had informed and revised pre-existing efforts to control the spread of infectious disease. Bacteriology had illuminated the role played by healthy carriers, while field and laboratory research had exposed the role of insects in the transmission of other ills. Laboratory insight had helped make water purification more than a rough empirical procedure and justified pasteurization of milk, even lowered the cost of food by helping rationalize the processing and preservation of foodstuffs. All these effects were ultimately to play a role in altering disease incidence and thus the experience of medical care.[35] Physicians and hospitals encountered fewer cases of typhoid, for example, even though they were still without an effective treatment for those cases that did occur.

These new ideas about disease and the role of science helped undercut traditional styles of practice even before (as in the case of typhoid) the laboratory provided the physician with effective therapeutic tools. An understanding of the patient's physiological individuality was to seem less and less important, an understanding of the disease from which he or she suffered more important. In this sense, patients were inevitably seen in terms that transcended their individuality, as instances of more abstract, yet somehow more real syndromes that manifested themselves in countless other men and women. Prognosis and therapeutics turned increasingly upon identification of the ailment that assailed an individual patient and not upon a nuanced evaluation of his or her biological and psychological individuality. The doctor began to treat diseases, in the words of a familiar aphorism, not patients.

We must be careful not to overstate the abrupt and categorical quality of this change. In earlier generations, physicians often practiced in rote cookbook fashion, while twentieth-century physicians have not uniformly lost sight of the patient as individual. Nevertheless, there is clearly an element of truth in this particular truism. The pathology-based and legitimated picture of disease grew increasingly prominent in medical thought, and the traditional emphasis on individuality and idiosyncrasy faded proportionately.

The hospital had, moreover, always provided more impersonal medicine than had private practice, an inevitable effect of class relationships and staffing ratios as well as the episodic quality of institutional care. The very impersonality of hospital treatment and the accident of its being provided by a physician ordinarily unknown to the patient made it vastly different from the general pattern of late nineteenth-century medical care. Private patients and their families were still treated by a familiar physician in the home.[36] Emphasis on disease specificity and "objective," laboratory-aided diagnosis may well have exacerbated unpleasant institutional realities for the poor. But they had never expected much in the way of individual attention. It was the middle-class patient who was to face a very different sort of experience in the twentieth-century hospital.

With the gradual acceptance of disease specificity, it became increasingly easy to see and treat patients as exemplifications of those categories. Hospital records indicate this in a number of ways: the increasing uniformity and studied impersonality of written records, the growing emphasis on specific diagnosis, and a corresponding rejection of terms describing general physiological states.[37] Admitting diagnoses such as "senility," "failing," or "marasmus" gradually disappeared in the 1880s. They had already become uncommon in self-conscious advanced institutions. At New York's Roosevelt Hospital, for example, a minority of patients were still admitted in 1878 with diagnoses such as "constipation," "destitution," and "debility from various causes." In 1882, significantly, the hospital's aggregate admission figures did include an entry for "debility," but it was followed by the words "diagnosis uncertain." The addition of those telling words encapsulates a fundamental aspect of the new-model hospital. Diagnosis—and the admission process—could be understood and legitimated only in terms of "objective" disease entities.[38]

Objectivity was no new goal in clinical medicine, but physicians had never possessed the tools to implement that elusive ideal. For the first time in man's history, it appeared in the late nineteenth century that "instruments of precision," as Philadelphian S. Weir Mitchell termed them, would allow the physician to measure the body's activities in health and disease, to make clinical medicine increasingly a science, less and less an art.[39] The personal equation was increasingly a factor to be reduced to its component mechanisms, not romanticized.

The late nineteenth- and early twentieth-century hospital was in part being transformed by new diagnostic tools. The clinical laboratory and x-ray promised to raise prognosis and diagnosis (if not therapeutics) to new levels of consistency. The physician would no longer be entirely dependent on the patient's appearance and subjective perceptions. By the beginning of the present century, he or she could call upon the results of chemical and bacteriological tests, the appearance of x-ray plates, the findings of microscope, stethoscope, opthalmoscope, and otoscope. Such tools were not applied routinely in private practice and, in most areas of internal medicine, could do little to guide an effective therapeutics. But they played a far more important symbolic role, representing to both doctor and patient the increasingly scientific character of medicine. In regard to the hospital, they were crucial, cumulatively suggesting that it was an appropriate, in fact necessary, site for the provision of medical care to all Americans and not just the urban poor.

The Rise of Clinical Technology

Physicians had always sought to see beneath the skin. What was it that constituted health and disease and what were the physiological processes that explained, perhaps constituted, life and death? It is no accident that traditional medicine should have concerned itself with the appearance of urine and feces, of drawn blood, of the tongue and eyes. All offered evidence of mechanisms otherwise opaque and supplemented the patient's own rendition of his or her symptoms. After death, the postmortem room could provide additional insight by revealing lesions that had caused symptoms during life. Knowledge of gross pathology began to accumulate from the seventeenth century on, but it was not until the nineteenth century that medicine began to find an array of tools that allowed it to begin the systematic investigation of the mechanisms that underlay the felt symptoms of disease.

Physical diagnosis provided one kind of insight, allowing the acute clinician to use his own senses, his fingertips and hearing, and to learn something of the state of a patient's heart and lungs, or of a fetal heartbeat. The stethoscope provided a further enhancement of those senses. By the 1870s, hospital physicians were generally familiar with the stethoscope and physical diagnosis—although they tended to use these techniques in only certain categories of illness, such as diseases of the chest.[40] The meaning of this more abundant sensory data was inevitably construed in terms of gradually accumulating postmortem findings.

Another path to medical insight grew out of chemistry. It was natural enough for traditional humoral ideas to shift gradually into chemical guise. The components of the body, the process of digestion, even the mechanisms that underlay disease could often be seen in chemical terms. The albumin in the urine of a patient suffering from Bright's disease, the sweetness in a diabetic's urine, the altered composition of the urine of a patient suffering from gout all pointed toward the promise of medical chemistry.[41] "Great discoveries," as one enthusiast put it in 1871, "in therapeutics and physiology are to be made only by renewing the bond which makes the Physician and Chemist one: and may we not truly say that if every chemist is not a doctor, every doctor must be a chemist, if he would march in the van of the great army of those who by searching would find out the truth."[42]

Such hopes implied the need for cooperation between the ward and laboratory. As early as 1842, for example, a small laboratory and two connecting wards at Guy's Hospital in London had been set aside for the clinical and chemical study of patients suffering from chronic kidney disease.[43] This arrangement was by no means typical; even in university hospitals it was not to become commonplace until well into the twentieth century. Nevertheless, the allure of laboratory-defined certainties was very real, even in an Anglo-American medical world in which government, universities, and private philanthropy had yet to provide support for clinical investigation.

Efforts to bring systematic scholarship into the nineteenth-century hospital were, in fact, most pervasive in the area of pathology.[44] Pathology was the most intellectually exciting frontier of medicine in the 1830s and 1840s, reflecting the prestige and accomplishments of the French clinical school during the first third of the century. A nucleus of eager young clinicians returning from medical study in Paris had sought to duplicate in a small way facilities they had enjoyed in the French capital. Medical staffs of the older and better-established hospitals worked to found pathological cabinets—collections, that is, of representative, rare, or atypical pathological specimens. Such collections, like a hospital's library, had been used since at least the late eighteenth century as instructional aids and signs of an institution's aspirations and accomplishments. A minority of ambitious attending physicians and house officers had also sought—with varying degrees of enthusiasm and effectiveness—to maximize the number of postmortem examinations performed at their institutions.

Even an unpaid position as pathologist or curator of a hospital's pathological cabinet might allow zealous medical men the opportunity to utilize "pathological materials" provided by the institution's charity patients. It was a professionally appropriate stop on the path to intellectual distinction and institutional security.

But the relationship between institutional preferment and intellectual achievement was neither consistent nor predictable. The structure of nineteenth-century career options dictated that such intellectual interests could be most appropriately pursued in the odd moments of a young man's career or cherished as a badge of elite status in an older practitioner's spare hours. The ordinarily unpaid office of pathologist was normally vacated by young men as they rose in the hospital's clinical hierarchy. It was a plausible and possibly advantageous way of marking time and occupying a lower rung on a well-understood ladder of advancement—but not a career in itself. Unpaid and lacking the status connected with membership on a hospital's clinical staff, incumbents ordinarily resigned pathology posts when private practice grew demanding. In 1855, for example, a committee of New York Hospital physicians urged the Board of Governors to pay a small salary to the curator of their pathological cabinet. A series of young men had held the position for short periods of time and, "Receiving no pecuniary remuneration they could not afford to forgo opportunities of professional advancement . . ." The results had been unfortunate. In retrospect, however, the attending physicians' justification for their request is even more significant than its occasion. "Humanity and true Medical Science alike," the staff committee argued, "demand that provision should be made for the support and increase of a collection like ours which may be made to contribute in so important a way to the elucidation of the nature of disease and the instruction of the medical profession." Even in 1855, such arguments had an immediate appeal: how could one not be enticed by the prospect of solving the mystery of disease or opposed in principle to the clinical training of physicians?[45]

Most of the older American hospitals did make gestures in the direction of recognizing such interests in the first half of the nineteenth century, usually by creating a pathological cabinet and appointing a curator. In the 1870s and 1880s, appointment of a hospital pathologist became increasingly common.[46] (Trustee support of systematic postmortems was, as we have seen, a good deal more problematic.) In few institutions, however, did the work of such pathologists or microscopists amount to much. So-called laboratories were often dark and dirty rooms, almost bereft of equipment and tucked into basement or attic corners. Short tenures and lack of specialized training almost guaranteed that pathologists would produce little.

Hospitals were hard-pressed to pay the costs of patient care (heat, light, and food) and could spare little to support scientific frills. And frills they certainly did seem to be. The insights of the postmortem room and microscope offered little to the practicing clinician. It might be interesting to establish the characteristic appearance of a diseased liver that killed one's patient, but such knowledge offered little guidance in treating similarly afflicted patients in the future. The Pennsylvania Hospital Board of Managers was only typical, if ingenuously candid, when it congratulated itself on creating the unsalaried position of Pathological Chemist in 1870; "where we can promote the cause of science," they explained, "without any expense on the part of the Board we consider it our duty to do so."[47]

But there was always a minority of staff members eager for increased laboratory facilities. Even in the mid-nineteenth century a handful of attending physicians were already urging the establishment of chemical laboratories and the appointment of microscopists.[48] They sought to enlist these new laboratory tools in the aid of diagnosis and treatment—to add an understanding of the disease process in life to the retrospective insight provided by the postmortem. "If pathology is to merit the title of the science of medicine," as one prominent medical editorialist argued in 1871, "it must be in its bringing together, in one connected series, etiology, diagnosis, and morbid anatomy—an exhibition of the phenomena of disease from its inception to its close, . . . Mere dead-house pathology" was clearly inadequate.[49] No clinical history could be considered complete, another enthusiast charged in 1868, ". . . while in a large number we can hardly be considered as having performed our duty as physicians, without a microscopical and chemical examination of the blood and more important secretions and excretions of the body."[50] Chemistry and the microscope had already provided a battery of procedures that could be applied to urine, blood, and even tissue samples. But such tests remained in fact academic curiosities; only the thermometer and a few urine analyses had become an accustomed part of hospital routine before the end of the century.

It was not until the late 1890s that the clinical pathology laboratory became part of everyday patient care even in America's most self-consciously advanced hospitals.[51] And medical schools had done little to build laboratory skills into curricula. Nevertheless, medicine's technical resources increased steadily, with much of such innovation coming from Germany's fertile laboratories. By the First World War, diagnosis of an individual patient might be aided by serological tests, careful temperature readings, chemical and microscopic evaluation of blood and urine, and by x-ray examination, where relevant. The laboratory's findings, as the New York Hospital's medical board contended in 1903, could now deal "not only with the problems presented by the dead body but also contributes to the solution of problems presented by the diseased but living body."[52] Yet, as some turn-of-the-century critics contended, the abundance and ingenuity of available tests was not matched by their relevance to everyday practice. Costs also discouraged many hospitals, even the comparatively modest expense of laboratories in a period of simple technologies and low-paid or volunteer labor. At first, the laboratory seemed only a drain on already tight budgets: scientific diagnosis did not automatically translate into financial returns for America's voluntary hospitals.[53]

Even private patients were accustomed to paying a single daily charge that included every aspect of care (except private-duty nursing and a physician's fee). It was only gradually that hospitals began to bill separately for blood and urine tests, x-ray plates, anesthesia, the use of operating rooms—and thus underwrite the cost of operating a laboratory. With the ability to define costs and charges, it was inevitable that the laboratory would become a "profit center" well before that now omnipresent term came into use. Such facilities were at first suited only to large urban institutions; they did not become general in smaller and more isolated institutions until the second and third decades of the present century.

Nevertheless, a growing minority of early twentieth-century physicians was enticed by the laboratory's promise—even while its relevance to everyday practice remained questionable. The test tube, microscope, and Petri dish offered ambitious young men new and reassuringly positive tools for use in studying disease and in doing so the opportunity to "accomplish some work of an original character."[54] It is no accident that the term "clinical investigation" became widely accepted in this period. Although the great bulk of early twentieth-century and late nineteenth-century clinical research might seem crude and simplistic in retrospect, it provided a new kind of credential, helping separate the specialist-oriented and intellectual young man from his less elevated peers. At first, such investigation had more to do with the definition and elaboration of academic careers than with care of the sick. For the medical profession more generally, the availability of scientific tools and procedures legitimated an impressive new style of medical identity: that of master of laboratory science and "instruments of precision" as contrasted with the more traditional ideal of wise and intuitive manager of elusive and idiosyncratic clinical situations.

In this sense, the new tools of diagnosis "worked" in their capacity to inspire the medical man with self-confidence and his patients with a parallel faith in his ministrations. Ultimately, of course, they were to help provide an increasingly substantive understanding of the biological mechanisms that underlie many clinical syndromes.

But this was a gradual and elusive achievement. The alliance between science and clinical medicine remained shaky and ambiguous before the First World War.[55]

Even as the elite in medicine grew increasingly enamored of what it called medical science, this new source of knowledge had in fact provided little beside aseptic surgery to change the hospital's therapeutic options. A bright young Johns Hopkins resident might be able to demonstrate characteristic white-blood-cell counts in lobar pneumonia, but still do little to treat the unfortunate patient. Before 1900, only diphtheria antitoxin seemed to offer the possibility of intervening decisively in the course of an acute nonsurgical ailment. One of the consequences, in fact, of an increasingly positivistic and reductionistic spirit in medicine was a growing skepticism in regard to the efficacy of aggressive therapeutics. Nursing, rest, and diet were highly valued by every sophisticated *fin de siècle* practitioner— even as he or she prescribed the modest doses of cathartics or analgesics patients expected. Digitalis, quinine, and especially opium and its derivates remained the profession's most effective drugs at the end of the century, as they had been a half-century earlier.[56] Pasteur's prophylactic treatment of rabies (1885) and Behring and Kitisato's diphtheria antitoxin (1891) remained atypical. And both, especially rabies, had little immediate impact in reshaping broad patterns of morbidity or mortality. The introduction of serological tests for typhoid (1897) and syphilis (1906) were impressive achievements, but were more relevant to prevention than treatment.

These discoveries did have an enormous effect on public opinion, however. One need hardly emphasize the social impact of a rabies treatment, for example, even if its effect on mortality rates was trivial. Like polio in the twentieth century, the emotional prominence of rabies belied a less formidable demographic reality. A similar observation can be made about diphtheria. Here was a disease particularly fatal in children and with an extremely high (if erratic) mortality rate. Then in the 1890s, it became clear that Behring's serum could be injected into a sick child and make the difference between life and death. The discovery had an enormous impact. Physicians differed about appropriate levels of antitoxin and the clinical situations in which it was most effective. Public health authorities experimented with the production of antitoxin. Skeptical historians question its actual efficacy in the 1890s, but the public was left with an image of the physician as healer, as capable of intervening in the course of a life-threatening illness. Pasteur's treatment for rabies and Behring's diphtheria antitoxin burst into the public consciousness, moreover, soon after the debates on antiseptic surgery and Koch's discoveries of the tuberculosis and cholera organisms (1882 and 1883). At one stroke, the German bacteriologist had demonstrated the cause of the century's most widespread and mortal endemic disease (tuberculosis) and its most fearsome epidemic ailment (cholera). The laboratory was coming to be seen as the source of medicine's new explanatory powers, while the great majority of laymen were incapable of making a consistent distinction between the laboratory worker, the practitioner who applied the laboratory's findings in patient care, and the epidemiologist or public health worker who sought to use knowledge in halting the spread of infectious disease.

The hospital, like the practitioner, gradually assumed a new image of technically based efficacy, but the reshaping of the hospital as a living social institution was to be a far more difficult undertaking. Middle-class patients were slow to enter hospitals, no matter how enthusiastic their response to medicine's new capabilities. And aside from aseptic surgery, there was no reason to assume that any of the then available diagnostic or therapeutic devices implied hospitalization. The hospital might be associated in a general way with technical progress in the 1890s, but this did not mean that middle-class Americans assumed it had anything to do with *their* medical care.

The hospital itself changed slowly and grudgingly in its orientation toward scientific medicine. The late nineteenth- and early twentieth-century hospital remained a fickle home for the pursuit of scientific medicine and the training of a new generation of medical men. Until the last decades of the century, there was simply no place for the would-be medical scientist in America's hospitals (or in general in its medical schools). The laboratory could still be seen as a will-o-the-wisp, leading young men astray from the clinical work that would necessarily be their bread and butter. Science was still regarded as a young man's mistress, clinical practice his wife: few could afford the demands of both. Even such pragmatic tools as the x-ray and clinical pathology were slow to find a secure home in many of America's poorly endowed hospitals, and no physician could realistically hope to attain professional security through the mastery of such technical skills alone.[57] At the beginning of the twentieth century, American hospitals offered only a handful of paid staff positions. Almost all medical school faculty members earned their bread as practitioners; attending physicians at even the most prestigious hospitals still served without pay and fit ward rounds into a busy clinical schedule. The conflict between ideals of research and the mundane realities of practice had existed for generations; they could only intensify at the end of the century as the achievements and allure of research increased.

The Grail of Science

American society provided virtually no support for the would-be medical researcher. The governmental support enjoyed by French and German professors could hardly be expected on this side of the Atlantic. Even the meaning of "science" and "medical research" remained unclear. Yet since at least mid-century, an energetic if tiny minority of English and American physicians had sought to bring change to medicine through "original investigation." It seemed probable, as an English advocate of research put it in 1855, ". . . that all future improvement in the treatment of disease must be based upon a careful and minute investigation into its nature, . . ." A knowledge of the natural sciences was thus as important to surgery and medicine as an understanding of grammar to a study of the classics, but he concluded that such work could at present in England, "only be effected by the careful private study of different members of the profession."[58] Conditions in America were if anything less congenial to original work.

Nevertheless, a cadre of young men accepted the validity of such demands, contrasting the ephemeral nature of material success with the more lasting rewards of scholarly achievement. It was embarrassing to travel in Europe and realize that many prominent American practitioners were unknown to the leaders of French and German medicine. It was not what a man earned but what he wrote that made a permanent reputation.[59] But for the generation of Americans who came of age before the Civil War, practice provided the only real option for professional survival. Yet success in practice inevitably "robbed" science of workers it could not "easily spare."[60]

More than a lack of support hindered the development of medical research. Definition of scholarship had to change as well: the traditional library mastery of a subject matter was no longer adequate. "Investigation" implied disciplined hours spent in the laboratory, the autopsy room, or hospital ward. The growing dominance of German medicine in the last third of the century underlined the inadequacy of an exclusively clinical and private practice orientation. A love of acquiring new knowledge for its own sake and the willingness of society to accept and support that devotion set German medicine apart from the Anglo-American professions. In England and America, as the eloquent William Osler put it in 1890, ". . . the young man may start with an ardent desire to devote his life to science, [but] he is soon dragged into the mill of practice, and at forty years of age, the 'guinea stamp' is on all his work."[61] By the end of the nineteenth century such arguments had become commonplace among an elite minority of American physicians.

Obviously, their arguments and attitudes were not those of the average practitioner, but advocates of medical science argued that even the commitment of a minority to investigation would benefit the entire profession. By the 1870s, prescient reformers were predicting that an increasingly enlightened public would in time learn that science set the regular profession apart from its sectarian competitors: had homeopaths or botanic doctors ever made an important discovery?[62] And by the end of the 1870s, a few conservative, and equally prescient, medical men were already alarmed at the growing prestige of research and an increasingly technical style of practice. "The desire of the time," one such nay-sayer warned in 1879, "seems to be to make students histologists, pathologists, microscopists, rather than sound practitioners, full of the humble but necessary knowledge of the practical departments of our art and science."[63] More petulant than accurate, this warning does indicate the steadily growing power of science as image and goal—if not as yet reality.

The hospital was inevitably to be a battleground for such differing views of medicine's appropriate role. If systematic clinical investigation was to be accomplished, the hospital's wards and postmortem room would have to be the profession's laboratory. Medical progress, as a Philadelphia editorialist contended as early as 1874, ". . . rests largely on the use which men make of hospitals, since very little valuable study of disease can be done in private practice." Americans had thus far acquitted themselves with little honor in attaining this goal: ". . . the prestige of a city which claims to be called, . . . a great medical centre, must always depend upon the amount of original work which it evolves; and it is just this which everywhere in America has been sadly wanting."[64] The same editorialist urged those planning the University of Pennsylvania's new hospital to accept as a matter of principle ". . . that all proper facilities for original work should be furnished, and that the performance of such work should be a recognized part of the duty of the staff."[65]

Hospital trustees and laymen generally had long accepted the idea that the institutions they supported and administered had a twofold function: care of the dependent sick and medical education. Now a small but vocal group of reformers sought to instill a third goal: the use of the hospital as a laboratory for clinical research.[66] They endeavored as well to recast traditional definitions of the hospital's long-accepted functions along more "scientific" lines: without modern laboratory facilities neither care nor teaching could be properly undertaken. "The hospital wards should furnish the material," a Harvard physician-bacteriologist contended, "the laboratories the means for study," if medicine's most intractable problems were to be solved.[67]

Without greater endowment, however, the hospital would never be able to take advantage of its unique research asset, its patients. The occupants of a hospital's beds could be regarded, as one outspoken reformer put it, as ". . . Nature's experiments with poisons cunningly elaborated in the tissues of the body, or with viruses coming from without, upon blood and bone, muscle and brain."[68] By the turn of the century, the stakes had risen and the demands of reformers grown more assertive. Recent findings in bacteriology and immunology had grown out of investment in laboratory research they contended; greater investment promised further returns to humanity and prestige for the discoverer. It also promised an improved status for the hospital that supported such work.[69]

Clinical research could no longer be conducted, an American Medical Association (AMA) spokesman argued in 1901, with "a few test-tubes, an alcohol lamp, and a microscope . . ." Such work required a fully equipped laboratory and "the use of exact methods and of the instruments of precision of physics, chemistry, and biology." The task of the hospital was equally to cure the sick and increase the profession's store of knowledge; ". . . where the second duty is not or can not be performed properly, the first also suffers neglect." Research did not conflict with the interest of individual patients; on the contrary, it helped guarantee first-rate care.[70] A handful of elite institutions had even begun to redefine their traditional responsibilities in a new hierarchy of effort. The care of individual patients could be seen, on balance, as less important than "the science of the prevention of disease."[71]

The stakes for staff members at elite hospitals were changing as well. As individuals, they also sought to do more than treat the assortment of sufferers their ward or outpatient duties brought to them. "We desire to do a great deal more in connection with our services," Boston neurologist J.J. Putnam explained in 1911, "than simply to attend to the most pressing needs of the patients. Investigations of one sort or another, or the need of a specifically prolonged and careful examination of some particular case are continually suggesting themselves to our minds. . . . we shall work with more zeal and interest," Putnam promised, "through having the feeling that the work accomplished is of such a sort as the community expects from us scientifically as well as practically."[72] Academic physicians disagreed as to its precise content, but all could join in invoking the values of medical science.

Science in fact continued to be more rhetoric than reality for the great majority of hospitals and medical men. The hospital remained, as it had been in the mid-nineteenth century, a place to earn prestige and accumulate clinical experience (some of which could be translated into the unsystematic clinical reports that still made up the bulk of medical publication) while progressing securely along the track that led to a successful consulting practice and a not unrelated academic status. By the beginning of the twentieth century, however, the voluntary hospital was becoming a place for surgeons and consultants to earn fees in practice as well. Despite brave words, it was in general no place for the laboratory scientist or, for the most part, the clinical investigator.

It was, however, a place for the academic consultant, the specialist, and specialist teacher. Both S. Weir Mitchell and J.J. Putnam spoke as neurologists when they endorsed the claims of scientific medicine. And it was in this guise that most ambitious American physicians advanced their careers—and in doing so helped reshape the hospital. Unlike laboratory science, clinical eminence provided both an avenue to intellectual distinction *and* access to the opportunities in practice that could support such ambitions. In 1910, few "laboratory men" could hope to gain hospital preferment or clinical reputation, at least while remaining in the laboratory. The leaders of American medicine were the surgeons, the prominent consultant-teachers, and the specialists who filled attending positions, became chiefs of clinical services, and taught a new generation of medical students.

CHAPTER 7

A Marriage of Convenience: Hospitals and Medical Careers

Mid-nineteenth-century medical careers were nurtured in a system of professional choices well understood by those Americans who had had to find their way among them. Every ambitious young physician sought to increase his chance of success in practice by cultivating influential patrons, selecting the most appropriate educational opportunities, and competing for desirable hospital positions. Although all physicians made such decisions, not all documented their calculations. Clarence Blake was one who did.

Blake was born in 1843, attended Harvard's Lawrence Scientific School and Medical School, then served in 1864 on the first house staff of the new Boston City Hospital. His father was a prosperous industrial chemist and businessman. After volunteering as a surgical assistant in the last year of the Civil War, Blake sailed for Europe in the fall of 1865. He was to spend almost four years on the Continent, preparing to enter Boston's competitive medical world.

Blake was meticuously self-conscious as he sat at his desk in Vienna and evaluated professional options, explaining them carefully to "mater" and "pater" in Boston. At first, he had explored the possibility of studying analytic chemistry in conjunction with clinical training. Chemical pathology had offered important new insights and the possibility of consulting work; but it soon became clear that the laboratory was no viable choice for a would-be physician. "I cannot see any opportunity of uniting chemistry with medicine," he concluded in the spring of 1866, "and am every day less and less inclined to practice any other than the medical profession."

Chemistry and clinical medicine might be intimately related so far as intellectual progress was concerned, but they stood "widely apart in practice. If it were possible to unite chemical knowledge with some particular branch of medical investigation and make a remunerative specialty of it I should very much like to do so, but as yet do not clearly see an opening which will lead to the desired end."[1] There was the possibility of an appointment in "Chemical Pathology" at the Boston City Hospital, but it would never lead to a secure practice; one had to be either a laboratory man or a clinician.

Specialization was one obvious resolution of the dilemma facing a young man who sought both intellectual distinction and a successful practice. It was a choice that Blake was to embrace with enthusiasm. America was a new country, he argued, and oversupplied with physicians. And, although conservatives in the profession viewed specialization with disdain, it seemed clear that rapidly accumulating knowledge, allied with the rather more sordid need to achieve visibility in a crowded and competitive urban marketplace, pointed toward a deep if narrow, rather than broad, clinical competence. Such comprehensive understanding was in fact no longer a possibility; there was too much to be learned and too little time in which to learn it.[2]

The German academic and hospital system pointed in the same direction. Vienna's General Hospital was, the ambitious young provincial explained, "a small town of 3200 inhabitants," with almost 9,000 births a year and "living specimens" accustomed to being pushed, shoved, poked and, finally, dissected. "A year here," he assured his parents, "is worth more than many years of private practice at home."[3] Foreign credentials were highly useful to an aspiring practitioner and a "Vienna degree is worth more than any to be got at home."[4]

After a flirtation with midwifery (made enticing by the abundance of "clinical material" and its centrality to practice) and neurology (his parents' suggestion and a field that seemed to be growing rapidly among the wealthy), Blake fastened on otology.[5] His decision came only after "a careful study of the ground and a calculation of probabilities" and a weighing of "inclinations, expediences and possibilities."[6] It was a novel specialty, perhaps something of a gamble, but it combined technical skill, a certain amount of science, and the promise of immediate professional visibility. Without such a specialty and the reputation, the referrals, and the consultations it promised, even an able and well-connected "young man might wait 10 or 12 years before getting anything like a remunerative practice."[7]

When he contemplated a return to Boston in 1869, Blake's first step was obvious. What he needed was a position as "Aurist" at the Massachusetts Charitable Eye and Ear Infirmary; perhaps, Blake suggested to his father, cousin Percy could put in a good word with board members. "When I get home," he explained, "such a position will give material for study and be the best possible opening to practice as an Aural Surgeon."[8]

The hospital was a necessary stage for acting out the ambitions of those who would play an elite role in an increasingly competitive medical world—competitive in intellectual as well as economic terms. A hospital position would provide Blake not only with immediate professional recognition and an opportunity to hone his skills and make professional contacts, but access to the pool of charity patients that provided indispensable raw material for scholarly work and publication. If he could "get charge of a clinique shortly after returning to Boston," Blake explained to his father, "it will be the best possible introduction to practice and to further opportunities for study and observation."[9]

Blake was to play a prominent role at the Massachusetts Eye and Ear and at Harvard Medical School for some forty years. As part of a circle of like-thinking contemporaries, many of them German-trained, Blake became a force for change in Boston medicine. His career was hardly characteristic of physicians generally, but it was entirely typical for a member of his generation's hospital-connected medical elite.[10] What is particularly revealing for the historian is Blake's self-consciously explicit evaluation of the choices that faced him as he sought to make a career in Boston medicine—and the meaning implicit in Blake's successful transformation of his family's material resources into professional "capital for my practice at home in shape of study and buying books. . . ."[11] Like the conservation of energy, the convertibility and "conservation" of social advantage remained a key aspect of elite medicine. On an individual level, it allowed young men from good families to contemplate a set of choices very different from those available to their less fortunate contemporaries. In a more general and schematic sense, it provided for a relatively smooth and gradual transition from an early nineteenth-century elite, defined largely by birth and social position, to one based increasingly on knowledge and formal credentials.

No institution was more central to this transition than the hospital. The integration of evolving medical careers into the hospital's day-to-day work was one of the most intricate yet fundamental aspects of the institution's history. It was of equal significance to the profession; in addressing the staffing problems necessitated by increasing patient demands, hospital trustees were to play a fundamental role in the institutional development of American medicine.

The Dilemma of Specialization

At the beginning of the nineteenth century, special practice was seen as a style of quackery.[12] Practitioners alleging a peculiar competence in treating one disease or body part were defined as no more than underhanded competitors preying on the pain and ignorance of laymen. Special competence was a contradiction in terms. If all parts of the body were inextricably related, then physiology and pathology denied the advantage—and legitimacy—of specialization. And in fact, traditional medicine had known a variety of specialists of various sorts in areas defined as marginal to mainstream medicine: pox doctors or would-be specialists in venereal disease, eye doctors, experts on ills of the rectum, and bone setters. But such individuals could not aspire to eminence in regular medicine.

One manifestation of special practice had been well established in England and France by the mid-eighteenth century; that, of course, was the formal distinction between surgeon and physician. A consistent distinction in practice, however, was limited to certain urban practitioners—in England, largely to London and, in London, to those who treated the small minority able to pay the licensed physician's honorarium or surgeon's fee. The bulk of medical care was in fact provided by general practitioners, whether their formal status was that of apothecary, surgeon, or physician. (Some sought and won dual qualification, but this was not a necessity.) Outside the largest cities, medical men turned their hands to minor surgery, delivered babies, wrote prescriptions, and treated the poor at the expense of local authorities.[13] In America, there had never been distinctions between different types of physicians, even in the largest cities, yet social, educational, and locational differences had created a hierarchical profession, although such realities were not reflected in titles or formal credentials.

In America's pioneer hospitals the situation had always been closer to the English model and rather different from practice in the community. Hospital staffing had usually reflected a distinction between medical and surgical appointments. This was not to say that individuals who served as attending surgeons limited their practice to surgery outside the hospital. That would have been self-defeating. They did, however, pursue a well-accepted, if nonexclusive specialization based on their hospital work and related consulting in private practice. A handful of largely urban surgeons and "man-midwives" were seen as possessing special skills that justified referrals. Surgery, as we have seen, demanded manual dexterity and an appropriately dauntless temperament. Every practitioner, especially the rural and isolated, would have to perform minor surgery and deliver babies; it could hardly be avoided. A few, however, were comfortable with the handful of demanding procedures that defined the hospital surgeon's particular domain. Throughout the nineteenth century, hospital appointments reflected an unquestioned division between surgical and medical competence. Attending surgeons and physicians served as equally powerful chiefs of service in their respective wards; surgeons especially could offer their students and house officers a technique-oriented ward training.[14] Medical school faculties reflected the same casual assumption; even when there were only three or four professorships, surgery (often connected with anatomy) was one, and medicine was a second.

Midwifery and diseases of children tended to be a third. As early as 1810, for example, T.C. James was appointed "physician to the lying-in department" at the Pennsylvania Hospital.[15] Every physician had to manage childbirth and infancy if he were to be successful in family practice—and this very lack of specialization ironically created a demand for specialists to train the vast majority of generalists. Medical apprentices could rarely learn from their preceptor's private obstetric practice, so that insofar as it was not taught from books and mannikins, nineteenth-century obstetric instruction was entirely dependent on hospital and dispensary patients. Student desire for midwifery experience and the staffing needs of those hospitals and lying-in dispensaries that provided obstetric services implied the need for attendings with special expertise. And such men would naturally be called as consultants in difficult and protracted deliveries in private practice. Thus, a handful of experts gained reputations as consultants and teachers in obstetrics while still practicing general medicine.[16] Ophthalmology and orthopedic surgery were also fields in which a few American specialists were active by mid-century and in which pioneer hospitals and dispensaries had already been established.

But these were tentative beginnings: With the exception of a handful of prominent, almost always urban, consultants, antebellum American medical practice remained largely undifferentiated. However, the situation began to change in the middle third of the century. French and German clinicians had begun to cultivate the surgical specialties and probe deeply into delimited areas in general medicine; in Paris, Vienna, and Berlin, men earned reputations as experts on particular organs, diseases, or procedures.[17] A growing interest in local pathology and the desire for academic achievement (and a not unrelated success in private practice) provided motivation for ambitious young ophthalmologists, dermatologists, and venerealogists, otologists, orthopedic surgeons, even experts in mental illness. Pragmatic considerations allied themselves with an increasingly self-conscious commitment to systematic clinical investigation.

It was in the German-speaking countries that specialization first attained this new maturity. Or at least so it seemed to the many young Americans who flocked to study there in the last quarter of the nineteenth century.[18] "A German specialist is a true specialist," one alert American reported to his peers, "he treats no cases whatever not in his own peculiar branch." German publications were based on careful study of long series of cases, not elaborations of a priori theory or unsystematic reflections on a single patient. Science and the scientific spirit were, he explained, becoming synonymous with specialization.[19] It was equally obvious that this scientific spirit had been nurtured in hospital wards and could not well thrive outside them.

Yet, in the English-speaking world, specialists did not always have an easy time during the 1870s and 1880s. In both Britain and the United States, hospital and medical school establishments resented and resisted these new claimants to authority. Attending physicians and general surgeons jealously guarded their power over hospital wards; professors only grudgingly allowed specialty courses into the curriculum (first often in the form of summer electives). To grant the new specialties regular faculty status was to narrow the domain of regular chairholders; to grant them beds was to concede a key element in hospital power.

Gradually specialization did find a place in the Anglo-American hospital. England, and especially London, led the way. Bright young men, frustrated at their inability to make a place for themselves in the elite of general hospital attending physicians, found laymen willing to support the establishment of specialized dispensaries and hospitals—ophthalmology, orthopedics, obstetrics, pediatrics (with a strong orthopedic component) all appealed to philanthropists. By 1860, "there were in London alone nine special hospitals for lying-in women, seven for diseases of the eye, six for idiots and lunatics, five for deformities, four for diseases of women and children, four for diseases of the chest, two for diseases of the ear, and one each for cancer, fistula and fevers, and one Lock [venereal disease] hospi-tal—forty-three altogether. . . ."[20] Such institutions had flourished despite the antagonism of established physicians and surgeons who attacked them as little more than advertisements for the clinical services of ambitious young men, unwilling to wait with appropri-ate patience and humility for their turn in the succession to attend-ing positions.[21]

In the United States, there was less open conflict; there were also fewer specialty hospitals and these were, of course, limited to the largest cities.[22] Specialization first made a place for itself in general hospital outpatient services and independent dispensaries, which began to organize themselves into "classes" or specialized clinics. By the 1870s, most hospitals were beginning to recognize this new style of practice in the organization of their outpatient departments.[23] For example, even the conservative Massachusetts General Hospital established clinics in dermatology in 1869, nervous diseases and throat in 1872, and ophthalmology in 1873. Appointments to such outpatient services were a way of rewarding well-connected and useful young men without allowing them a full role in hospital governance. Hospitals could also appoint specialists as consultants, without offering them control of beds or a place on the institution's board of attending (and decision-making) physicians. Thus, while gaining a foothold in practice, a young man could fashion a de facto specialty residence during a few hours of his working day. He could also use his clinic stint to earn extra income tutoring medical stu-dents with no access to small-group training in their formal under-graduate curricula.

As we have seen, however, attending physicians and surgeons

tended to draw a line at providing specialists with inpatient beds. A ward was the attending physicians' fiefdom, and they were loath to fragment the professional capital provided by its clinical resources. Control of wards meant control of informal, but often lucrative, teaching opportunities, of clinical decision making, of the raw material for articles and books. It is no accident that nineteenth-century hospital bylaws often specified that house officers could not publish without the permission of their superiors. General surgeons were particularly resentful of the surgical specialties that impugned their competence while threatening to diminish their caseload. Attendings often resisted calling in specialist consultants, even when diagnostic problems demanded expert skills in the use of otoscope, laryngoscope, or ophthalmoscope.[24]

But concessions were gradually made. Specialists found their way on to hospital boards, and special outpatient clinics proliferated. At other than the most prestigious hospitals, well-trained specialists could simply refuse to serve in outpatient and consulting roles without the quid pro quo of access to inpatient beds.[25] Even more important was a gradual acceptance of the technical superiority of special practice. By the 1880s, it was generally understood by both laymen and physicians that the highest quality of care and competent teaching could only be guaranteed by men "such as have attained more than ordinary proficiency in one or more of the special departments of medicine."[26] It did not seem right that primary responsibility for patient care should be left to the less qualified, even if their skills should gradually improve while on the job. "The ideal hospital," as a prominent Boston clinician expressed this consensus in 1900, "is a place where the poor can have the benefit of the highest skill and attainment in every branch of medicine—a beneficent trust in which specialists are associated and work harmoniously together."[27]

The number of specialty hospitals increased, but perhaps more important, general hospitals gradually assigned beds to specialty wards or guaranteed a number of beds for particularly "interesting" cases that appeared in outpatient departments. Students and attendings could now follow cases more carefully and systematically.[28] By the first decade of the twentieth century, hospitals had begun to operationalize their acceptance of the specialist's intellectual primacy; staff rules might, for example, require that ophthalmologists be summoned to surgical or medical wards when a patient's eyes demanded attention.[29]

Specialization was gradually integrated into the hospital's organizational structure without fundamentally changing it. Medical boards made grudging room as did medical school faculties, but the nature of decision making changed little in this period. By assimilating an array of specialists, however, hospitals could lay claim to the intellectual prestige and public confidence already associated with these new clinical fields. Patients asked for specialists, referred themselves to specialists, naturally associated them with institutional settings. Private patients found the limited and technically defined services of small specialty hospitals less stigmatizing and easier to accept than general hospital admission, while urban working people turned naturally to the reassuring authority embodied in a "professor" at the specialized outpatient clinic or dispensary.

At the same time, general hospitals were to exert a significant influence on specialization; they served as home, as training ground, as rationale. By the second decade of the twentieth century, the urban hospital had become an important site for the specialist's private practice. In a period before board certification or formal residency and fellowship programs, hospital and dispensary posts and appointments served as equivalents (supplemented, of course, by European sojourns). "One cannot learn practice from books," an American wrote home from London's Royal Ophthalmic Hospital in 1880. "My one year's experience here amounts to at least 20 years of private work. It will be expensive but I think it will be money well planted."[30] The agricultural metaphor was aptly chosen. One had to invest money and time in order to reap the harvest of professional success. Clarence Blake's European education took place somewhat earlier and lasted longer than that of most of his compatriots, but was otherwise typical of the path followed by America's late nineteenth-century clinical elite.

It was no accident that the German-speaking world figured so prominently in the plans of these young men. As we have seen, these countries offered the most advanced and self-consciously "scientific" training in clinical medicine. It was, of course, hospital-based and it was to this model that ambitious young Americans looked in the last third of the nineteenth century. German styles of training and practice were not transferred intact across the Atlantic, but the ideological prestige of science and systematic clinical investigation were. Specialization exemplified and exacerbated a more general tendency of medicine toward the reductionist and technological; its existence helped justify and act out the powerful image of the hospital as scientific institution.

In addition, a new group of specialties—clinical pathology, anesthesiology, and radiology—grew directly out of hospital needs and largely in hospital contexts. Specialization and the hospital seemed to fit naturally and easily together. When board certification of specialties and specialty-training programs were gradually established in the twentieth century, it was only natural that the several certifying boards should have been organized by nuclei of men hospital trained and, almost always, hospital connected. Board certification retrospectively mandated and formalized already well-established patterns of training, staffing, and practice.[31]

Hospitalizing Medicine: The Ladder of Preferment

The road to hospital preferment was clearly marked. As an ambitious and well-connected young man entered the late nineteenth-century profession, he sought contacts with hospital wards and outpatient departments; it was almost a necessity in a period when formal clinical training remained inadequate. Summer externships, for example, provided one foothold for undergraduate medical students, assisting in outpatient services another. After graduation, the more fortunate might compete for internships, then regular outpatient appointments, perhaps supplemented by substitution for senior attendings who, along with their patients, fled the cities' summer heat. Such services plus a good many years of patience, deference, and the support of a well-placed patron might in time bring membership on a hospital's senior attending staff, a "circle of men," as a prominent Bostonian recalled, "who then seemed little less than gods."[32]

Patrons were indispensable if one were to achieve these heights. Such sponsors could be lay trustees or medical men, but in the long run one could hardly hope to succeed professionally without medical patronage. It was natural enough for a whimsical New Yorker to refer to a group of ambitious clinicians as "orphans" because they had "no uncles in the New York Hospital. . . ."[33] Young practitioners often worked as library and clinical researchers for older men,

served as stand-ins (and potential inheritors) in their private practices, assisted and gave anesthesia in patients' homes. The benefits
were reciprocal; the aspiring young man could offer valuable services to his older and more established patron, providing informal
support services within the hospital setting and the functional
equivalent of it in the homes of wealthy patients. Each youthful
participant in the system hoped that years of such self-effacing
service would be rewarded by succession to an attending or teaching
position and lucrative referrals in private practice.[34]

The first step, of course, was securing a house officership. "Like
kissing," a Philadelphia editorialist chided in 1873, "the appointments to medical residentship in the hospitals with us go by favor. . . ."[35] The courting ritual was both obligatory and distasteful.
No contemporary expressed his negative feelings more acidly than
the young William James. "The present time is a very exciting one
for ambitious young men at the Medical School," he wrote to his
sister in December of 1866,

. . . who are anxious to get into the hospital [MGH]. Their toadying the
physicians, asking them intelligent questions after lectures, offering to run
errands for them, etc., this week reaches its climax; they call at their
residences and humbly solicit them to favor their appointment, & do the
same at the residences of the ten trustees. So I have sixteen visits to make.
I have little fears, with my talent for flattery and fawning, of a failure.[36]

Such demeaning solicitations continued throughout the century.
Would-be house officers at Philadelphia's Episcopal Hospital in the
1880s were "expected to call on each one of the twenty-five members of the Board of Managers." At the same city's municipal hospital, political connections were almost a necessity.[37] As late as 1910,
the superintendent of the Pennsylvania Hospital warned applicants
without suitable Philadelphia connections that it would be fruitless
to apply.[38] A mixture of academic accomplishment, social advantage, and the tenacity needed to piece together an ad hoc assortment
of part-time and short-term clinical appointments were elements
that brought professional success.

This made for a less uniform career pattern than we have come
to accept today. Physicians might graduate, practice for some years,
then apply for hospital officerships; others might switch from field
to field and institution to institution. Lengths of appointments were
inconsistent and clinical responsibilities diverse—no matter what

formal titles might imply. In 1901, for example, George Wilkins applied for a post as assistant resident at Boston's Long Island Hospital. A Harvard Medical School graduate of 1899, Wilkins had spent thirteen months during his four undergraduate years working in hospital outpatient clinics. He then served as house officer in the Carney Hospital's surgical service before beginning a six-month term as house physician at the Boston Lying-In Hospital.[39] This was a typical résumé for an ambitious would-be resident at the turn of the century; it records a clinical training rather different from the well-structured and explicitly mandated track that has since come into being.

Nevertheless, there are striking parallels between the elements of an *elite* career in the late nineteenth century and a *normal* late twentieth-century medical career. One continuity lies in the centrality of the hospital. Would-be members of the elite were bound to it as students, as house officers, as junior staff members (the functional equivalent of modern senior residents or fellows) while they accumulated years of service in wards and specialized outpatient departments. And for the intellectually ambitious, institutional patients provided the "clinical material" that could alone provide the basis for publication and the accumulation of an academic reputation. So long as they sought such reputation, aspiring physicians would be critically dependent on access to hospital beds. Most late nineteenth-century practitioners, however, had little or no contact with hospital medicine—excepting perhaps the few score hours spent in an impersonal amphitheater during their student days.

Obviously, wealth and family position were not the only requirements for success, even in the class-conscious years before the Civil War. Intelligent and energetic men like Samuel Gross in Philadelphia (born on a farm near Easton, Pennsylvania) or Southerners, such as T. G. Thomas, Thomas Addis Emmett, and J. Marion Sims in New York fought their way into the specialist elite, although not without opposition.[40] But these were white males from respectable, if provincial, families.

Most Americans had no real access to the hospital system. No women held formal medical credentials before the midnineteenth century. And in the second half of the century the small but earnest vanguard of females with medical school degrees were generally excluded from house officer and attending positions. Females who sought clinical training were limited to a minority of relatively low-status medical schools and a handful of hospitals for women and children.[41] Blacks were of course excluded.

For both black and female students, the need for clinical training and their teachers' and clinicians' desire for hospital privileges were central and well-understood motives in the founding of hospitals for their particular "communities."[42] Thus, for example, the founding of the New England Hospital for Women and Children (1862), the New York Infirmary for Women and Children (1860), New York's Lincoln (1882), and Harlem (1887) hospitals, Philadelphia's Douglass (1895) and Mercy (1907) hospitals, and Chicago's Provident Hospital (1891). In each case, the need for student and practitioner access to hospital practice was as important as the desire to provide clinical services.

The older urban hospitals remained strongholds of well-entrenched elites, both at the trustee and medical staff levels. Immigrant physicians had to find alternative paths to success in hospitals and dispensaries supported by their particular religious and ethnic groups.[43] German-speaking physicians whether Jewish or Christian might find attending positions in German and Jewish hospitals. Homeopathic physicians, conscious of a need for formal training and the credentials that certified such training, demanded places in established hospitals; failing that, they set up their own.[44] In the midwest and far west, with a shorter history and more open institutional life, hospital founding had been associated from the first with immigrant groups—particularly the Catholic church and its nursing orders.

Not surprisingly, hospital staff members were resented by the majority of practitioners who had never had an opportunity to climb the ladder of professional achievement. They had always resented the places held (most would have said monopolized) by a "ring" of well-placed hospital physicians. "These favored few," one less favored medical man argued in 1894, "of all the great medical body have a monopoly, so to speak, of the material provided by the wealth of the charitable rich and the misfortunes of the suffering poor, for becoming and remaining leaders in medical thought and action."[45] The average practitioner resented both the status and intellectual condescension of the "hospital men."

And such privileged competitors threatened their livelihood as well as their self-esteem. A hospital title was construed by a city's less-privileged practitioners as no more than an effective form of free advertising. Like the specialist's claims, such badges of institutional status seemed to demean the ordinary practitioner's skills. Laymen were impressed by such credentials and might in consequence forsake their regular family doctor in moments of need.[46] Much of such rank-and-file hostility was expressed in attacks on what contemporaries termed hospital and dispensary "abuse," the gratuitous institutional treatment of patients able to pay for care. The proliferation of outpatient clinics and inpatient charity beds seemed to many urban practitioners to reflect in good measure the selfish desire of medical school and hospital physicians (often one and the same) for a generous supply of "clinical material." The lack of a consistent factual basis for these complaints should not obscure the perceptions and motivations of the numerous physicians who reiterated such charges in the half century between 1870 and the First World War.[47]

These were arguments of the dispossessed. The hospital was a resource of the privileged—a place in which the upper stratum of medical men could accumulate status, connections, and perhaps a solid publication record, professional capital that provided a competitive advantage in the practitioner's crowded marketplace. To shut most practitioners out of wards and operating theaters was to denigrate them, to erode their skills, to make them less able to make a living in the practice of medicine, or so two generations of bitter urban practitioners contended.

The hospital was, to look at it another way, all too precisely integrated into medical careers and professional status relationships. It was an integration that began with medical school at the beginning of a young man's career and continued on through private practice. This was a reality unquestioned by contemporaries—those who advanced within the hospital system as well as those shut off from its advantages.

Medicalizing the Hospital: Evolution of the Medical Staff

There was a radical inconsistency, as we have suggested in a previous chapter, between the nominally comprehensive authority of nineteenth-century attending physicians and their actual presence on the wards. Some staffs were more responsible than others, and hours of attendance generally increased as the century progressed; yet in no hospital did attendings attend with notable regularity. Only at the very end of the century and in a few self-consciously academic hospitals did senior men spend more than a few hours a day in the wards; in some they appeared only a few times a week. Summers, of course, prompted a general exodus of all those able to leave. Valued private patients were away, and senior attendings fished, hunted, and traveled. Theirs was a comfortable niche and much resented by the junior men who performed the bedside tasks that had still to be done. One such staffer expressed his feelings in wry, and prudently anonymous, verse, whimsically attributed to a senior attending.

> Let others auscult or percuss,
> Examine all sorts of secretions
> Of ill-smelling patients who fuss,
> Prescribe building-up and depletions.
>
> Let others work hard and perspire,
> Pant, struggle, e'en fall in the race,
> While we pack our traps and retire,
> Assured in advance of a place.
>
> While we roam the hills or the waters,
> Intent upon pleasure or gain,
> Let them stay the slaughter of paupers
> Who in the hot city remain.
>
> To them be the privilege given
> Of hospital work without stint;
> Let them lay up riches in heaven,
> *But give us the credit in print!*[48]

Age and position brought deference and sometimes covert resentment, but young men had little choice if they hoped to rise in the hospital. The time might come when they too would enjoy the ward's perquisites and avoid its less pleasant duties.

The system was ill suited to the consistent delivery of care or clinical training and the situation was only exacerbated by the almost universal system of rotation. Although it had been criticized since at least the 1820s by medical men concerned at the lack of continuity it implied for patient care, the practice of alternating clinical responsibilities among attendings remained alive into the twentieth century. It spread the equity of hospital place-holding, perhaps moderated resentment among potential attendings, and limited as well the time demanded from busy practitioners. The system's advantages were substantial enough to preserve it; rotation was entirely functional in a period when senior staff received no salary and ward rounds had to be tucked into the odd moments of a home-oriented and time-consuming private practice.

As the nineteenth century progressed, however, hospital staffing needs changed. Admissions soared, while an ever-larger proportion of those admissions involved surgery. Such procedures implied more house staff and nursing hours per case, and some of these hours would have to come at night. This increase in surgery allied in many institutions with parallel increases in proportions of acute medical cases (and the availability of gas and then electric light) meant a growing demand for twenty-four-hour staffing; in the period before 1880, hospital work had been in large measure limited to daylight. At the turn of the century, moreover, private patients began to be found in significant numbers in all except municipal hospitals. Their presumed sensibilities and the hospital's desire to cater to their needs also implied an increased number of house officers.

Medicine was becoming more active and intrusive, and attitudes toward appropriate levels of care had changed as well; no longer were ratios of one house officer to as many as seventy-five patients seen as adequate, even in large municipal hospitals. Small community hospitals began to seek resident house staff, for even a handful of surgical or typhoid patients might demand twenty-four-hour attendance, an attendance that busy admitting physicians could not provide. All these factors implied a changed doctor-patient ratio. A reform agenda gradually coalesced around this very need for more adequate staffing, and, not surprisingly, medical men provided both rationale and leadership.

Critics grew impatient not only with inadequate house staff ratios, but with the organization of the house officers' tenure. It had always seemed unfair that youthful medical graduates, often with no bedside training, should be assigned primary care responsibilities. "The men immediately after graduating are placed on duty in the wards," the resident physician at Philadelphia's municipal hospital argued in 1886, "and are expected to treat the patients satisfactorily. Now nine out of ten have never prescribed for a patient, and they are not only greatly embarrassed, but truly do not know what to do."[49] Learning on the job in a randomly-assigned ward or wards did not answer the educational purposes implied by the house officer's role, while it guaranteed erratic care. One answer was the gradual development of graded house officerships, another the evolution of an identifiable residency out of its less differentiated short-term progenitor. Since the mid-nineteenth century, moreover, reformers had urged that objective examinations replace the lobbying that had traditionally determined the selection of house officers.

By 1900, many large hospitals had become critically dependent on their senior medical and surgical residents, often chosen from among each "class" of interns completing their term.[50] The need for full-time service in admissions was one factor explaining such dependence; the need for supervising novice house officers another. Specialty residencies had begun as well. The demands of an increasingly sophisticated surgery were particularly important; it is significant how quickly other institutions accepted the chief residents carefully groomed at Johns Hopkins's pioneer program in the 1890s and early years of the twentieth century, and how easily most were able to institute at least aspects of the Hopkins's system in their new institutions.[51] Surgical specialties, such as ophthalmology, gynecology, otology, and orthopedics, were established in their own hospitals or wards in large general hospitals.

The hospital-based specialties soon found a niche in the residency system. Anesthesiology and clinical pathology were functions that had at first been seen as part of house officers' everyday duties (to spare hospital budgets and as preparation for careers in which they would be running their own urine and blood tests, administering anesthesia to private patients and those of their friends). By the time of the First World War, however, these skills were assumed to be too demanding for the odd moments of busy and inexperienced house officers, even if supervised by more experienced part-timers.[52] The need for reliable care coupled with a growing demand for instruction of medical students and junior house officers implied the gradual establishing of residencies and staff appointments in these "service" fields. As private patients came to accept hospital care, the need to provide state-of-the-art clinical facilities for these desired clients strengthened the rationale for residency programs, although anesthesiology and clinical pathology remained much lower than general medicine and surgery in the hospital's status hierarchy. Radiology underwent a parallel evolution. After the introduction of x-rays in 1896, a mixture of pho-

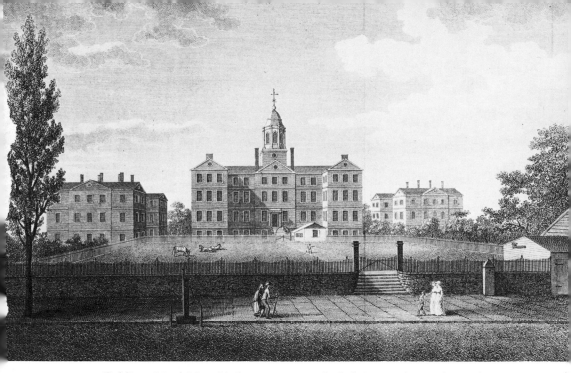

ABOVE: Public-spirited New Yorkers were proud of their new hospital—as they were of their new nation. Its architecture expressed and embodied a sense of order and social responsibility. ("View of the New-York Hospital," *An Account of the New-York Hospital* [New York: Mahlon Day, 1820], frontispiece. Author's collection.) BELOW: But the reality of prebellum hospital life could be rather different—especially in municipal hospitals. Whether or not such scenes represented an accurate picture of life in New York's Bellevue, they exploited and reinforced popular fears. (*Harper's Weekly.* Library Company of Philadelphia.)

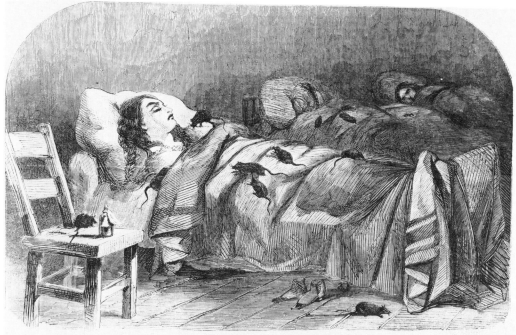

THE SICK WOMEN IN BELLEVUE HOSPITAL, NEW YORK, OVERRUN BY RATS

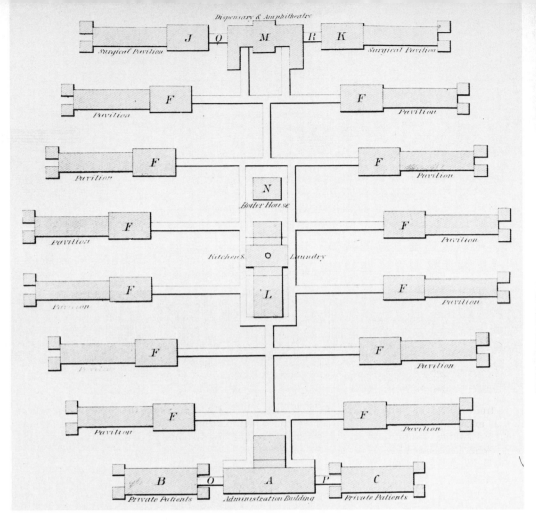

Mid-nineteenth-century efforts to reform the hospital and banish infection invoked a new architectural and etiological consensus. Like many other authorities, John Shaw Billings envisaged a pavilion-style hospital in which ventilation would be maximized and patient density minimized. ("Sketch Plan of Arrangement for Johns Hopkins Hospital, with One Story Pavilions, Temporary or Permanent. By Dr. J. S. Billings U.S.A.," Trustees of the Johns Hopkins Hospital, *Hospital Plans. Five Essays Relating to the Construction, Organization and Management of Hospitals, . . .* [New York: William Wood, 1875], Author's collection.)

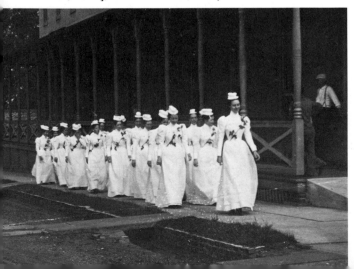

Against a revealingly shabby background, a hospital-trained and disciplined nursing staff represented a new force in the hospital, bringing order and efficiency to the ward's sphere of more traditional values. ("Nurses on Parade," Philadelphia General Hospital, circa 1895. Historical Collections, College of Physicians of Philadelphia.)

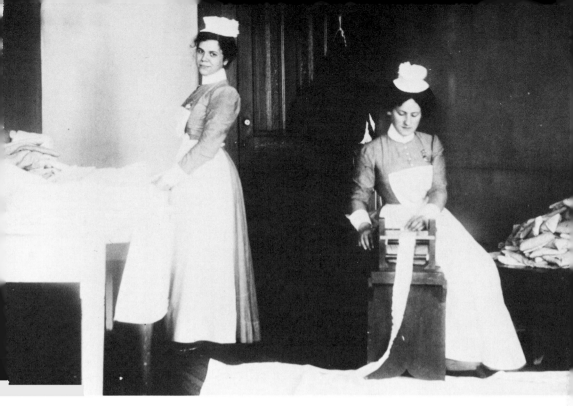

Nurse training in its formative years was characterized by boredom and long hours of physical labor as exemplified in such routine tasks as those pictured here. ("Student Nurses Rolling Bandages and Folding Laundry [1890]." Center for the History of Nursing, University of Pennsylvania, School of Nursing.)

In the post–Civil War years, youthful house staff members were issued military-style uniforms indicating rank and, by implication, expressing authority and responsibility. ("Resident Staff, Blockley [Philadelphia General Hospital]," circa 1885. Historical Collections, College of Physicians of Philadelphia.)

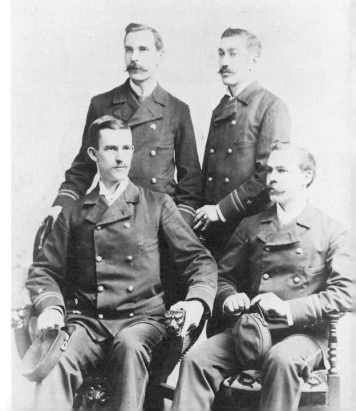

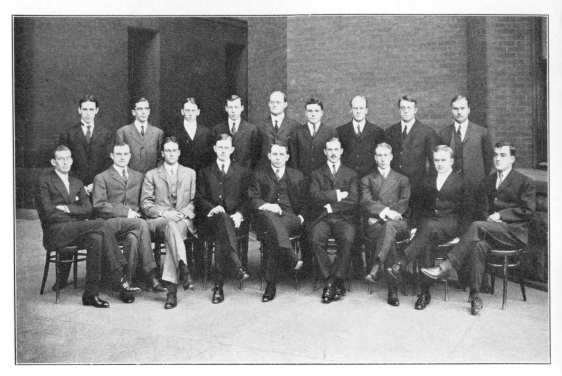

In the half-century after the Civil War, house staff numbers increased, and they were no longer encumbered by quasimilitary garb. One thing remained the same, however. Elite hospital house staffs continued to be made up of white males exclusively. ("House Staff, 1907," Presbyterian Hospital, New York, *Annual Report for the Year Ending Sept. 30, 1907.* Author's collection.)

Excluded from elite medical schools and hospital staff positions, women formed their own—parallel—institutions. Without clinical experience, female physicians could not well compete with their male contemporaries. "Internes at the Women's Hospital of Pennsylvania, 1903–4," P-498. (Archives and Special Collections on Women in Medicine, The Medical College of Pennsylvania, Philadelphia, Pa.)

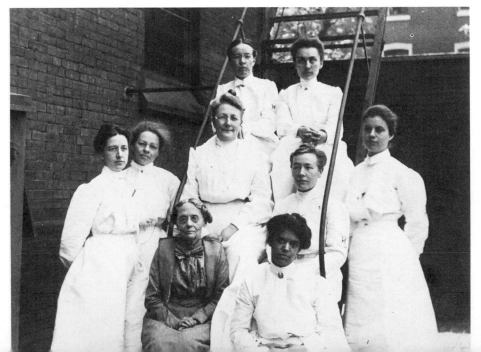

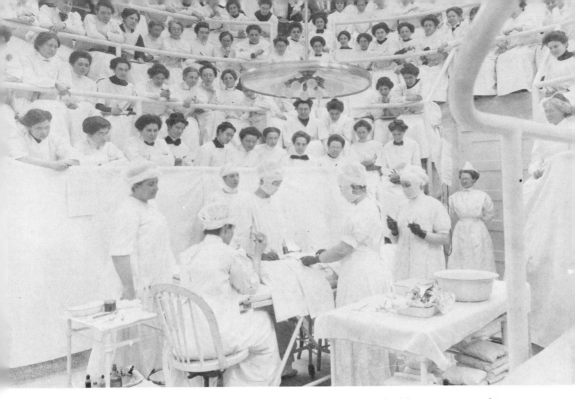

ABOVE: Throughout the hospital's history, the surgical amphitheater had been a center of instruction and a source of emotionally resonant collective experience. After the advent of asepsis, surgery became far more important to the hospital's burden of care. ("Operating Room Scene [1911] of the Woman's Medical College," P-1603. Archives and Special Collections on Women in Medicine, The Medical College of Pennsylvania, Philadelphia, Pa.) BELOW: Changes in attitude and expectation helped make well-to-do Americans contemplate hospital care. Hospitals vied with each other in furnishing and advertising enticing private rooms. ("Private Rooms, Germantown Hospital," *National Hospital Review* 10 [June 1907], p. 37. Historical Collections, College of Physicians of Philadelphia.)

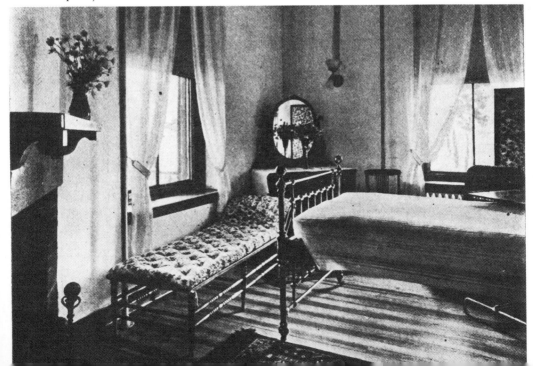

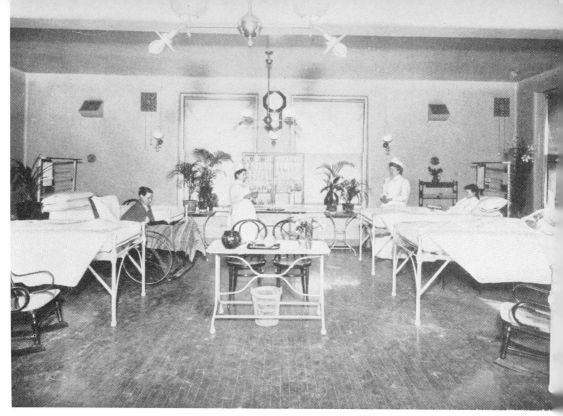

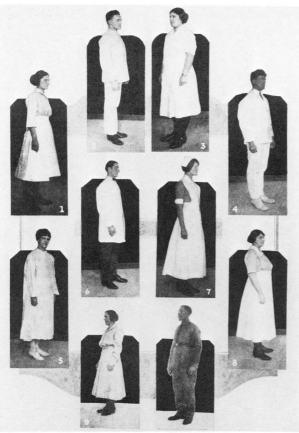

ABOVE: Hospitals soon became aware that patients able to pay for private rooms were in short supply. They had long been aware that respectable working people and members of the less affluent middle class objected to the demeaning democracy of the large charity ward. One solution, as illustrated, was the creation of smaller pay wards in which numbers were limited to four or eight, and the fees maintained at a modest level. ("Private Surgical Ward," Presbyterian Hospital, New York, *Annual Report for the Year Ending Sept. 30, 1897.* Author's collection.) LEFT: As hospitals became more self-conscious in regard to "efficiency" and bureaucratic order, administrators sought to control every aspect of hospital life. Uniforms provided an obvious way to express status and function. ("Uniforms for Hospital Workers," *Modern Hospital* 20 (April 1923), p. 377. Historical Collections, College of Physicians of Philadelphia.)

RIGHT: By the turn of the century, a growing dependence on technology had stimulated a flourishing hospital supply industry. ("The Hospital Supply Co." Advertisement, *National Hospital Record*. Historical Collections, College of Physicians of Philadelphia.) BELOW: Despite much talk of elaborate and novel technology, many hospitals—especially community hospitals and dispensaries—provided only modest facilities. ("Department of Surgery," *Union Mission Hospital Reports, May, 1894,* facing p. 16. Author's collection.)

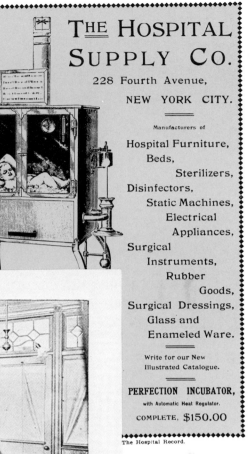

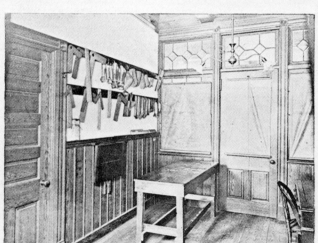

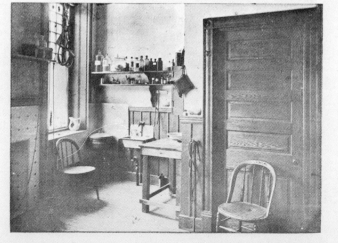

DEPARTMENT OF SURGERY.

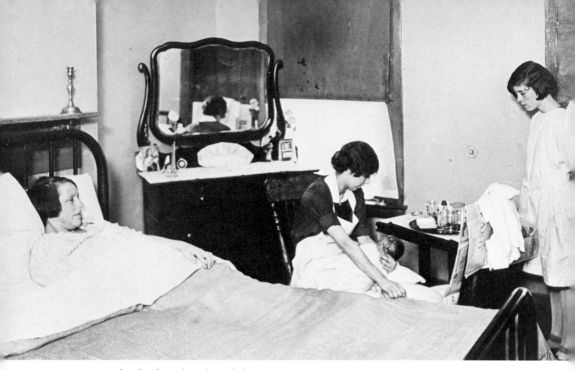

ABOVE: In the first decades of the twentieth century, public health nursing seemed an important and promising alternative to the expensive and increasingly acute care-oriented hospital. (Visiting Nurse in Tenement Home [1905]. Visiting Nurse Association of Boston.) BELOW: Hospitals and public health authorities both sought to overcome lingering public distrust of inpatient care. Pictures such as these aimed to quiet parental anxieties. ("Hospitals Take Care of Cardiac Children and Adults During an Acute Illness" [1915]. H. C. Carpenter Slide Collection, Historical Collections, College of Physicians of Philadelphia.)

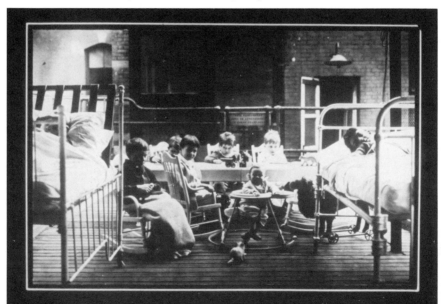

tographers, clinicians, and technicians at first took charge of this new technology, but it soon became clear that radiology demanded specialized skills—and capital costs too great for most practitioners. The hospital became the setting for training and a good proportion of radiological practice.[53]

Residency programs grew increasingly formal as well as more diverse.[54] The internship, for example, became a standard prerequisite. As early as 1890, the Johns Hopkins Hospital demanded that candidates for resident physician, surgeon, and gynecologist have had at least eighteen months "in a well-ordered hospital or an equivalent experience."[55] By 1910, such requirements had become universal at large hospitals.

Another reform demand applied to senior attendings; it called for the end of rotation and the institution of "continuous service." This meant that attending physicians would be responsible throughout the year and not just for three- or four-month terms. But this reform was not accepted without a struggle, for it drastically reduced the number of attending appointments in medicine and general surgery and implied longer hours on the ward, although it did facilitate teaching (and integration of hospital and medical school). The German model of salaried, full-time clinical staff was never a real option in late nineteenth-century America. Hospitals were largely dependent on unpaid house officers and attendings, and government did not see the need to underwrite such costs. No matter how able the clinician or how gifted he or she was as a bedside instructor, private practice had necessarily to come first, hospital work second.[56]

A final aspect of staffing reform was a more self-conscious integration of appointment and examination schedules with medical school terms. Throughout most of the nineteenth century, hospitals had hired house officers at their convenience on some traditional date unrelated to the medical school year. Now terms of house officers began to assume a uniform starting time in the late spring or summer; young men could move directly from graduation into the next stage of their professional training. These developments in hospital staffing were all cumulative and gradual. Naturally enough, hospitals differed in their willingness to change traditional practices and to assume the increased costs demanded by more generous staffing ratios. Nevertheless, by 1910 the basic mechanisms of twentieth-century hospital training were in place; large urban institutions had evolved de facto internship and residency programs—options that appealed strongly to that increasing proportion of medical graduates able and willing to invest their time.

The great majority of house officers were not paid; only the more senior residents with substantial administrative responsibilities received a salary. Hospital staffing was based on a kind of barter; the would-be practitioner paid with his time and intelligence for the clinical opportunities and credentials received in exchange. Yet, despite the long hours, the deferral of marriage, and the lack of substantial compensation, an ever-increasing number of young men sought those opportunities. A gradual upgrading in levels of aspiration and education made them anxious to spend a year or even more on a hospital house staff.[57] The growing appeal of special practice only intensified these demand-side pressures.

Specialization, the internship, and residency had all come into being before they were recognized as indispensable aspects of medical training and practice. By the 1920s, career choices available only to the elite in midnineteenth-century American medicine had developed into options—and in the case of internship, requirements—for every regularly trained physician. The hospital house staff had through creative inadvertence and in response to day-to-day clinical demands become a kind of pilot program defining and domesticating patterns that we have come to accept as fundamental to twentieth-century medicine.

An Invisible College: The Shaping of an Academic Elite

A small minority of early twentieth-century American physicians had wanted more, however. They sought careers in which dependence on private practice could be subordinated to a concern with clinical teaching, publication, and systematic investigation. The example of the German professoriate was powerful; one did not have to study in Germany to assimilate the ideal of scholarship and the vision of medicine becoming a scientific enterprise. Such would-be academicians saw no ultimate conflict between their goals and those of the hospital and the individuals treated in its beds, for they never doubted that a teaching hospital guided by a research-oriented senior staff would necessarily provide high-quality care while helping accumulate a store of knowledge that might bring healing to countless others in future generations.

For these members of what they themselves saw as a "movement," the hospital was an indispensable objective. "The hospital," as one put it, "is after all a great laboratory that only awaits the hand of the scientific sculptor to mold it in whatever shape he will." These were the words of Simon Flexner, director of the Rockefeller Institute, written to Lewellys Barker, soon-to-be chairman of medicine at Johns Hopkins. What these men needed was "a way of obtaining material which we may control."[58] That need for control implied that institutional tactics could not be divorced from intellectual strategies.

Lewellys Barker was in many ways typical of this highly motivated group of coconspirators. Trained at Toronto, Johns Hopkins, and in Europe, Barker was interested in using the tools of the laboratory to reduce the phenomena of disease to mechanisms that could be studied objectively. "Perhaps the most significant movement at present observable in medicine," he wrote in 1900, "is the beginning of the application of the newer ideas of physics and chemistry to the solution of biological questions."[59] Within the hospital, he sought to integrate the laboratory and bedside, facilitating a new style of clinical investigation—and the training of a new cohort of like-thinking investigators. But such goals were not easily attained, even at the Johns Hopkins Hospital. The great majority of medical men found it difficult to forge the kind of career this budding professoriate envisioned. And even when aspects of their program could be undertaken, they had to be justified in terms of immediate clinical relevance.

"Endowments must be found," one would-be research scholar explained his dilemma, "for such workers as choose to follow out investigations . . . which do not bear results having commonsensical value." How enviable it would be to work ". . . without the necessity of producing salable (sic) merchandise . . . free to labor for the single purpose of revealing some of the mysteries of nature."[60] But few members of this generation could enjoy such luxuries. Dedication to scholarship did not necessarily bring hospital appointments. "It really is bitter to me that we have no place for such a man," William Councilman, another Hopkins associate, wrote Barker from Boston where he had sought unsuccessfully to place Joseph Pratt, a promising clinical scholar, in the city's rigid hospital hierarchy.

"The only hope for a young man here," Councilman explained, "is to secure an outpatient position in a hospital, follow closely the traditions of the past and at the age of fifty when enthusiasm is a tradition with him, he obtains a position of some usefulness."[61]

The hospital was, in other words, a necessary aspect of the would-be medical academician's career; but its carefully evolved relationship with a practice-oriented profession had produced an institutional system ill adapted to such ambitions. The career ladder so effective in staffing the hospital and training practitioners was far less suitable to the scholar. House officers and residents worked too hard to do much in the way of investigation; it was not their job. Senior attendings were busy in their private practice, while few of even those most committed to scientific medicine were trained in modern research techniques. Nothing, for example, was more fashionable in the first decade of the twentieth century than ventures into biochemistry that promised to reduce clinical findings to their, presumably, underlying biochemical mechanisms.[62] Yet few hospitals could support laboratories; even those facilities dedicated to routine clinical pathology inched along on parsimonious budgets in the early years of this century, before it was discovered that they could be made to pay for themselves. Promising titles such as neuropathologist or bacteriologist were often belied by a far less impressive reality: poor or nonexistent laboratory facilities and a harried young man with a few hours to spare each week. Would-be investigators without a firm clinical niche were forced to seek hospital-based patrons who could provide access to wards and the "material" they contained.[63] An intense localism, as reflected in Councilman's bitter comments on Boston, also characterized hospital personnel decisions. Such localism could rarely be consistent with the cosmopolitan values and research orientation of that small minority of publishing scholars attuned to the international world of learning.[64] Yet, just as a Clarence Blake saw the future in specialization in the 1860s, so a cadre of ambitious young men a half century later felt that the future of medicine lay in the creation of a class of research-oriented, full-time, and salaried, teacher-clinicians.

Henry Christian was one such figure, as self-conscious in his analysis of academic strategies in the first decade of the twentieth century as Blake had been in the 1860s. Christian was a Hopkins-trained clinician who was to become first chief of medicine at Harvard's Brigham Hospital and dean of the Medical School. When recruiting resident physicians he was careful to emphasize that the successful candidate would not be burdened by clinical routine. "The Resident Staff," he explained, "will be expected to devote practically their entire time to investigation, utilizing the resources of the Hospital for this purpose." At the end of a year, Christian encouraged, the young man might want to spend a year in studying chemistry, "or some one of the fundamental sciences for, say a year, then come back into the clinical work, . . . and from that work into some visiting capacity in connection with the Hospital."[65] Christian had already sought to associate prominent physiologist Walter B. Cannon and biochemist Otto Folin with the new hospital.

It might be argued that such career tracks were highly uncommon in the first quarter of the twentieth century and that even the Brigham was far more successful in training skillful clinicians than in bridging the yawning gap between laboratory and bedside. However there is a perhaps more important point. And that is the fundamental agreement as to the nature of an ideal program for advancing medicine and the value associated with that program. We are dealing not simply with a group of well-connected academic careerists, but with a community of believers—whose belief turned on the transforming and transcendent role of science in medicine.

"The man of the future," Harvard surgeon R. H. Fitz had written to Christian in 1906, "ought to be good in experimental physiology—chemistry—pathological anatomy and bacteriology—in the meantime we must make such shift as is feasible." Fitz went on to dismiss a candidate by describing him as ". . . honest and earnest but does not seem to have the celestial fire and may be obliged to devote himself to sordid practice."[66] These were hardly typical words; nor did they describe typical careers, but they did express a seductive promise for both medical men and their patients.

At least some ambitious and well-connected young men were beginning to create a new kind of academic career track in compliance with such goals. Just as the midnineteenth-century elite followed an educational path very different from that of the great majority of their peers, so their counterparts a half century later pursued options unavailable to or disdained by all but a very few of their generation. Francis Peabody, for example, was one of the applicants for resident physician at the Brigham; his résumé or "Lebenslauf," as he termed it—the use of the German word was hardly accidental—indicated that he had already published ten articles. Peabody attended Harvard College and graduated in 1903, before receiving his Harvard medical degree in 1907. He interned at

Massachusetts General Hospital in 1907–1908 and then served at the Johns Hopkins Hospital as assistant resident (1908–1909) and fellow in pathology (1909–1910). Peabody studied chemistry at Berlin in 1910 and, when he applied to the Brigham in 1912, was serving as assistant resident physician at the new Hospital of the Rockefeller Institute.[67] Academic credentials and the mastery of a body of esoteric knowledge, not family connections alone, had defined Peabody as a young man of promise.

This new elite was hardly significant in terms of delivering care. The overwhelming majority of American physicians, in and outside of hospitals, practiced a rather different style of medicine and had been trained in vastly different and rather more casual fashion. Routine medical practice had changed little in the previous half century; only in surgery could systematic cognitive activity lay claim to having transformed everyday practice patterns.[68] But in some sense the comparative handful of scientific medical men felt and expressed a sense of legitimacy and entitlement that their far more numerous professional colleagues could not. All the majority did was treat sick people—that would go on no matter what, sometimes better and sometimes worse, but change and improvement could only come through the linked revelations of the laboratory and clinic.

This was an argument that was used with effect by scores of academically oriented publicists as they appealed for support among laymen and in the profession. If the trustees of the Johns Hopkins Hospital had lacked vision, as one such advocate contended: "Baltimore would have had a large hospital for the sick poor of the ordinary American type whose usefulness would have scarcely extended beyond the boundaries of the city." Yet as a result of their foresight the hospital had played another and far more important role. "They built a pathological laboratory so large and so well equipped for teaching and research that it must have seemed an unwarranted expenditure of hospital funds to many 'practical men,' lay and medical." Yet history had already demonstrated the prudence of that innovative decision; three of the four men who had discovered that mosquitoes transmitted yellow fever had been trained in that very laboratory. "If the trustees had built a vast hospital for the sick poor," the author reiterated, "instead of a teaching hospital of the highest type, there is small chance that the United States would be building the Panama Canal to-day."[69] The author of these words was Joseph Pratt, the same clinician William

Councilman had sought to place in Boston's rigid medical establishment a decade earlier. Not entirely surprisingly, Pratt urged that university hospitals create paid assistantships for young men who could divide their time between routine ward work and research. "Many bright young fellows would gladly devote all their time for a few years to this work if they saw any chance for an academic career."[70]

But such posts were hardly routine in the years before 1920. Even university hospitals did little to create special opportunities for the would-be researcher. Conflict between care and research was very real; the relationship between laboratory and bedside still problematic. Equally problematic was the continued gap between the academic and consulting elite and the great mass of ordinary practitioners who sought to make an often precarious living in general practice.

The ideology of science-oriented reform was to provide one basis for reconciliation of such diverse interests. Scientific medicine promised status and economic stability to the regular practitioner, healing to society, and increasing freedom for the elite to pursue their own goals. It provided legitimacy for regular medicine's war on the ill trained and the sectarian. It was a program that appealed to educated laymen and the well-meaning practitioner, who could look forward to a future in which he or she practiced a more effective medicine in a less competitive environment. The hospital became even more central to the mid-twentieth-century profession, smaller and more uniformly educated. The prestige of scientific medicine helped make the hospital a more consistently and self-consciously medical institution, while the medical profession became more intensely hospitalized. Perhaps most important, the hospital had become the classroom for a new generation of practitioner.

CHAPTER 8

The Ward as Classroom

Education had always played a prominent role in the American hospital, but it was not until the twentieth century that a stable relationship between care and learning evolved. The key elements in that now familiar symbiosis developed gradually and almost imperceptibly in the half-century between the 1870s and the First World War.

When Benjamin Franklin called upon fellow Pennsylvanians to support a hospital in 1751, he argued that it would not only heal the sick, but "the Multitude and Variety of Cases" would also "render the Physicians and Surgeons . . . more expert and skillful." The hospital's wards would serve as the classrooms in which they could pass those skills on to a new generation of practitioner.[1] Franklin was only expressing his generation's enlightened wisdom. The goals of providing care and educating physicians seemed entirely consistent.

The objects of charity who filled a hospital's beds could hardly refuse to cooperate in clinical teaching; it was the principal way in which they could repay society for the gratuitous care they received. The poor were, in fact, particularly apt teaching aids; "their theories and caprices are not so troublesome," a contemporary English clinician put it, "as those of people in higher life; . . . Nothing hinders the physician from following his own reason and experience in the cure, and he is responsible to his own conscience alone."[2] In eighteenth- and early nineteenth-century private practice, of course, patients might be from a social class equal or superior to that of the physician, even those prominent urban practitioners who held hospital appointments. The "tact"—if not humility—so necessary in dealing with such patients and their families was obviously not required in the managing of hospital patients. The ward was an excellent setting for clinical instruction.

The hospital's teaching function also fit neatly into the hierarchical structure of the medical profession. America's earliest hospitals, like their English predecessors, were founded on the practical assumption that they would provide a place in which the medical elite would practice and in which their students and professional successors would be taught. It was a mechanism, like an eminent practitioner's elevated preceptorial fees, that helped guarantee that "respectable" young men would maintain a status in medicine consistent with that of their families in the larger society. The initiation of such youths into the world of medical practice was, as we have seen, very different from the casual training accumulated by the vast majority of practitioners. In antebellum America, any physician with even minimal training could call himself "doctor" and enjoy the same legal rights as his social and educational betters; but such equality was no more than formal and only magnified the significance of informal mechanisms in creating and legitimating a medical elite. The hospital was perhaps the most important of these mechanisms.

The century and a half following Benjamin Franklin's shrewd fund-raising efforts on behalf of the Pennsylvania Hospital brought extraordinary change in medical thought and institutional arrangements. These developments steadily increased the centrality of the hospital's educational role. The introduction of physical diagnosis, of diagnostic tools such as the ophthalmoscope, otoscope, and laryngoscope, and the greater role of surgery cumulatively underlined the need to learn medicine in small groups at the patient's bedside, in the operating theater, and in the clinical laboratory. By the end of the nineteenth century, no serious student of medical education doubted the need for bedside teaching and thus access to hospital patients. Although only a small minority of medical schools were in fact able to provide an adequate clinical experience, few forward-looking faculty members questioned the desirability of such training—a judgment affirmed by medical students and recent graduates who clamored for increased teaching in hospital wards.

As the physician's voice grew more commanding in hospital management, it was inevitable that in at least some institutions self-consciously academic medical men should impose their wishes for greater student access and larger house and outpatient staffs on increasingly malleable boards. The teaching hospital as we have come to understand it, with its tight integration of hospital routine and medical school curriculum, did not become a regular feature of medical education until after the First World War. However, the hospital's training function had gradually increased through the previous half century, especially in the postgraduate years. The acceptance of the internship and residency were developments with educational as well as narrowly institutional implications. Specialty hospitals and wards, specialist outpatient services, summer and small group tutorials all played a role in medical and specialist education—and in the hospital. The tightly bound relationship between the hospital's internal order, patient care, student and house officer education, and the structure of medical careers was already well established before 1910 and publication of the landmark Flexner Report on medical education—with its famous and eloquent call for just such integration of ward and classroom.[3] The reluctance of most institutions before the First World War to allow undergraduate medical students to assume hands-on responsibility for individual patients on hospital wards, the so-called clinical clerkship, should not obscure this gradual expansion of clinical training in the hospital. Educational goals had become increasingly important in staffing decisions (and thus patient care), while staffing needs had already helped transform medical education.

The patient's role in medical education, however, changed little in the years before 1920. Need and social class were still fundamental in determining the likelihood of an individual's serving as "clinical material." And an ever-increasing amount of teaching almost certainly enhanced the likelihood that any particular ward patient would be caught up in the educative process. Paying patients had no reason to fear the student's prying eyes and brusque hands; their fees and presumed status guaranteed a measure of privacy. Even as it became more scientific in its rationale and more effective in its technical capacities, the hospital remained an institution in which community values and presuppositions could not help but act themselves out. The presumed sensitivities and perquisites of class were prominent among those assumptions.

From the medical students' or house officers' point of view, the hospital constituted a powerful collective experience, an initiation into the culture of medicine etched in their emotional response to the ward and surgical amphitheater and legitimated by an ever-more elaborate and demanding body of knowledge. The hospital helped fuse emotion and generation-specific ideas into a compelling blueprint for behavior. By the 1920s, education at the hospital bed-side had become a mandatory aspect of every physician's training.

Walking the Wards: The Origins of Hospital Teaching

Only a small minority of antebellum physicians ever held hospi-tal positions. A far greater number, however, "observed the prac-tice" in the wards or, more often, attended clinical lectures in a hospital amphitheater. Most urban medical school matriculants were offered at least some opportunity to observe, if not actually practice, hospital medicine.

The system worked best for the personal students of hospital attending physicians, who could follow their preceptor on his rounds. The fee-paying pupils of attending physicians at the New York Hospital, for example, served in the formal capacity of "walk-ers" and "dressers" in its medical and surgical wards. At other hospitals, the pupils of visiting physicians could attend clinical lec-tures and "witness the practice" on the wards without any payment to the hospital. Use of the terms "witness" and "observe" in con-temporary descriptions emphasizes the passive quality of the stu-dent's experience. With the exception of surgical dressers, students did not actually manage patients themselves. Although attending physicians were not paid a salary, the use of the wards in their care by small fee-paying tutorial groups was ordinarily considered a legitimate perquisite of office.[4]

Even those matriculants unable to afford the attending physi-cian's tutorial fees had some opportunity to learn in the hospital. Students at local medical colleges might be urged, or at times re-quired, to attend a hospital's clinical lectures; the charges were modest and they could and often did attend. Even at the Phila-delphia Almshouse Hospital, where the struggle between politically oriented lay managers and medical school teachers was particularly intense and where all teaching was banned for a dozen years at midcentury, special facilities for lecturing had been arranged as early as the 1820s and small clinical wards for "interesting" medical and surgical cases had been established in proximity to the clinical amphitheater, wards in which cases for "demonstration" had been chosen by the lecturers.[5] Even earlier in the same institution's history, members of the almshouse staff had requested permission to have a "select class" of students follow them on their rounds. As we have seen, lay trustees and administrators had always assumed that the hospital should in some measure serve as a "nursery" for physicians. The problem lay in implementing that assumption.

Ideally, moreover, some portion of hospital training should take place at the bedside and not in a large amphitheater exclusively. Students should observe and make their own clinical evaluations, not simply see an occasional patient in the form of semidecorative prop in a formal lecture. Since the early eighteenth century, influential clinical teachers at Pavia, Leiden, Edinburgh, and Vienna had demonstrated the possibility and urged the necessity for bedside teaching. Maximilian Stoll (1742–87), for example, had placed individual patients in Vienna's General Hospital under the care of his advanced students who would present them when the professor made his rounds. At the end of the eighteenth century, Edinburgh medical students were expected to keep careful clinical histories of patients at the Royal Infirmary. Hospitals had already come to serve as the foci of medical and surgical education in London.[6]

Hospital training was not simply an ideal endorsed by English and European authorities, but a practical necessity. How might the youthful aspirant to a successful practice acquire skills that would allow him to diagnose, to make confidence-inspiring prognoses, to prescribe—and to prosper? "How many young men are there in this country," a Charleston physician complained in 1835, "who have been embarrassed, and mortified at their want of practical information when they have entered into life?" Medical education was incomplete without hospital training.[7] "Chemistry requires a laboratory," the prominent New York physician Samuel Bard argued in 1819

botany a garden; and anatomy a theatre and subjects; and above all, the nature of diseases, and the practice of medicine, cannot be taught but in a public hospital. . . .

The student must see, and hear, and feel for himself. The hue of the complexion, the feel of the skin, the lustre or langour of the eye, the throbbing of the pulse and the palpitations of the heart, the quickness and ease of respiration, and the tone and tremor of the voice, . . . Where can these be learned but at the bedsides of the sick? and where shall a young man, who cannot be admitted into the privacies of families, or the chambers of women, acquire the necessary information, but in a public hospital, which is not only intended as an asylum to relieve the complicated misery of poverty and sickness, but as a school of medicine, to contribute to the public welfare.[8]

It was only to have been expected that ambitious physicians should have played a leading role in calling for the founding of America's first voluntary hospitals: Thomas Bond in Philadelphia, for example, Samuel Bard in New York, and James Jackson and J. C. Warren in Boston. Competition between cities and schools only sharpened the demand for adequate clinical facilities. The dominance of Philadelphia was, for example, one of the arguments used by Boston physicians in urging establishment of what was to become the Massachusetts General Hospital.[9] The hospital, medical teaching, the intellectual life of medicine—even urban rivalries—were inextricably bound together.

Although America spawned a goodly number of small town medical schools in the first half of the nineteenth century, these so-called "country schools" always operated at a significant disadvantage. The city and its hospital wards constituted an irresistible lure for any young man who could afford the somewhat higher costs. "The fact is," a Dartmouth medical student confided to his journal in 1809, "a student cannot be benefited by practice, at any medical college, unless he has the advantage of attending a hospital." His reflections had been prompted by the spectacle of his eager classmates following their professor of surgery seventeen miles into the country to watch him operate. "A dollar or two expended, a day's study lost, themselves fatigued, and six-cents worth gained."[10] In a hospital such operations—if no daily occurrence in this period—were still part of expected clinical routine. It is hardly surprising that in competing for matriculants the faculties of urban medical schools always emphasized proximity to hospitals.[11]

From the novice medical student's point of view, the hospital constituted an emotionally resonant theater, and surgery was central to the hospital's impact. Major operations were often advertised in advance and spacious amphitheaters constructed for spectators. In the days of surgery without anesthesia or antisepsis, the surgeon himself occupied, in fact cultivated, a self-consciously dramatic persona. The operator did indeed require "the heart of a lion and the daring of an eagle" as he sought with a few bold strokes to complete a procedure before his patient died from shock and loss of blood.[12] Medical school circulars and advertisements boasted of the number of operations performed in local hospitals, while hospitals might cooperate by giving priority in admissions to patients with severe and incapacitating surgical ills. When the Massachusetts General Hospital opened in 1821, for example, Harvard Medical School began almost immediately to boast of the surgical opportunities it would offer. Prospective students were reassured that "indigent patients, from any part of the continent, requiring surgical operations, are received, supported, and attended gratuitously at the Hospital, particularly during the winter months." (The winter months constituted most of the early nineteenth-century medical school's brief term.) At the same time, the hospital's attending staff were able to assure the institution's trustees that the "knowledge of surgery has been extended and its grade in the scale of those arts essential to our community has been distinctly elevated."[13]

Medical students were entranced. "I tell you," a Virginian observing surgical practice in Philadelphia wrote to a rural friend in 1842, "this is the place after all—the patients are never tied nor do they suffer or even grunt."[14] Like obstetrics, surgery was a skill that every ambitious young physician sought to master. The realities of contemporary practice demanded that he undertake to treat any of those periodic crises that might face one of his families; to confess inability was to risk losing clients to another, more confident or experienced practitioner.[15] Medical rounds and presentations or the routine of surgical dressings could not compare in drama to the surgeon's swashbuckling incursions, yet they provided a valuable exposure to the everyday realities of physicianship.

The hospital experience changed little for medical students during the first three quarters of the nineteenth century. James Post, for example, a medical student in New York in 1792 visited the hospital each day at twelve, "to see the Physicians visit the patients and hear them prescribed for." Usually rounds were brief, but some days he could not leave for lunch before two, "as [the professor] who is to give us clinical lectures is preparing cases for us," which demanded "rather more attention than is commonly bestowed on hospital patients." The sights and sounds and smells of the hospital made an ineradicable impression. As in the case of most other medical students, surgery made by far the deepest impression on Post. He was horrified, for example, to watch surgeon Richard Bayley, ". . . operate on one Baldwin for a fistulous ulcer in the groin. But so great was the irritability and anxiety of him, that it was impossible unless throwing him into an absolute fit of phrensy. . . ."[16] In the pre-anesthetic era, every medical student who spent time in a hospital had necessarily to share this same initiatory experience. Almost forty years later, another New York City medical student felt a parallel horror when first witnessing surgery. "But, oh, how my feelings recoiled at the sight," he confided to his diary after observing an amputation:

To behold the keen shining knife drawn around the leg severing the integuments, while the unhappy subject of the operation uttered the most heart-rending screams in his agony and torment, . . . to hear the saw working its way through the bone, produced an impression I never can forget.[17]

Most hospital experience was rather less intense, but of marginal usefulness to that great majority of medical students who could neither afford the tutorial fees of staff physicians nor compete for the handful of resident house officerships.

Students complained of the crowding, of the swarms of their peers who followed the professor through the wards and filled the amphitheaters; little could be seen in the crush. In the second quarter of the nineteenth century, as physical diagnosis became better understood and accepted, passive observation itself came to seem increasingly inadequate as a way of learning clinical medicine; auscultation, percussion, and use of the stethoscope could only be learned by doing, not watching. At the same time, contemporary students often criticized the medical school's regular diet of didactic lectures, sometimes intoned from texts already in print. One such student referred to himself as the "passive recipient" of "garbled plagiarisms."[18] Thus, even when relationships between antebellum hospitals and medical schools were relatively placid, conditions for learning in the hospital were far from ideal. They consisted of either a formal set-piece in a large auditorium or a crowded cluster of medical students pushing and craning their necks to catch a better view of an intimidated patient being questioned and examined by an unapproachable attending physician. The inadequacy of such instruction only increased the value of those informal tutorial arrangements that allowed at least some medical students to work in small groups on the wards after the brief school year came to a close.

To medical school faculty and prominent urban physicians generally, the antebellum hospital was always a real or potential teaching
tool, but one never entirely responsive to their needs. Yet, even
when specific faculty requests for teaching privileges remained
unmet, such requests were marked by a revealing consistency. What
clinical teachers always wanted was clear enough: access to patients,
the construction of clinical amphitheaters convenient to wards, increasing influence in the admission and discharge of patients, autonomy in the selection of house staff, the right to charge tutorial
fees for teaching small groups in hospital wards. As early as 1791,
for example, Benjamin Rush, in his capacity as University of Pennsylvania faculty member, suggested such a program to the Pennsylvania Hospital's Board of Managers. The university hoped to create
a professorship of clinical medicine, but it could hardly do so without the hospital's cooperation.

To render such an institution useful it will be necessary that the Patients
who are to be the subjects of the clinical lectures should be lodged in a
room by themselves, to be called the "clinical ward" where they will be
visited at the usual hours on hospital days by the clinical lecturer, who will
be at the same time one of the attending physicians of the hospital. The
patients lodged in the ward will be accessible at all times (except when
they are visited by the clinical teacher) to all the students of medicine. The
prescription book will be likewise open to them—but it will be proper to
restrict attendance upon the clinical patients when they are visited, &
examined by the clinical teacher, only to those students who are his
pupils.[19]

Although a few antebellum hospitals did allow the creation of clinical wards, few if any medical school faculty members enjoyed all
those privileges Rush specified. But although circumstances
changed gradually in succeeding decades, teaching proposals remained consistent in their desire to expand contact between students and patients.[20]

Hospital trustees, as we have seen, were not eager to surrender
their responsibilities and prerogatives to medical school faculties,
while a particular hospital's attending physicians, who might or
might not be faculty members, saw no reason to endorse such requests. Medical schools played the role of supplicant as they sought
the clinical access so important in attracting students. During the
late 1840s, for example, when the Philadelphia Almshouse Hospital

was closed to clinical instruction, the University of Pennsylvania School of Medicine found itself without a senior surgeon on the Pennsylvania Hospital attending staff. They were forced to negotiate with Jacob Randolph, surgeon at the Hospital—finally offering him the position of clinical Professor of Surgery at a salary of $500 per year—but only so long as he continued to hold his visiting position at the hospital.[21] Both Pennsylvania and its chief competitor, Jefferson, were so anxious to find "material" for their eager classes that they authorized payment for patients at nearby boarding houses so that they might be available for operations. Similarly, arrangements with outpatient physicians at a city's dispensaries might provide illustrative cases for teaching (and serve as stakes for dispensary physicians to play in hope of ascent in their community's medical establishment).

As mid-century approached, medical school faculty members increased the urgency of their demands for clinical facilities. In a smaller city like Charleston, for example, the Medical College of South Carolina had exploited the limited clinical opportunities offered at the community's almshouse and marine hospital and strongly supported the creation of a city hospital—one in which purely medical cases could be treated outside the demeaning confines of an almshouse. In the 1850s, the New Orleans School of Medicine established a free dispensary to attract patients to be used in clinical instruction; its students already had some access to patients in the city's Charity Hospital. The University of Maryland Medical School had created its own dispensary in Baltimore even earlier. Indeed, medical schools began not simply to importune hospital authorities as they had for decades, but, like the Medical College of Virginia, to create their own inpatient facilities.[22]

It was in the largest cities that the stakes were highest and the infighting most tenacious. One solution, favored by ambitious but still junior physicians, was the founding of small clinical schools or classes that ordinarily met after the regular medical school lectures concluded in the spring and provided supplementary anatomical and clinical teaching for young men able to afford the time and tuition.[23] But such ventures did not greatly increase access to hospital patients beyond that already available through the teaching privileges enjoyed by attending physicians.[24] (Although the apprenticeship system of the eighteenth and early nineteenth centuries was moribund at mid-century, these tutorial arrangements preserved an opportunity for individual bedside instruction.)

Such privileges were ordinarily circumscribed by lay authority. There always remained a substantial gap between hospital policies and the professional ambitions of clinical teachers. In some cases this was exacerbated by differences between attending staffs and the faculty of local medical schools. New York Hospital's attending staff, for example, nurtured a grievance against several of the city's mid-century medical schools that festered for decades.

Anxious to provide teaching materials for their students, the medical colleges had been busily establishing outpatient clinics and even inpatient beds. In a period when one could open a dispensary in a storefront or a hospital in an ordinary brownstone, it was tempting for medical school faculties to create and advertise such ad hoc facilities (sometimes in fact closing them when classes were not in session). These "dispensary exhibitions," as one caustic New York Hospital physician described them, provided neither adequate training nor appropriate care; both patient and student were inevitably exploited. Yet competition for patients became only more intense. Seven years later, another New York Hospital physician complained that the city's medical schools plotted with ever-increasing ingenuity to siphon off illustrative cases for teaching. The faculty, he contended,

connected with these private enterprises have, at times, been so anxious for attracting patients to themselves, that they have had their agents at our public dispensaries, and even at our own institution, for collecting the materials for display at the colleges.[25]

The "materials" to be "displayed" were an important prize in a complex and multisided struggle for prestige, for achievement in the form of publication, and for financial reward in the form of increased tuition fees. Hospital and dispensary appointments, as we have seen, like medical school professorships, were equities to be prudently managed in a complex and demanding marketplace.

Quest for Control: The Reform Consensus

Medical teachers in the last third of the nineteenth century conceded that American medical education was sorely in need of closer ties between ward and classroom. The rapid growth of hospitals only expanded such instructional opportunities and underlined the gap between bedside teaching as it was and as it might be.

Marketplace pressure was at least as important as pedagogical conviction. Prospective students wanted and expected some exposure to clinical practice, and medical schools always emphasized the number of beds accessible to their matriculants. The gradual acceptance of physical diagnosis in the second quarter of the nineteenth century had underlined the long-felt need for clinical teaching, and professional developments after the Civil War intensified both the logical rationale and student demand for bedside instruction. The growth of ophthalmology, of otology, of neurology, of antiseptic surgery all urged the importance of procedure-oriented small group teaching in medical education—and thus by implication a place for the student in wards and outpatient clinics.

The parallel growth of a dependent urban population and of hospitals to serve it provided in a rough-and-ready way, as we have seen, for the educational needs of the best prepared and financed among a new generation of medical men. As occupants of the increasing number of residencies and internships, they turned the hospital's staffing needs into educational opportunity. And these were the same young men who had been able to afford summer courses and tutorials before applying for house officerships.

But these opportunities for the elite did not solve a more general student demand for clinical training. Medical schools lacked access to hospital wards, and where that access could be obtained, it had to be cautiously negotiated. In the years immediately after the Civil War, the medical schools still did not possess the social influence to control hospitals nor did the universities with which many were nominally connected possess the endowment—or commitment to medical education—that might have led to their sponsorship of university-owned clinical facilities.[26] Even the most privileged medical students had to contend with a formal curriculum frustratingly devoid of clinical experience. A good many young practitioners hoped, moreover, to accumulate some specialist skills in order to compete with their peers, if not to undertake an academic or consultant's practice. Yet even when aggressively advertised, medical school clinics and amphitheater lectures often disappointed the would-be practitioner. As a Louisianan studying in New York reported in 1878, "Notwithstanding the large amount of clinical material furnished by these institutions, the lectures are for the most part didactic, and at the clinics the patient is simply exhibited to the students."[27] Medical school boasts of abundant clinical resources were more a reflection of student demand and institutional competitiveness than of pedagogic reality.

This state of things seemed increasingly intolerable. By the late 1870s, a reform consensus had been firmly established. Since its founding in the late 1840s, for example, the American Medical Association had concerned itself with upgrading medical education and the indispensable role of the hospital in providing such training.[28] Critics of the prevailing system were fond of a clichéd analogy between the teaching of medicine without bedside instruction and chemistry without experiments or anatomy without dissection. Exclusive reliance on lectures seemed the primary villain; a prominent woman physician referred to it in 1872 as "an enormous anachronism, a legacy of the times of medieval darkness, when original scientific study was unknown. . . ."[29] Large amphitheaters should be subordinate to the bedside and hospital design should reflect this goal; small classes of thoroughly trained students ought ultimately to replace formal and impersonal presentations. "The time for large lecture classes," one hospital planner argued in 1876, "we trust has passed never to return; that *quality* is henceforth to be considered rather than *quantity*."[30]

Yet would-be reformers of medical education encountered a number of persistent problems: one was the intransigence of lay hospital authorities, another the lack of endowment and absence of a strong academic tradition in the medical schools themselves. They also faced the resentment of ordinary physicians. Such practitioners had seen the hospital and dispensary as unfair and unwelcome competitors; and they associated advanced credentials and hospital training with elite prerogatives. At some level, the raising of standards meant greater difficulty in entering the profession and an acceptance of the values and privileges of an upper stratum of medical men. But reformers held out a compelling inducement for rank-and-file physicians, threatened from below by the quack and the ill trained. Raising standards and decreasing numbers—the argument for quality rather than quantity—would set the regularly trained physician apart from such competitors. "The hospital is not," as one advocate of a more demanding medical education placated in 1892, "in any sense, the rival or antagonist of the practitioner. Their lines are parallel, and far above the mercenary level on which the charlatan reaps his harvest." The hospital was a potential ally not an enemy. When every medical college had a four-year curriculum and each state enforced licensing requirements, there would be an abundance of patients for all.[31] American medical schools graduated too many casually trained physicians; it was hardly surprising that so many left the profession within a few years of entering practice.[32]

Regular arrangements between hospital and medical school would also avert the undignified maneuvering that accompanied urban rivalries for ward access. Such tactics only demoralized respectable urban practitioners and provided ammunition for the profession's critics. Where accommodation could not be reached, controversy fractured the local medical community and provided evidence for those laymen who saw the profession as greedy and manipulative. "The Cincinnati Hospital," a local editorialist could write in 1872, "has always been a carcass of contention among the medical crows of the Cincinnati colleges. Its control by the faculty of either gave that great advantages over the others in the way of demonstrating the killing, cutting, and curing art before its students."[33]

What could medical schools do to provide clinical teaching for their students? One obvious tactic was to convert the informal clinics and dispensaries of mid-century into full-fledged hospitals in which the medical school would specify attending appointments and admission policies—and thus control not only access to beds but the particular occupants of those beds. At the University of Pennsylvania, for example, where a pliant state legislature provided funds for hospital buildings and operating expenses, the medical school was able to open a new hospital in 1874, one in which the chiefs of the several clinical services were faculty members and in which the school's full professors filled seven of the eighteen seats on the Board of Managers.[34] The medical school's half-century-old battle with Philadelphia's municipal hospital authorities and their more clubby, yet not always smooth, relationship with the genteel managers of the Pennsylvania Hospital were by no means ended, for the new hospital could not provide enough clinical material for the school's enormous classes. But some teaching access could now be guaranteed and a number of clinical and part-time teaching positions created (including four new clinical professorships). Afraid to fall behind in the competition for students, Philadelphia's Jefferson Medical College opened its own hospital in 1877, and the city's homeopathic Hahnemann Medical College followed suit in

1887.[35] These were by no means the first example of medical school controlled inpatient beds. The University of Michigan, for example, eager to provide teaching material for its medical students established a small hospital as early as 1869.[36]

Every urban school faced similar difficulties. The Philadelphia example was typical in the desire of competing local institutions to provide clinical faculties, atypical because of the state legislature's generosity and the scale of their operations (Pennsylvania and Jefferson were two of the largest American medical schools). The less well-known case of Richmond provides a more characteristic example. Pressed by competition from Philadelphia, the Medical College of Virginia organized an infirmary as early as the 1850s. Its announcement for 1860 advertised private rooms for white patients and ample accommodation for slaves and those ordinary citizens who could not afford private rates.[37] The school's infirmary also served as the Marine Hospital for the Port of Richmond, while prospective students were assured that they might enjoy some access to cases at the city's almshouse. Nevertheless, the medical school planned to build a seventy-five– to one hundred–bed hospital with state support.[38] Later in the century, Richmond's medical schools followed a similar pattern, making contractual alliances with a succession of local hospitals, always seeking a quid pro quo in which the faculty bartered medical attendance—and where necessary, financial support—for control of wards to be used in teaching.[39] The Richmond story had parallels in other middle-sized cities. University of Louisville faculty members paid fees for the use the City Hospital's amphitheater, ostensibly to defray the costs of constructing an amphitheater.[40] When faced by a looming debt and necessary repair bills, the Albany Hospital was rescued by its medical staff in 1879; they organized a fund drive to retire the debt and paid for improvements in drainage and ventilation themselves. Not surprisingly, the clinics were open to students at the local medical college, where many of the attendings also taught.[41] In Charleston, the Medical College of South Carolina had, as we have noted, sought to use almshouse and marine hospital facilities where it could, urged the establishment of a general hospital, then negotiated a contractual arrangement with the city hospital to staff the institution in exchange for teaching privileges.[42] In this and all similar arrangements, lay authorities were careful to specify that patient rights should be protected. Throughout the nineteenth century, voluntary and municipal hospital authorities retained some degree of suspicion—at times animosity—toward those medical men who sought to use hospitals for undergraduate instruction.

As late as 1910, a recent historian has emphasized, only two American voluntary hospitals had worked out arrangements with medical schools that provided anything approximating the patient contact twentieth-century medical educators would consider adequate to clinical training. What seemed particularly radical—and offensive to lay values—was a responsible role for students in the diagnosis and care of individual patients.[43] Trustees guarded their independence (and, they felt, patient rights); medical school faculties might often enjoy nominal university connections, but not the resources to build their own clinical facilities. At the same time, student demand and a growing consensus among medical educators called for at least some hands-on patient contact as part of the regular curriculum. By the 1890s, forward-looking physicians had begun to accept the idea that a medical school without effective hospital connections would be an anachronism in the twentieth century. It is not surprising that medical school faculties and hospital staffs pressed everywhere for such arrangements. "The chief warrant for our future existence among teaching bodies," as the faculty of Philadelphia's Woman's Medical College put it in 1897, when urging their board to expand clinic facilities, "must be the control of ample clinical material available for purposes of systematic instruction."[44]

One solution to the problem would have been the creation of hospital-based medical schools in which an institution's senior staff served as faculty. Despite compelling English precedents for this system, however, it never became a significant aspect of American medical education. A few nineteenth-century schools did in fact develop in this fashion: Long Island College Hospital and Bellevue in New York, for example; for a brief period Cincinnati General Hospital also offered its own "Clinical and Pathological School." But such programs remained in the minority as did independent institutions such as Jefferson and Hahnemann that began as medical school faculties and then founded subordinate hospitals. To some extent, moreover, American physicians explicitly rejected the oligarchical English system in which social and institutional power was concentrated in a few hands.

Students and graduates still asked for more than the schools could provide. Until the twentieth century, the total number of house officerships, like opportunities for small group teaching, was inadequate for all those who sought them. When the American Medical Association conducted its first hospital survey in 1873, only 309 house officerships were available in the United States.[45] Some graduates, of course, accumulated or possessed the resources to study in Europe (a substantial portion of whom had already served as house officers in American hospitals or volunteers in outpatient clinics). Between 1860 and the First World War, roughly fifteen thousand Americans studied at German-speaking universities—the vast majority at intensive brief specialty courses in such clinical centers as Vienna and Berlin.[46]

Those who could not afford such status-enhancing trips might still be able to attend a short course at one of the postgraduate schools that sprang up in large cities in the 1880s, catering to the would-be specialist and self-improving generalist who felt his (or less frequently her) clinical training to have been inadequate. "A few years ago," the New York *Medical Record* noted in 1884, "there was some excuse for a doctor graduating and going into practice without ever having seen a case, except perhaps from the back seat of a large amphitheater. Now, with our well-supplied clinical schools, it is unpardonable that such a thing should happen."[47] In the early twentieth century, these postgraduate programs were gradually deprived of their reason for being as regular medical schools upgraded the clinical training offered their undergraduates and as hospital expansion provided a steadily increasing number of house officerships for those able and willing to undertake them.[48] But in the 1880s and 1890s, they played an important role (also offering teaching positions to individuals who might have remained marginal in the status systems of the more established schools). Even at the Johns Hopkins Hospital, revealingly, courses in eye and ear, throat, skin, children's, neurological, and genito-urinary diseases were offered in the hospital's clinics as soon as the institution opened—and four years before the Johns Hopkins Medical School accepted its first student.[49]

Education had moved into the hospital in a gradual, yet inexorable way. The absolute number of house officerships had increased steadily, as we have seen, and the timing of internship appointments had been coordinated with medical school schedules. Although clinical clerkships did not become a standard part of every undergraduate medical curriculum until after the First World War, a good many medical students were concocting equivalents—if more informal and often inadequately supervised—as externs and summer replacements. At the same time, hospitals began to allow an increasing amount of small group teaching on the wards, decreasing their emphasis on the traditional showpiece amphitheater lectures. "While each year shows a diminution in the number of students attending general clinics," the Philadelphia General Hospital reported in 1904, "continuous advance is made in bedside instruction and lectures to small classes." Over 27,000 student visits had taken place that year, as opposed to roughly half that number in 1903. The new system seemed advantageous for both student and hospital: "Bedside instruction and ward rounds by students accompanied by members of the staff, have increased and become more thoroughly organized. The method by which the student performs as nearly as may be, the duties of a resident physician, seems to most effectually hold the interest of the student and to have the greatest teaching value." The trend continued. In 1909, medical students paid almost exactly 50,000 individual visits to the hospital; 39,000 were in the form of small group bedside instruction.[50]

Teaching had implications for patients as well. At one level, of course, it shaped admissions decisions wherever medical men had the power to do so. Hospitals might reduce rates or offer free treatment in an effort to attract "patients available for teaching."[51] Admission policies might even shift during the academic year so as to provide illustrative cases for undergraduate teaching; two Philadelphia general hospitals, for example, that forbade tuberculosis admissions during the rest of the year, allowed them "during the winter season for purposes of class demonstration. . . ."[52] In other instances, hospitals established services for explicitly didactic purposes, often to provide a full range of clinical opportunities for student physicians and nurses.

Charity patients did not relish being used in such clinical exercises. Despite frequent medical reassurances that patients welcomed the attention, I have found no institutional data to question the abundant evidence that patients did in fact fear the invasion of their bodies and privacy by student hands and eyes. Constantly reiterated warnings by governing boards that patients could not be used without their permission (and even complaints that medical staff might be more interested in using their wards for teaching than for providing care) constitute evidence more of a persistent conflict between lay and medical attitudes than of the effectiveness of these ritual admonitions in guarding patient sensibilities.[53] But such lay anxieties seemed increasingly the relics of ancient and irrational attitudes, not to be tolerated in an era of scientific medicine.

To medical men, the situation appeared in a very different light. First-rate medical care for society's dispossessed was impossible without a medical school hovering nearby and guaranteeing state-of-the-art care. The truest philanthropy turned on the ability to provide care of equal quality to poor and rich alike. "I feel very keenly," the influential policy maker Ray Lyman Wilbur wrote in 1923:

that the medical situation in Los Angeles will not be satisfactory until a first-class medical school is developed there, which will bring to the care of the indigent sick and the dependent poor men who are thoroughly trained and deeply interested in the welfare both of the patients and of medicine itself. The way to insure the best of medical service for the poor is to have medical students under guidance study their problems.[54]

Patient complaints were subjective and misleading; they might well obscure the excellent technical quality of the care provided in America's best teaching hospitals.

The more thoroughgoing of early twentieth-century reformers realized that the hospital itself would have to change, to reflect a new kind of academic spirit in teaching—one that paralleled the laboratory and research ethos that was also transforming the small but influential world of academic medicine. "So far as the healing art is concerned," Harold Ernst, a Harvard bacteriologist and advocate of full-time teaching appointments, argued, "its methods are now learned and taught in the hospitals . . ." Students learned how to treat patients on the wards; teaching no longer took place in private practice. It had been the case since the midnineteenth-century demise of the apprentice system. And the next step was both logical and radical, Ernst continued: "as a matter of fact the treatment of patients—the practice of the art of healing—is more perfect to-day in any good hospital than in a home."[55] A hospital was the best place to practice as well as learn medicine; there was, in fact, no distinction between the two.

This was a far cry from previous generations when it was assumed that practice in a home setting was in its essence a very different matter from hospital medicine. This argument enshrined the scientifically oriented academician and at the same time emphasized a reductionist view of disease and therapeutics. The role of the family, of personal interaction between doctor and patient—relationships that had been so important in medical theory and to the practitioner's self-image a half century before—began to seem marginal, if not inconsequential. It is not surprising that Ernst called for the creation of full-time clinical positions, analogous to those of laboratory scientists appointed in university departments.[56] This was still an extreme position, but in some influential circles a decisive one. The Harvard bacteriologist was as prescient as he was aggressive.

Flexner and After

Most physicians, if they know anything of recent medical history, know of the Flexner Report—the source, in conventional wisdom of everything good or, depending on one's viewpoint, bad in contemporary medicine.[57] A key aspect of that report was a particular view of the physician: he or she should not be expected to be a practicing scientist but should have nevertheless been trained to think scientifically in the laboratory and in clinical clerkships at the bedside. Yet as we have seen and as recent scholarship has emphasized, the Flexner Report is most appropriately regarded as a culminating incident in a much older reform program; it reflected and incorporated a widely understood elite consensus that had been forged in a half century of frustrating experience with existing teaching arrangements. It was hardly the beginning of a movement; it was the end of a beginning. When he undertook the Carnegie Foundation's charge to investigate medical education, Abraham Flexner expressed a longstanding elite consensus.

A clinically oriented medical education had gradually evolved; it had not been imposed by foundation fiat.[58] That evolution grew out of an intricate symbiosis between hospitals constantly in search of staff, on the one hand, and on the other, physicians who sought clinical training and status. Without central planning, parallel needs and parallel values helped structure recurrent patterns of institutional behavior. Like Topsy, medical education had just grown in the years before 1910—but along predetermined paths. Residencies and internships came into de facto existence before national boards and formal certification of internship and residency programs. As the nineteenth century drew to a close and as the medical curriculum expanded from two to three (and in a few cases four) years, small group teaching at the bedside had changed from an individually arranged privilege of the wealthy and ambitious into an integral part of the curriculum at America's leading medical schools. At the same time, as we have seen, with the rapid growth in hospitals, a larger and larger number of aspiring practitioners were able to supplement their still shaky formal clinical curricula at both the undergraduate and graduate levels. A quiet revolution in clinical education had already taken place. By 1914, more than three-quarters of medical graduates were taking an internship, and five medical schools had begun to require a year's house officership for the M.D. degree.[59] And in a number of influential institutions, medical schools had just made or were in the process of forging tight links with teaching hospitals. Our hospital-based system of teaching clinical medicine had already come into being. "Subsequent changes," as the leading historian of this movement concludes, "were of degree, not of kind—continually adding to the student's work and responsibilities, not questioning whether students should be given responsibilities in the first place. With the appearance of the teaching hospital, training that in the nineteenth-century had been available only for the very good or very lucky students became mandatory for everyone."[60]

The hospital's practical needs had created an armature around which medical ideas and careers could be articulated and supported. Increasingly, late nineteenth- and early twentieth-century physicians of any respectability sought hospital connections—no matter how casual and tenuous. In Philadelphia in 1900, there were almost 1,000 institutional staff appointments among 1,954 medical men. At the same time, the number of teaching positions had increased from 50 in 1860 to 372 in the city's six medical schools by 1900. There were some 445 staff appointments at hospitals and dispensaries associated with medical schools; almost one-third of the city's regular physicians engaged in some aspect of medical education.[61] For most, it was a minor time commitment—a clinic two afternoons a week or block of time serving as bedside or laboratory instructor—yet it served to integrate medical education into the hospital, on the one hand, and on the other, into the ongoing realities of a profession structured around private practice.

Yet, in 1910, the great majority of hospitals still guarded their autonomy, while most medical schools still sought vainly for control over wards, appointments, and admissions. Many of the reformers' goals were not to become reality until the interwar period. There were only the smallest beginnings of a salaried academic professoriate in the hospitals and clinical chairs at related medical schools.[62] The integration of science and clinical medicine was even more problematic, both as an intellectual and organizational task. The researcher still had a difficult and often obstructed road to travel.[63] The ideals of medical reformers had still to transform either medical practice generally or the hospital as a social institution particularly. But enlightened and influential men within and outside the medical profession had come to accept the desirability of greater and greater cooperation between hospital and medical school—with the goal being a profession composed of fewer but more scientifically trained physicians. In 1910, this was still primarily a consensus of attitudes and expectations, not of policy. Nevertheless, this consensus was a significant agent of change; the key to its power lay in a particular configuration of ideas about the appropriate nature and ultimate capacities of medicine—and the promise of healing that these anticipated abilities held out to society. Central to these assumptions and expectations was the transforming role of science in medicine, of hands-on training in medical education—and of the hospital in both.

But just as the medical profession had changed in the half-century between 1870 and 1920, so had the hospital in which that profession played so prominent a role. It was not only a larger and more genuinely national institution; the hospital had also become more self-consciously medical and bureaucratic. Medical needs and medical perceptions had played a pivotal role in shaping and legitimating that change, but medical men and ideas were only one element in a complex and interconnected hospital reality.

CHAPTER 9

Healing Hands:
Nursing in the Hospital

We are all familiar with the legend. Professional nursing began with the lady and her lamp—Florence Nightingale bringing skill and enlightenment to a realm of besotted ignorance. Like many reformers, Nightingale and her followers inspired a usable, if somewhat less than accurate, history, one that emphasized the contrast between their new dispensation and a past in which hospital nursing had been the exclusive prerogative of alcoholics and prostitutes too feeble to practice their more ancient profession. Hospital nurses, in Nightingale's own words, "were generally those who were too old, too weak, too drunken, too dirty, too stolid, or too bad to do anything else."[1]

The nursing reform movement deployed an ideology as well as a history (if the two can be regarded as distinct). This founding ideology incorporated attitudes toward gender, toward class, and toward the nature and treatment of disease. Perhaps most important, it played upon the contemporary assumption that there was a necessary and laudable conjunction between nursing and femininity; the trained sensibility of a middle-class woman could alone bring order and morality to the hospital's grim wards. In this generation, sickness and health were still related inextricably to environment, and, as we have seen, Nightingale and many of her contemporaries could not distinguish between the moral and the material in their understanding of that environment. Nursing was at least as important as the physician's drugs and instruments in preserving and restoring health.

And the training school movement did indeed flourish, beginning in the 1860s in England and 1870s and 1880s in the United States. By the end of the century, American nursing leaders were demanding increased classroom work, decreased hours on the ward, a lengthened curriculum, and postgraduate certification. Until recently, most historians of nursing in America were trained in this reform tradition, accepted it, and celebrated it in their work; they chronicled a laudable progression from the pretraining school era of slovenly ignorance to a period of increasing respect, skill, and professionalism.

Students of nursing history have become more skeptical in the past generation.[2] They have, for example, construed the hypothetical attributes of femininity as constraints which helped limit nurses' professional aspirations and not a basis for their vocational legitimacy. The physician's intellectual authority has seemed to such revisionist historians a mask for exploitive paternalism, and the nurse's abnegation of self, a crippling false consciousness. But these ideological visions and revisions in some ways obscure the origin of modern nursing in a specific reality—the mid-nineteenth-century hospital.

Nursing Before Nurses

In 1849, nurses at Massachusetts General Hospital worked from five in the morning to nine in the evening. Before leaving duty, they communicated any special orders from the house staff to the "watchers" responsible for the wards at night. Ordinarily, one such watcher ministered to twenty patients; the pay was fifty cents for women and a dollar for men. Males were "not generally appointed."[3]

Hospital nursing was long, hard work. It was performed by both men and women and conformed in organization to a ward structure in which at least a score of patients normally occupied the same large room. Nurses lived in the hospital, often in odd cubicles tucked in attics, in basements, or, at times, immediately adjacent to the ward. Antebellum nurses were by no means recruited from among the depraved and infirm alone. Although they often learned on the job, many ward nurses were highly skilled, enjoyed long tenures, and exercised considerable responsibility.[4] They dressed wounds, administered drugs and enemas, prepared special diets, as well as scrubbed, dusted, and made beds. Ward nurses supervised the work of one or more assistants as well as the casual, if often indispensable, efforts of convalescent patients.

The size of the ward dictated nursing's organizational structure; there was too much work for one nurse and too little money for more than one, but someone had to be in charge. Contemporary mores and the sexual segregation of wards also implied that men nurse men and women nurse women. Nursing was a more dignified occupation in private than almshouse hospitals; almshouse nurses had often begun as "inmates," but even as they gradually progressed from convalescent helper to assistant nurse to ward nurse, they never escaped inmate status.[5] In every hospital, however, a traditional paternalism guaranteed that employees would be treated as minors in need of control. Both paternalism and the need to ensure stability in the ward's supervisory structure encouraged trustees to reward long-term employees. At the New York Hospital, for example, wages were increased 50 percent after "a faithful service" of five years, another 33⅓ percent after ten years, and after twenty years an annuity of $25 and ". . . in case of need, . . . support in the hospital during life. . . ."[6]

The line between nursing and domestic service could hardly be drawn in the mid-nineteenth century. Male and female nurses worked with their hands and ministered to their patients' most basic needs. Emptying bedpans, cleaning and cooking, changing sheets, and removing vomit and bloodstains were all tasks that guaranteed a humble status in this class-conscious society. And in many cases, nurses had in fact risen from more humble service jobs in the hospital. But the lack of secure and stable work—especially for women— guaranteed that at least some hard-working Americans would trade the freedom (and better, if less predictable, pay) of the noninstitutional labor market for the more secure, if paternalistic, world of nursing. Others moved back and forth between work outside and inside the hospital's walls.

Thus the inconsistency of many late nineteenth- and early twentieth-century accounts of hospital nursing; their authors were well aware that some mid-nineteenth-century nurses had been responsible, stable, and dedicated, even if others had been casual, filthy, and unreliable. "Of the evils of the old system," a chronicler of New York's Charity Hospital wrote in 1904, "no one of the present day can form the slightest conception. Helpers of every degree of unfitness and immorality had been employed to care for the sick." Most nurses and servants were, in fact, workhouse prisoners who remained after serving their terms, "receiving no wages but a pretty liberal allowance of whiskey...." Yet many of these unpromising recruits, he conceded, "although uneducated in nursing, illiterate and even depraved, did faithful service as far as their ability permitted."

No nobler character ever existed than old John Collingan, head nurse in the fever pavilion—a man whose self forgetfulness and never ceasing kindness to those under his charge brought many a desperate case of typhoid fever to a favorable termination. Although an ignorant Irish peasant, he was by instinct a gentleman and a born nurse, with the tenderness of a woman and the motives of a saint.[7]

It was into a well-established world of hospital work and authority that the Nightingale movement intruded with the promise that it would create a more intelligent, skilled, and reliable nursing corps, as well as a new level of order and efficiency predicated on the existence of these trained nurses.

Individual institutions, and especially their medical staff members, had sought to upgrade the quality of nursing throughout the century. They were well aware of the steps that needed to be taken: better wages, minimizing the use of patient labor, and reducing the amount of menial work were clearly the ways to attract and keep first-rate nurses. In 1840, for example, attending physicians at the New York Hospital urged their Board of Governors to raise wages and to seek to recruit better educated and more temperate nurses, to avoid the use of convalescent patients, and to limit the nurses' duties as much as possible to patient care. The board, significantly, decided that wages for female nurses were adequate; with respect to male nurses, however, the board conceded that wages were too low to "command the services of men of good character" and agreed to raise the wages of men—while forbidding female nurses from taking in needlework or engaging in other employment to supplement their salaries. The board also promised to employ night nurses and to restrict the nurses' duties to patient care.[8] But these good intentions were short lived. The later history of the hospital, like many of its sister institutions, makes clear that the problems of inadequate night nursing and unrelenting demands for menial work continued until the end of the century.

Even if America's first nursing schools were not established formally until 1873, nurse training had been discussed much earlier. In 1851, for example, Philadelphia Episcopalians had suggested that nurse training would be one of the benefits of a proposed denominational hospital: "An apprentice system," as they described it, ". . . which will in time produce a corps of well-instructed and faithful individuals, capable of serving the public as paid or as gratuitous attendants upon the sick."[9] Founders of women's hospitals before 1873 often saw as one of their goals the training of nurses for the community, especially for women in childbed.

The 1850s were a period of heightening interest in nurse training. The Crimean War and consequent prominence of Florence Nightingale had made American as well as English philanthropists and physicians conscious of nursing and the hospital as fields ripe for reform. In calling for an upgrading of nursing at New York Hospital, for example, staff surgeon Willard Parker urged in 1860 not only an increase in numbers, but the replacement of male with female nurses. Men, he explained to the Board of Governors, "even if they be of the best quality, cannot meet the demands of the sick. They have not the instinct for it. They are consequently awkward, untidy, and out of their proper sphere."

It seems to me the cause of humanity, the Reputation & welfare of the Hospital demand some change. What are physicians & Surgeons without efficient, educated Nurses?

Permit me to suggest an arrangement by which two efficient Female Nurses should be furnished to each of the large Wards, Except the Syphilitic, and a Male *Ward Man* or scavenger, who should at all times, be subject to the call of the Nurses.[10]

Every aspect of the nurses' task should be evaluated and improved: "The position of Nurse is very responsible," Parker argued, "& I wish we could raise up some Florence Nightingale."

Experience during the Civil War seemed only to underline such convictions. No hospital, civil or military, as one medical man put it, could be well managed without "a corps of female nurses. Nursing is as absolutely the peculiar province of women as any branch of house-wifery. The qualities of a good nurse are vigilance, discretion, and gentleness; and these are her special qualities."[11]

Despite such sentiments, the exigencies of war temporarily halted nursing reform in civil hospitals just as it slowed efforts to recast the institution's physical structure. In the long run, however, the Civil War emphasized the need for trained nurses. It is no accident that America's first formal nurse training schools were founded in the decade after Appomattox—and that a number of nursing's influential advocates had played an active role in military hospitals.

An Ideology of Legitimation

It seemed obvious to most contemporaries that women were better suited than men to nursing; their innate sensitivity would bring warmth and reassurance to the patient as it brought cleanliness and order to the ward. This was as well a generation when much social activism reflected and was motivated by a secularized evangelicalism; lives were not to be wasted but dedicated to morally appropriate vocations. Such justifications were particularly important to that minority of respectable women who sought a socially acceptable sphere of activity outside the home.[12] Even Florence Nightingale, although no orthodox believer, saw her crusade in similar terms; choice implied responsibility and responsibility, action. There could be no compromise with the imperfect. More pragmatic arguments for nursing—that it provided respectable work for women and a skilled nursing force for homes and hospitals—supplemented and intensified such transcendent imperatives.

This complex of ideas regarding social activism and women's appropriate role was also consistent with many aspects of mid-nineteenth-century medical thought. An increasing skepticism toward much of conventional therapeutics (or at least the tendency to see such interventions as merely supportive of the body's natural healing processes) logically emphasized the importance of nursing—along with diet, cleanliness, and rest. Nightingale explicitly attacked the traditional notion that "to give medicines is to be doing something or rather everything; to give air, warmth, cleanliness etc. is to do nothing." In treating such acute ills as fever or cholera, medicine had demonstrated only its impotence and underlined the need for careful nursing.[13] Medical therapeutics could aid but not replace innate healing mechanisms.

Florence Nightingale was not alone in her rejection of disease specificity. As we have seen, sickness was understood by many of her contemporaries to be a general state of the body, a failure of adjustment to its environment. But that environment could be manipulated and the patient aided in the process of readjustment which constituted healing. This was a persuasive point of view in a period when holistic assumptions characterized medical thought, when lay persons and physicians assumed that every aspect of the individual's physical and psychic environment could interact to produce health or disease. It was only natural for nursing advocates to magnify its potential contribution within this holistic context. "I use the word nursing," Florence Nightingale explained, "for want of a better. It has been limited to signify little more than the administration of medicines and the application of poultices. It ought to signify the proper use of fresh air, light, warmth, cleanliness, quiet, and the proper choosing and giving of diet—all at the least expense of vital power to the patient."[14]

The Nightingale movement also mobilized these views in justifying an autonomous female role in the hospital. As she originally conceived it, the nursing superintendent, a woman of class and breeding, would control nursing in the hospital, subordinate only to the institution's governing board. The prerogatives of female sensibility and class identity helped legitimate such novel demands. But this was only a part of Nightingale's argument; she assumed that femininity in itself did not guarantee nursing competence. Technical instruction was required. The knowledge needed to manage a ward or hospital does not "come by inspiration," she argued caustically, "to the lady disappointed in love nor to the poor workhouse drudge hard up for a livelihood."[15] The Nightingale program wedded intuitive moral capacity and intellect, piety and efficiency, and promised hospital trustees and administrators a stable and relatively inexpensive labor force along with improved internal discipline and lower mortalities. It constituted a powerful and well-calculated appeal for public and medical support.

Not surprisingly this aggressive demand for hospital-based nurse training mobilized opposition as well as support. Many English hospital physicians were dismayed by such strident claims; some indeed preferred the older style of nursing in which ward nurses had been and would remain subordinate to the attending staff who had sponsored their careers. They were particularly unhospitable to the notion that a female nursing superintendent should enjoy direct access to a hospital's governing board.

American hospital reformers reiterated all these contentions in the formative years of trained nursing. Nursing was particularly suitable for women; it was a key to controlling the hospital's internal order and promised an efficient and unrelenting surveillance of every aspect of ward life, from cleanliness to discipline to diet.[16] It is ironic that all these arguments, so plausible in their mid-century context, were to become increasingly inconsistent with the profession's future aspirations.

Expanding the Training School and the Feminization of Nursing

The demand for trained nurses and attempts to provide a supply of such women in fact antedated by a generation the founding of America's first three nursing schools in 1873. The work of religious women constituted the most conspicuous precedent for trained nursing—as it did in England and on the Continent. The Catholic orders (particularly the Sisters of Charity and Mercy) had organized and staffed hospitals for decades. Even Protestant women had begun to make their way into hospital work, following precedents such as those that influenced Nightingale herself. In New York's St. Luke's, Boston's Children's and Philadelphia's Episcopal hospitals, for example, "lady volunteers" began to assume the responsibilities that had formerly been those of ward nurses—aided by paid assistants of less elevated social origin.[17] Women's hospitals too were especially receptive to the idea that nurse training was one of their natural responsibilities. When, for example, the Woman's Hospital of Illinois was organized in 1871, one of its stated aims was the training of "intelligent, conscientious women" as nurses; diplomas were to be issued to those who should "prove themselves possessed of the necessary amount of judgment, kindliness, tact and efficiency, . . ."[18]

Offering such a varied assortment of benefits, one might have expected to find this new social institution spreading even more rapidly than it did. The 1880 census located only fifteen nurse training schools with three hundred-odd graduates.[19] There are some obvious reasons for the hesitancy initially displayed by many hospitals. One, of course, was the fear that establishing a nurse training school would demand a large initial outlay of scarce capital. Another rested in the assumption that the nursing of men by women was morally compromising (and often physically taxing). In addition, the Nightingale movement's demands for nursing—and female—autonomy alarmed a good many attending physicians and board members who took their cues from English counterparts. Finally, well-established ward nurses and their supporters (especially in municipal hospitals) had no intention of dividing, let alone abdicating, their accustomed authority to newcomers who shared neither their values nor their experience—yet expected an appropriate deference. Some pioneer nurses met active opposition from such well-entrenched opponents. Linda Richards, a genteel training school pioneer, recalled with horror her first encounters with ward nurses in the early 1870s. These "indigenous" nurses were addressed by first name by everyone in the hospital, Richards recalled; they had been recruited from the "same class" as the patients and, "when asked to do so, showed me about the wards with an air of insolence not pleasant to remember."[20] At Bellevue, Cook County, and Philadelphia General Hospital, for example, entrenched nurses defended their wards against the imposition of training school authority.[21]

This initial opposition soon dissolved. The number of nurse training schools grew steadily in the 1880s and 1890s, and by century's end they had become a necessary part of every large and not a few small hospitals. The reasons for this rapid acceptance are not hard to understand: they were functional to the women who became nurses, functional to the hospitals, functional to society in providing skilled workers for home and hospital in a context consistent with that society's cultural assumptions.

Perhaps most important was the role of nursing schools in the hospitals' political economy. Nursing students provided a relatively inexpensive, stable, and disciplined workforce. It was a stability based not on the long-time service of particular individuals, but on the continued viability of the school itself. America's handful of midcentury urban hospitals had been able to make do with a cadre of long-term ward nurses and a less reliable pool of aides and assistants, but with increases in scale and a changing sense of appropriate ward behavior such traditional makeshifts would no longer have answered hospital needs.

It is true that almost every nursing school paid its students a modest sum (after they left probationer status), ostensibly for uniforms and books. This was typically ten dollars the first year and twelve during the second of the training school's two-year program.

But this expenditure guaranteed the services of young women who worked a minimum of sixty and, more frequently, seventy hours a week on the wards—and who accepted a discipline that could not easily have been imposed on an equal number of men. Not only the ingrained assumptions of paternalism and female deference, but the threat of expulsion (and thus denial of the school's diploma and the livelihood it promised) provided a leverage more than adequate to discourage potential defiance by the great majority of student nurses.[22]

Both economics and the desire to impose order dictated that hospitals seek to minimize the number of graduate nurses they employed; graduates were far more expensive than students and less amenable to discipline.[23] Ratios of ten students to one supervising graduate nurse were typical in American hospitals at the end of the nineteenth century. At Philadelphia General Hospital, eight "permanent head nurses" supervised eighty-seven students in 1889; in 1897, the Worcester Memorial Hospital employed one graduate nurse to supervise eighteen pupils; Atlanta's Grady Hospital in 1899 employed three head nurses and nineteen students, while one of those students acted as night supervisor and another took responsibility for the children's ward.[24] Well-run hospitals sought to establish a prudent ratio of student nurses to patients, but this was more easily intended than accomplished. Critics were as aware of the situation as hospital governing boards; neither effective teaching nor optimum patient care could be expected in such circumstances.

The staffing logic of the ward was at first little altered by the introduction of formal nurse training; the table of organization looked very much the same before and after the establishment of training schools—except that probationers and students replaced the assistants and ambulatory patients who had previously been supervised by the ward (now graduate or senior student) nurse. Descriptions of the tasks assigned assistants before the training school period read very much like those describing the work performed by students under the supposedly new training school regime.[25]

Education and the credential it legitimated had become both inducement and part payment for a key segment of the hospital's labor force. This was an economic logic too compelling to be ignored. Both hospitals and prospective nurses were capital poor; it was only natural for the two parties to barter: work for diplomas. Even hospitals far too small to offer adequate training hastened to establish nursing schools, for training schools guaranteed small-town institutions a cheap and reliable labor supply. "Schools" with a student body of as few as four or five were established without a second thought. Community hospitals almost always operated with minuscule budgets and sought inevitably to save dollars and pennies wherever they could. In many such hospitals, indeed, student nurses not only provided unpaid labor, but became a source of much needed income when sent out on private duty assignments (usually, but not always, during their second year). Their fees were, of course, paid to the hospital. At the Elliot Hospital in Keene, New Hampshire, for example, twenty-two pupil nurses performed 330 weeks of private nursing outside the hospital in 1905; they earned $3,176.13 in a year when the institution's income from all sources was $13,260.96—and of this only $1,749 was paid nurses.[26] Hospital administrators felt few qualms; private duty nursing seemed an appropriate part of nurse training when it was assumed that the vast majority of Americans would never see the inside of a hospital. Student nurses needed to learn the skills necessary for dealing with private patients in their homes.

The logic underlying the feminization of nursing was at least as much economic as ideological. From the very beginnings of the American hospital, men had always been paid more than women for the same work; only the traditional assumption that certain tasks had necessarily to be performed by men justified the expense. Antebellum hospitals, moreover, were ordinarily small, and amounts budgeted for salaries modest. The cost of maintaining a higher scale for an institution's few male nurses was trivial. After the Civil War, however, hospitals grew in size and number and became increasingly cost conscious.

With the coming of the training school, the economic logic of minimizing the number of men employed on the wards soon became apparent to hospital decision makers. Contemporaries were also aware that male nurses were often unwilling to take orders from a woman. The only men on their wards, the superintendent of the Johns Hopkins Hospital reported in 1891, were aides who worked under graduate nurses in the male wards. "They are not trained nurses," he explained, "and I should hesitate to introduce such here for fear of unpleasant clashing in the discharge of duties."[27] Nursing, in addition, offered no opportunities for ambitious men; the important administrative positions were all defined as female. Feminization discouraged men as it attracted women.

The training school also offered hospital administrators noneconomic advantages. This was the everyday presence of a disciplined corps of nurses in the ward—nurses recruited from very different sources than the hospital's urban, working-class patients. They were women who could be subjected to a very different style of socialization. Two kinds of student filled early training school classes. A minority were of middle-class origin inspired by the desire to make a career outside the family. A far greater number were women who desperately needed the opportunity and the few dollars of income each month that went with it. In either case, training school administrators could impose a grueling work schedule and constricting discipline. And no matter what their social origin, student and graduate nurses did not identify with their ward charges as earlier generations of nurses had; their intimidating, uniformed presence made it far easier to impose a due order on the ward and its working-class and often immigrant denizens.

If the training school was functional to the hospital, it was equally so to the women who were its products (and in some sense its victims). The options for dignified employment were few for women in postbellum America; nursing and teaching were two exceptions, soon to be joined by office and sales work. And among these choices, nursing boasted the conspicuous advantage of allowing the prospective nurse to contribute her labor as the cost of entering a credentialed vocation. After two years of exhausting work the nursing graduate could look forward to a lifetime of respectable self-employment. Even so, recruitment was constrained by the fact that the poorest families could not spare the work and possible income of daughters—while those daughters would in any case have been at a competitive disadvantage in the nursing schools.[28] For hospital and nursing superintendents entertained firm ideas of those social characteristics they sought in nurses. These included sensitivity, breeding, and intelligence—code words for middle-class in style of life, education and self-image. Nursing school records indicate a consistent bias against women who appeared "coarse," "like a servant," "direct."[29] The reform of nursing was in some measure the substitution of middle-class for less elevated attitudes and behaviors. Well-brought-up purveyors of mercy and rationality were often shocked when they first walked city hospital wards in the 1870s and 1880s; the indigenous nurses were a particular source of dismay. "Does the nurse taste the sick man's food before him with his spoon to see whether it is right . . . ?

Or put down a heavy quart jar of milk commenting 'Here is your dinner' when the patient was clearly too weak to lift it?"[30] Nurse training schools would presumably put an end to such inappropriate behavior.

Consistently enough, nursing schools were preoccupied with the moral and social characteristics of prospective students and relied heavily in admissions on letters attesting to the candidate's social acceptability. The New York Hospital, for example, explained to references that they were particularly anxious to know if the applicant was ". . . a woman of high moral principle, of fair educational advantages, of exemplary life, stainless name and repute, and refined by associating with people of good social standing. Is she worthy of implicit confidence and respect, in view of her character, antecedents and reputation?" No quality was more important than a student's ability to "conduct herself in a ladylike manner," as a San Francisco physician put it, although students might be rejected if they "seemed unsatisfactory as to grammar, fractions, neatness, etc."[31]

Later in their student careers, women might betray a fatal lack of tact, but such insufficiently passive young women were often from respectable backgrounds and able to surmount the original barriers that protected the "best" nursing schools from the crude and unlettered. In 1902, for example, the superintendent of New York Hospital explained why they had not allowed a particular young lady to advance from her probationer status despite her being a "good worker, of good antecedents and well educated." Unfortunately she lacked subtlety "in polish and refinement of manner and address. This, however, is only a suggestion. There was never any outward expression of it," the administrator conceded, "nor disobedience of orders. Possibly her long experience as a school teacher, wherein she exercised authority over others, may have made it difficult for her to submit. . . ."[32] Submission or at least its outward aspect was a necessary component of the nurse's skills.

Despite early hopes of attracting middle-class women, however, the majority of student nurses at even the most selective schools were not recruited from middle- or upper middle-class families. Many in fact hailed from farms or small towns; a good many were women "on their own" who had tried other work before settling on nursing.[33] Nevertheless, a minority of women from better social backgrounds did enter nurse training during the first half century of American nursing. Among them were daughters of professionals or businessmen, some boasting a solid secondary education as well as the appropriate social style. Day-to-day life in the training school could be difficult for such protected young women. "It is very trying," the superintendent of the Pennsylvania Hospital Training School noted in 1899, "and in some cases, a severe ordeal, for women of refinement to be obliged to share their rooms, more especially in a Training School as mixed as one of this size must necessarily be."[34]

It was such "women of refinement" who were selected from the first to be the supervisors and administrators in America's growing hospital network; the identification of this elite began with their first days as probationers. They were given the most responsible student positions (as night supervisors or acting headships of particular wards) and, of course, recommendations reflecting both their social origins and accumulated responsibilities. A de facto two-track system came into being with the founding of the first training schools. The less ambitious or less well educated were consigned to private duty, their better prepared sisters advanced to administrative positions.[35]

The latter group of graduate nurses could hope for a training school superintendentship in a large urban hospital or an executive position in a small community hospital (where the roles of administrator and chief of nursing were often filled by the same woman). It was a neat system, offering in nursing and hospital administration one of the few executive careers open to women from somewhat better homes—and in private duty nursing, a respectable trade for women with more limited prospects. Thus, despite its initial cost in work and independence, the hospital-based training school offered an option attractive to a variety of American women, and it grew steadily in the half century after the first schools were founded. The expansion paralleled and facilitated expansion of the hospital system itself. And the situation was encouraged by an expanding market; competent graduate nurses with administrative ambitions had little trouble finding positions into at least the early years of the twentieth century.[36] The demand for private duty nurses grew as well. Nursing registries and the supply of skilled private duty nurses expanded to parallel the growth in number and size of hospital training schools. It was a system that seemed to work.

Advocates of nurse training schools could, in general, congratulate themselves; they had supported an innovation that was useful to society in general and to the nurses in particular. Supporters and administrators of hospitals felt they were helping to provide an answer to the dilemma of "what a woman could do"—while providing skilled nursing care not only for hospital patients, but for that far larger number of Americans who would never have entered a hospital.[37]

The Training School: A Would-Be Total Institution

The training school itself reflected both the social assumptions and the relationships of power that characterized the generation of its founding—as well as the mundane advantages that made it so attractive an innovation to hospital administrators and trustees. Practically speaking, it meant an institution in which a rigid and paternalistic discipline shaped every aspect of the student's day and in which the need for ward work superseded every other pedagogic goal.

The aspiring student nurse normally began with a brief probationary period. If she fared well and exhibited no physical or mental weakness, she would be admitted to the regular program. This normally lasted two years, interrupted only by brief (most frequently two-week) vacations each year. The curriculum consisted largely of ward work—more an apprenticeship than schooling. Student nurses worked regular shifts, from seven in the morning until eight at night for day nurses, from eight to seven for night nurses. In practice this meant being awakened by a bell at six, followed by a quick visit to the lavatory and a "bracing cold bath" before breakfast was served at six-thirty. (The half-hour between six and six-thirty was particularly hectic, ". . . and is scarcely sufficient time for keeping the rooms in perfect order, and open for inspection, as they are required to be.")[38] Usually nurses were allowed some free time—at Haverhill's Hale Hospital, for example, one hour after one-thirty each weekday and four hours on Sunday.[39] Student nurses had to fit themselves into the normal ward routine; they learned on the ward and served, in fact, as the backbone of the hospital's work routine.

Most of the schools offered only a few hours a week of formal lectures, normally given by hospital staff members. Even here, the students were limited to a narrow and intensely practical assortment of subjects, taught in a style that recalled grammar school recitations (and reflected the limited academic preparation of a good many student nurses). Students were often expected to make fair copies of their lecture notes and submit them for inspection; content, spelling and grammar were all evaluated. The Hartford Hospital boasted, for example, that its student nurses spent one hour each day in recitation from "the text-book" used in the school; two days a week they received instruction in the diet kitchen, while the house physician gave two other lectures each week.[40] Most physicians believed that nurses were simply not capable of assimilating complex materials. "Experience," as a New York Hospital Medical Board communication explained in 1887, "proves that it is not possible to give any useful instruction to nurses in anatomy and physiology, and that it is as unwise as it is impracticable to teach them anything concerning the causes and effects of disease; nor is it necessary to do this to make them good nurses."[41] It was no accident of bureaucratic usage that decided student nurses were to be "trained," not "educated."

The great bulk of nurse training consisted of manual skills taught by example at the bedside. Abstract learning hindered as much as helped. Worcester's Memorial Hospital described the instruction provided its nursing students in 1895; it included the dressing of burns, blisters, and wounds, the application of leeches, minor dressings, and fomentations, the administration of enemas and baths. Nurses were taught to pass catheters, manage helpless patients so as to prevent bedsores, manufacture bandages, apply splints and bandages—as well as to observe and report their patients' symptoms.[42] Although much was said of the need to separate nursing from domestic service, the great majority of what the student nurse actually did during her long hours on the ward might as well have come under the latter heading. Students changed beds, folded and arranged laundry, swept and scrubbed, waited on patients, and bathed them, while gradually learning to change dressings, administer drugs, and take temperatures.

Given contemporary attitudes toward both cleanliness and order, an absolute distinction between domestic service and the provision of nursing care could not easily have been maintained. The worship of absolute cleanliness (enjoined by the apparent correlation between dirt, disorder, and disease) was a key element of the Nightingale reform position and antedated by a generation the establishment of formal nurse training schools. "Cleanliness," nurses in Troy, New York's Marshall Infirmary were enjoined in 1859, "must be strictly observed in the persons of nurses as well as patients and in the wards and halls as well as the sleeping compartments . . . *neither person nor place should be considered clean if they can be made cleaner.*"[43]

The germ theory only intensified such admonitions.[44] By the 1890s, practical techniques for maintaining cleanliness and order had become the central aspect of nurse training. "Cleanliness & good discipline go together. It is not enough to have an occasional house cleaning," a nursing student in Boston faithfully recorded her professor's admonitions. "This system is the fundamental work of hospitals. Order, system, Good Training, and attention to personal appearance."[45] This was a doctrine that emphasized character and internal discipline and ignored the problematic relationship between those attributes and intellect.

Discipline was severe and unremitting; it was in fact the fundamental training school subject matter. Nurses knew that their rooms might be inspected at any time of the night or day, that impertinence or carelessness might lead to immediate dismissal, that even talking with a house officer might incur the same penalty. (Sympathetic by reason of age and parallel subordination, interns and resident physicians could be outspoken in defending nurses who had been arbitrarily disciplined. Significantly, however, they often blamed female administrators and not male superiors.)[46] An undue familiarity with ward patients could also bring reprimand or even dismissal. Nurses were not allowed to wear jewelry or elaborate hairstyles, and were ordinarily required to purchase "common-sense boots with rubber heels." At most schools a pass was required if the nurse wished to leave the hospital grounds.[47] Paternalism (or maternalism in this case) never questioned its right to control every aspect of the nurse's life and work; it was in fact a necessary aspect of the responsibility that came with status. "The nurses are now well disciplined," a Raleigh hospital reported with satisfaction in 1902, "not allowed to leave the grounds without a chaparrone [sic], and required to be in their rooms by ten oclock at night." Having only a small student body, they added unselfconsciously, the students could not be spared "from the practical work of nursing long enough to have lectures."[48] Contemporaries doubted neither the practical advantages nor the morally appropriate nature of such authoritarian—and dubiously educational—relationships. Although some administrators questioned the hours and arduousness of nurse training, few challenged the structured subordination within which that work was performed.

Exploring New Options: The Goals of Nursing Reform

Nevertheless, increasingly egregious flaws in the world of nurse training were soon to become the agenda for a thoroughgoing reform program. An energetic and ambitious core of nursing superintendents, with the aid of like-thinking medical men, called for a recasting of nurse training, an improvement reflecting in attenuated form the parallel movement for reform in medical education. The intellectual content of nurse training was to be made more demanding, while as a necessary prerequisite, hours of ward work were to be curtailed and the course lengthened from two to three years. Physical conditions too needed improving; nurses should not be required to live in attics and basements with no access to facilities for study or recreation. Hospitals with only a handful of beds or limited clinical services should not be allowed to allege that they provided adequate training. The rapid development of careers in administration—as training school superintendents and community hospital administrators—required the creation of at least some postgraduate training programs. As a final step, most reformers urged that states institute the registration of nurses (in connection with the standardization of nursing school curricula).

The key irritant was clearly the nature of training itself: the long hours, the repetition of menial work, the lack of intellectual content, the inconsistency between programs. Henry M. Hurd, for example, superintendent of the Johns Hopkins Hospital, was one of the medical establishment's more prominent advocates of improved nursing education. Hurd contended that increasing knowledge and growing demands on the trained nurse implied that the standard training course be lengthened to three years of appropriately graded material. This was dependent, of course, on reducing work schedules. The Hopkins superintendent suggested a modest decrease to eight hours of ward work each day with two hours free for study. Smaller hospitals must, he urged, either close their so-called training programs or cooperate with other institutions so as to provide their students with adequate clinical experience; curricula could hardly be standardized when hospitals with as few as forty or fifty beds claimed to provide effective nurse training. Hurd was particularly scornful of institutions that sent untrained students out to work in private homes and then pocketed their fees. "The position of the nurse thus sent away from the school was akin to that of the tourist in the Cannibal Islands," he quipped, "who, when he was welcomed to a feast, found to his surprise that he was personally expected to provide the meal."

The effect of such a practice has been altogether bad. The nurse doubtless learns something of human nature by these semi-charitable excursions into the homes of the well-to-do; but . . . she loses far more than she gains. Orderly, systematic instruction under competent supervision is impossible.[49]

Hurd was not alone in such sentiments, but like most other elite critics he was well aware of the economic realities that made it so difficult for the great majority of hospitals to reduce hours on the ward and spare student nurses the repetitive round of scrubbing and washing that filled so much of their time. "At least ten hours a day," another medical man explained, the student nurse was "compelled to be upon her feet, constantly attending to the necessity and the whims of a sick patient. Ten hours a day she is compelled to do things that she has done time and time again. Ten hours a day she is compelled to smile and look pleasant under all circumstances." The belief was gaining ground, as one authority argued in 1911, that only those hospitals "which are willing that the school should be an expense rather than an economy" had the moral right to maintain a nursing school.[50]

No one aware of training school realities could ignore the often grim physical circumstances in which the first generation of professional nurses lived and worked. As early as 1888, for example, New York Hospital's Board of Governors confessed that their nursing staff occupied small, crowded, and low-ceilinged rooms originally designed for servants. High rates of sickness underlined the need to provide better facilities for student and graduate nurses. At the Cincinnati General Hospital, almost a sixth of the nursing force were on the sick list, proving that "working 12 hours in a crowded ward, and sleeping in small rooms immediately adjacent thereto, in many cases opening directly from the wards, requires a strength of constitution far above the average."[51] Such arguments were often effective, and by the First World War, most respectable nurse training schools boasted physically separate residences with facilities for washing, study, and recreation. But this steady progress toward improving physical amenities was an atypically successful—and noncontroversial—aspect of nursing reform.[52]

In retrospect the movement was doomed to only limited achievement. Attempts to raise the economic and social status and increase the autonomy of nursing were plagued by divided goals, external opposition, and an inconsistent and self-defeating public image. Every factor that had facilitated the creation of this novel enterprise conspired ultimately to limit and constrain its professional horizons.

The relationship between nursing and medicine was particularly problematic. Yet the fortunes of the two groups were indissolubly related; medicine's ever increasing authority did help legitimate the social claims of nursing, and individual physicians were in many cases advocates of nurse training and appreciative of the newly trained nurses' clinical skills. Nevertheless, the nature of their relationship presumed the subordination of nursing—in the hospital and in patient care generally.

It is no accident that commentators on the relationship between doctor and nurse were so fond of military and nautical metaphors; in each sphere the chain of authority was sacred. "When two generals with equal authority attempt to manipulate the same army," as one physician put it, "the battle is generally lost."[53] A ship could not be commanded by two captains nor a business by two managing directors. Most physicians felt that disciplined subordination was the essence of professionalism in nursing. When away from a patient, the physician saw through the nurse's eyes. "She is the passive agent." As a consequence, the physician had "the right to expect that cordial submissive cooperation which complete sympathy alone can insure, . . ." When her training "has been thorough" the nurse could be relied upon, unless she was "illy adapted to her work and self sufficient, self opinionated, . . ."[54] In the sick room especially, the medical man could tolerate no questioning of his authority; the patient needed to maintain faith in his or her practitioner— and physicians were often uneasy at the prospect of working with knowledgeable and opinionated trained nurses.[55]

Despite such qualms, most American hospital physicians were at first relatively supportive of training schools, although some had been skeptical from the first. Opponents were concerned that they might as a consequence of their need for skilled and reliable labor be tolerating the creation of a rival profession that would contest their clinical authority. The secular ward nurse could, before the Nightingale dispensation, call upon neither social status nor formal credentials to buttress her position in the hospital hierarchy. The aggressive demands of the early English reformers especially seemed to threaten an undermining of due medical control. Leading authorities on hospital administration, both English and American, united in their opposition to separate and autonomous female-headed training schools.[56] The training school might be tolerable, but only if subject to the hospital's superintendent and medical board.

The feminization of nursing promised at first an ambiguous equity for medical men. While women could hardly be expected to master the physician's cognitive skills and challenge that aspect of his authority, they could marshal a different kind of authority, that based on their peculiar capacity to function in a sphere of emotion and empathy less amenable to man's more analytic capacities. Especially when these attributes were united with high social status, the nursing superintendent promised to be a tenacious antagonist. But such fears were generally short lived.

Nursing was to attract few women of high social status, while the presumed attributes of femininity served on balance to underscore woman's necessary subordination in medical care. Sacrifice, devotion, and sensitivity, not intellect and decisiveness, were woman's appropriate contribution to the physician and nurse team. The formulas of conventional rhetoric were clear enough. "Truly," as one orator put it, "since God could not care for all the sick, he made women to nurse."[57] Fears that aggressive "new women" might come to dominate professionalized nursing were allayed by reassurance that, "her art is ancient history" and that nursing did not desex its practitioners, but was instead an ideal preparation for woman's "highest potential function in life"—marriage and motherhood. "What kind of a wife would a trained nurse make who did not abandon her calling?"[58] Hospital publications often boasted of their nurses' attractive appearance. "When one sees them in their dainty uniforms," a Richmond hospital promotional circular simpered, "the suspicion that they were selected with regard to their comeliness is hard to suppress."[59]

Not surprisingly, medical fears that trained nurses would prove restless in their subordination proved to have little basis in reality. Nevertheless, even sympathetic physicians were reluctant to expand the intellectual content of nurse education—perhaps the central demand of early twentieth-century nursing reform.[60] When in 1903, for example, the medical board of New York's Presbyterian Hospital endorsed reform in their institution's nursing curriculum, the board's goals were carefully and typically circumscribed. They resolved that "the scope of bacteriology, chemistry, and urinanalysis be limited and confined to practical instruction; and that instruction in chemistry, if possible, be given in connection with teaching the principles of diet and cooking." The report recommended as well that the hours devoted to anatomy and physiology "be restricted" and that "the study of materia medica be restricted to practical instruction in poisons, antiseptics and the preparation of solutions."[61] Too much knowledge was not necessarily a good thing. "A nurse may be over-educated," as one physician put it, but "she can never be over-trained."[62]

Upgrading the intellectual content of nurse training not only implied potential conflicts of authority, it conflicted directly with the hospital's labor requirements. A student in the lecture room or laboratory was not available to make beds, empty bedpans, and change dressings (or to be sent out on private duty). Such frills as physiology, pathology, or anatomy were in any case hardly appropriate to the better performance of such humble duties.

Even enthusiastic reformers conceded that most nursing skills would inevitably have to be learned at the bedside. Critics were equally well aware, however, that this aspect of nurse training could also be inadequate, no matter how many hours the student might spend on the ward. Even in the best-run hospitals, the number of graduate nurses was so small that they could rarely provide adequate instruction to their supposed apprentices. Increasing the numbers of experienced graduate nurses increased salary costs—for many institutions no option at all. In every hospital, students complained of the endless hours spent in the ritual performance of routine cleaning—meticulous folding of sheets and making of beds, the fanatical dusting of baseboards and windowsills.

Nursing reform was particularly threatening to community hospitals. The smallness of their scale implied a parallel fragility of budget and made them particularly dependent on students.[63] Yet the very paucity of their beds also made it almost impossible for such community hospitals to offer student nurses adequate clinical opportunities. Reform threatened to demoralize small hospitals; many conceded that they would not be able to continue without training schools.[64] A few responded by working out cooperative programs with other hospitals, but in the first decade of the century, most hoped that such reform efforts would simply go away.[65]

By the First World War, however, nursing reformers could claim that many of their educational goals had been attained. The three-

year curriculum was a reality in the better schools and the intellectual content of nurse training had been expanded as well.[66] Most
schools boasted separate residences for their student nurses and
admitted classes at regular intervals rather than on the basis of
mutual convenience. Hours of ward work were somewhat shorter
and in many of the better schools nurses were no longer paid a
salary, but instead provided uniforms or cut-rate fabric from which
to make them. Doing away with monthly stipends allowed the
schools to increase the number of students and supervising graduate
nurses. In 1904, for example, the Worcester Memorial Hospital
trustees decided to extend their training course from two to three
years, to shorten the hours of work, and to discontinue paying
salaries. They conceded that the inexorable increase in medical
knowledge demanded a parallel upgrading in the nursing course.[67]
The beginnings of nursing specialization were already discernible—
in operating room, anesthesiology, administration, and public
health.[68]

The movement for state registration of nurses provided another
occasion to restate the same reformist themes. For many licensing
proposals turned on accreditation of nurse training schools—and
thus the validity of existing curricula. But this new strategy for
expanding nursing autonomy mobilized immediate opposition.

When reformers turned to the states' power to improve nursing
education and legitimate the field, they were opposed by many
physicians who saw in the registration of nurses a threat to their
authority. If nurses were licensed, they would, as hostile practitioners put it, feel that they too were professionals and thus licensed to
contradict the physician as well as practice nursing. As one outspoken doctor put it, contemporary nursing was flawed by the idea
". . . which prevails to some extent among nurses that nursing is a
'profession' like that of medicine, law or theology."[69] Registration
would, as another physician argued at a public meeting to discuss
the question, be a "positive menace to the public good." It was
simply a mercenary scheme by hospital-trained nurses to monopo-
lize the field. "Isolated and individual opposition to the will of the
physician may be overlooked, but *organized opposition,* with a show of
legal authority to apparently justify it, must *command prompt and effective resistance!*"[70] Many nurses who had graduated from marginal
schools or failed to complete training programs at larger ones also
opposed registration. Advocates had to wage an uphill fight in state

after state before registration became a familiar and accustomed part of nursing's vocational landscape.[71]

Other aspects of the reform struggle were equally ambiguous, particularly the ideology that had originally helped legitimate the demands of midnineteenth-century nursing activists. Most ironically, the fact that nursing had quickly and effectively become feminized helped limit the potential for reform; contemporaries could hardly credit the intellectual and institutional claims of a female-dominated profession. Medical men who found it easy to support demands for improved living conditions in nursing schools found it less easy to endorse requests for more lectures or laboratory work. Not surprisingly, discussion of nursing's intellectual content often turned on its unique ability to provide order and efficiency in the ward and sickroom and not on discipline-specific cognitive skills. The efficiency argument, however, like the emphasis on female sensibility, was a double-edged sword. For efficiency also implied hierarchy; and order implied subordination, and if scientific knowledge and clinical responsibility legitimated medical authority, the nurse could only frame her demands for improved status in terms that reaffirmed her subordination to medicine and medical science. She could help apply but not master the knowledge that seemed increasingly to underlie medical status.[72]

Like the traditional emphasis on her essential femininity, emphasis on the nurse's ability to deal with emotions and environment now served to demonstrate her inability to gain mastery of the impressive new knowledge that had come to dominate the medical profession's understanding of disease causation and treatment. The holistic and antireductionist pathology of the midnineteenth century was no longer an appropriate style of legitimation for a profession that claimed scientific credentials, even reflected ones. Self-abnegation too was a double-edged sword, as nurses discovered when their economic demands were dismissed as materialistic if not indeed unionistic. "You will often be repaid by gratitude," as one prominent medical man counseled, "and if not, then repay yourself with thankfulness for opportunities for helpfulness."[73]

Nurses had attained a status somewhat higher than domestic help, but clearly beneath that of physicians and their private patients. It was natural for a hospital administrator in 1912 to make a division of the hospital's inhabitants into three groups: "(1) the help, (2) the nurses and ward patients, (3) the staff and private patients."[74] Similarly, a nagging problem in private duty nursing was the relationship between nurse and household servants; would the nurse, for example, eat with the servants? by herself? with the family?

Until the 1920s, the system seemed to work relatively well. Hospitals expanded dramatically; in 1923, there were almost seven thousand in America and roughly a fourth of them housed nursing schools.[75] Women still had comparatively few vocational options, especially ones in which there was some prospect of achieving administrative responsibility. The market for private duty nursing had expanded as well, if rather less rapidly. Thus, there were places in abundance in training schools and a promise of employment for their graduates.[76] For the most ambitious and socially oriented graduate nurses, public health work seemed to promise a new area of usefulness and autonomy away from the hospital's hierarchical constraints and the physicians' control.[77]

By the end of the 1920s, however, nursing was experiencing a sense of frustration and crisis. The hospitals, driven by their own needs (and able to draw upon a supply of women who sought a career away from the factory or office), were producing an increasing supply of nurses for a private practice market expanding far less rapidly. The number of families able to employ nurses in their homes was limited, and the hospital was becoming more and more central to medical practice, yet hospitals were only gradually adjusting to the need for employing graduate nurses. The expansion of public health nursing had come to an abrupt halt. Grudging support for public medicine and competition from physicians in private practice and the hospital had conspired to discourage this new style of nursing practice. The depression only exacerbated matters. Nursing assumed the shape that has led to several generations of anxious self-searching and reform proposals.

The germs of this crisis were present from the very beginnings of the field: the hospitals' hunger for a cheap, reliable, and orderly labor supply, the feminization of nursing, the very ideology that originally justified the creation of this new profession, all interacted to constrain the options available to nurses. The autonomy supposed to characterize professions has to some degree always escaped it; nursing has been in good measure a dependent variable in the equation of social and economic forces that created and shaped it.

CHAPTER 10

The Private Patient
Revolution

In mid-nineteenth-century America it was well understood that, aside from an occasional emergency, none but the truly indigent would voluntarily enter a hospital; the working poor preferred to pay a local practitioner if they could or tolerate a dispensary physician's casual visits. Only when length or severity of sickness overtaxed family resources would they consider hospital care; "there are large numbers of clerks, mechanics, and artisans, and strangers," the superintendent of New York Hospital explained in 1858, "whose needs require, but whose feelings revolt at the idea of a hospital."[1] It would be no easy task to overcome such fears.

By the First World War all this had changed. Respectable Americans were beginning to find their way into hospitals—especially, but not exclusively, for surgery. This change was taking place not only in established urban institutions, but in a network of hospitals that had mushroomed in thousands of smaller communities—many in areas where such institutions were a novelty and where a hospital stay had never carried with it the stigma of indigence. The hospital was being integrated into medical care as it already had been into medical education and the structuring of elite careers. To some extent this was a response to new technical capacities, but it was a response shaped by social and economic realities as well. Hospital budgets, physicians' practice patterns, attitudes toward science, charity, and the prerogatives of class—as well as the x-ray, antiseptic surgery, and clinical laboratories—interacted to transform the early twentieth-century American hospital.

As the new-model hospital became an increasingly important aspect of private medical practice, it changed both its social and economic profile. The nonprofit voluntary hospital ceased to be an embodiment of traditional urban paternalism and became ever more dependent on patient fees and thus the referrals of admitting physicians. Some older institutions were hesitant to enter the fee-for-service marketplace. In many private hospitals, however, the traditional vision of disinterested benevolence had never described the institution's actual operations. Limited endowments meant that the great majority of nineteenth-century hospitals had always sought to maximize income from patients just as they eagerly solicited the support of municipal, county, and state governments. In the early years of the present century a new factor emerged, a vigorous crop of private and proprietary hospitals that competed for fee-paying patients with unabashed and unambiguous enthusiasm.[2]

By the 1920s, the great majority of nonmunicipal hospitals had become dependent on income from patient care. Hospitals had become increasingly prominent in the medical care of ordinary Americans and in the practice of the physicians and surgeons who treated them. And those practitioners, on the other hand, whose referrals filled hospital beds grew increasingly prominent in hospital decision making. In alliance with the growing prestige of scientific medicine, these pragmatic realities had restructured the hospital's internal order. An uneasy equilibrium had been established that would last until the depression posed new problems and impelled new solutions. At the same time, the gap between charity and paying patients continued to shape relationships within individual voluntary hospitals and between municipal and voluntary institutions. Social relations still re-enacted themselves in the hospital's smaller world.

Making Do: Financing the Gilded-Age Hospital

A few postbellum American hospitals did have substantial endowments—such established institutions as the New York, Pennsylvania, and Massachusetts General hospitals and prominent newcomers such as Roosevelt and Presbyterian in New York, and Johns Hopkins in Baltimore. But the great majority of hospitals in the 1870s and 80s pieced together annual budgets with an eclectic mixture of contributions from local government, endowment income, the proceeds of community fundraising, and the fees of occasional private patients (as well as payments for individuals whose care could be billed to city or county governments).[3] Voluntary hospitals were always seen as clothed with the public interest even when their legal character was entirely private and their governing boards private and self-perpetuating. No sharp division separated the public and private sector, except insofar as those urban hospitals seen as *exclusively* municipal could not well compete for philanthropic support or the patronage of private patients.[4]

No American hospital in 1875 had an endowed income sufficient to underwrite the free medical care its community required. Even the century-old and atypically wealthy Pennsylvania Hospital, for example, found that its investment income totaled only $30,000 in 1867, when its annual expenses amounted to almost twice that much. In the previous decade, the hospital's endowment had covered almost all its current expenses.[5] Endowment tended, in any case, to be used in the purchase of land and construction of buildings. Few institutions had been successful in raising funds producing income equal to any substantial portion of their operating costs. Annual deficits had to be met by board members and appeals to the wealthy and benevolent. "Instead of securing a fund sufficient to guarantee a steady and permanent revenue to meet the probable current expenses," as one hospital explained its financial dilemma, "we are compelled to rely on individual benefactions, which unfortunately are too apt to cease with the emergency which prompts their bestowal."[6] Trustees of the generous bequest that established New York's Roosevelt Hospital were atypical in their far-sighted decision to reserve a portion of their endowment sufficient to support free care for half the hospital's beds; the other half, they assumed, would be occupied by "a class of industrious and worthy persons with small means, able and willing to pay for their support in a hospital."[7] It was an expectation that failed to survive a few years of discouraging experience; paying patients could help in a small way, but hardly make a major contribution to the budget of a large urban hospital in this period.[8]

Yet paying patients had often played a role in the optimistic financial scenarios of hard-pressed trustees. There was no time at which hospital boards had not sought to provide a few private rooms for that minority of patients who made use of hospitals as "convenient rather than as charitable" institutions and who would, of course, have been unwilling to be treated in common wards. "In a well regulated hospital," trustees of the Hartford Hospital argued at midcentury, there should be "private rooms for all those who are willing to pay for superior accommodations, at a comparatively small expense."[9] It made for better medical care as well as providing some income to the hospital (at least insofar as it allowed the institution to treat a larger number of patients without increasing income from endowment and donations). Even most municipal hospitals sought to provide accommodation for the occasional paying patient—"strangers, of means sufficient to defray the expenses of their sickness but without home or friends in the city" or "a few patients of the better class, who may be compelled by accident to avail themselves of hospital aid."[10] Hospital administrators were realistic and their assumed categories of potential paying patients were both limited and sharply defined.[11]

Religious and ethnic hospitals were generally more successful in attracting the elusive paying patient of modest means. Such institutions were often small and seemed to prospective patients very different from the impersonal, alien, and alienating general hospitals. To be treated by a religious woman and to pay a modest sum for one's room and board transformed a hospital stay for Catholics into something less painful and humiliating than it would have in a large, nonsectarian—that is, Protestant—voluntary hospital. And the nursing sisters' own vocation helped subsidize Catholic hospitals, their unpaid labor supplementing limited endowments. The mid-century medical board of Philadelphia's newly founded Episcopal Hospital were discouraged at the prospect of competing with St. Joseph's; the Sisters of Mercy, they reported, were "but a trifling expense . . . beyond their support." Most of the Catholic hospital's paying patients were charged three dollars a week, "which as their ordinary board in town is $2.50, they are put to a cost of only 50 cents per week additional, for which they receive medicines and medical attendance."[12]

Hospitals pursued a variety of tactics to support their work. One, of course, was lobbying; municipalities and some state governments such as Pennsylvania and Connecticut had a long history of providing annual grants toward current expenses or support for occasional capital improvements. Another widely employed fundraising tactic was that of soliciting endowments for free beds. This stratagem was particularly successful in the last third of the nineteenth century. Prospective donors were assured that an endowment of several thousand dollars would permanently support a free bed. At New York's Presbyterian Hospital, $5,000 endowed a bed in perpetuity, $4,000 during two lives, and $3,000 for one.[13] (Three hundred dollars was a figure generally agreed upon as approximating the annual cost of maintaining a free bed.)[14] Individuals or families providing such funds were often allowed to designate the bed's occupant as well. "The possession of the right," the Roosevelt Hospital assured prospective donors in 1872, "either for life, or in perpetuity, of having received and cared for, in such a hospital, any sick person requiring such aid, is certainly sufficiently desirable to induce any benevolent person to become its possessor."[15]

This relic of traditional paternalism was to become increasingly vestigial as the century drew to a close and as medical men and medical diagnoses increasingly dominated admission procedures. Endowments for specific beds were aggregated into general funds and admission decisions made by physicians on medical grounds alone. This change in the meaning of free bed sponsorship neatly symbolizes a more general transition from the personal and deferential benevolence of the late eighteenth-century hospital to the impersonal and bureaucratic relationships that were to become increasingly important in its successor a century later.

Free beds were only one of several devices that hard-pressed and resourceful hospitals employed to underwrite operating costs. Business firms sometimes paid for employees and beneficial societies for members' hospital expenses—usually at a per diem rate negotiated each year with the particular hospital.[16] Community churches could be organized to devote special collections on one Sunday each year to their hospitals.[17] Women's committees could also be an important source of funds; energetic ladies organized musicales and theatricals, canvassed door to door, and catered teas and garden parties in an effort to supplement limited hospital budgets. Their goals were often quite specific—purchasing an x-ray apparatus, for example, sewing new gowns, or outfitting an aseptic operating room.

Prepayment was another, less common, if prescient tactic for underwriting patient care. One form was indirect; benevolent societies might negotiate reduced fees for their members.[18] Other hospitals, especially ethnic institutions and surgical hospitals in timber and mining areas, organized schemes through which individual workers could prepay medical care by subscribing small sums each week or month. A consortium of fourteen midwestern Catholic hospitals, for example, sold certificates for $7.50 entitling the purchaser to treatment at any one of the cooperating institutions for a year from the date of sale. Brockton shoe-workers could pay a dollar for a certificate that guaranteed twelve days of hospital treatment in the following year; the payment of ten cents a month purchased one "day's hospital treatment for each monthly payment, within the year."[19] Such prepayment schemes were widespread at the end of the century; for sums ranging from ten to fifty cents a month, subscribers could ensure medical care for themselves, an employee, or family member at a variety of local hospitals.[20] But such arrangements seem more significant in retrospect than they were effective in practice; prepayment exerted only a small effect on the finances of most late nineteenth-century hospitals.

Even though budgets remained small and the cost per patient week remained under two dollars at most institutions, hospitals in the 1870s and 1880s were hard put to balance their books at the end of each year. The situation was only to deteriorate. Some aspects of the problem were diffuse and gradual, reflecting more general economic and technological change. By the end of the century, hospital physicians and administrators expected to have telephone service, electric lights, central steam plants, modern dishwashing and laundry plants, and ambulances (first horse-drawn, then electric, finally gasoline). Aseptic surgery demanded special facilities as did the x-ray and clinical laboratory; newer esthetic and hygienic standards required more frequent changes of linen and gowns. "This is an aseptic age of surgery," as one contemporary surgeon-administrator defended increasing expenditures: "It is easier to preserve health and to restore the crippled where absolute cleanliness is observed throughout every branch of the hospital." It was only to be expected that the cost of "maintaining a well-equipped hospital" would be much greater than that of a simple welfare institution.[21]

In actuality, however, costs relating directly to medical and surgical care remained a relatively small part of hospital budgets; food, fuel, and wages consumed the lion's share of hospital funds. Meanwhile costs of land, construction, and the consequent maintenance of larger physical plants increased steadily—as did the numbers of dependent patients. Aggregate outpatient as well as inpatient expenditures rose steadily, although costs per patient day remained relatively stable during the last quarter of the century.[22] Even with the "contributions" in kind of nurses and house staff reducing labor costs, no hospital could escape the inexorable pressure of rising costs.

The troubled economic years following what has come to be called the panic of 1893 only exacerbated the situation; hard times increased patient demand while making it more difficult to solicit funds.[23] At the Johns Hopkins Hospital, for example, expenses had increased by more than eleven thousand dollars in the year ending January 31, 1894, while receipts had declined slightly. The explanation was simple: the hospital had provided 6,293 more patient days, even though per capita costs had actually declined by eight cents a day. Such deficits could become cumulative. The Worcester Memorial Hospital, for example, reported in 1900 that its income had not equaled expenditures for the past half dozen years. Chicago's St. Luke's Hospital explained in 1898 that hard times had reduced expected income from its real estate holdings, along with its accustomed contributions from diocesan churches.[24] The immediate response, as it had always been in conservatively administered philanthropies, was to reduce expenditures. Well-run hospitals sought to monitor cash flow on a monthly or even weekly basis. Attending physicians were urged to cut the average length of patient stays and reduce the expense of drugs and surgical dressings.[25] Wages might be cut and food costs trimmed, while administrators importuned local governments and affluent board members with more than ordinary insistence. In extreme cases, hospitals might close wards (a severe measure indeed given steadily increasing patient demand). But none of these tactics seemed to offer a fundamental solution to the voluntary hospital's economic dilemma. There was a limit to the savings that could be attained through institutional belt tightening.

Outside the hospital, municipal governments were themselves trying to cut costs; city hospitals were in no better position than their voluntary counterparts. Even in the best of times, one constant in American hospital history had been the difficulty of forcing local and county governments to underwrite the full cost of caring for indigent patients at private institutions. Private hospital trustees and administrators were, moreover, hostile to the public sector and anxious to preserve the distance they had always maintained between themselves and their municipal counterparts. If things did not improve, the trustees of New York's Presbyterian Hospital warned in 1904, tax-supported municipal hospitals would inevitably take the place of "our present hospitals, which are private only in the sense that they were founded and have been supported by private benevolence." Such hospitals, the argument diffidently continued, were ". . . under the direction of managers recruited by natural selection from our best citizens, and not subject, as is too often the case with municipal hospitals, to political change or popular caprice."[26] For most urban hospitals, at least part of the solution to remaining viable and independent lay in maximizing income from private patients. For many smaller institutions it had always been a condition of existence.

Enter the Private Patient

Between 1880 and the First World War, respectable Americans began for the first time to consider hospital care a plausible option when they or members of their families fell ill.[27] "There is a growing belief," one hospital authority observed in 1911, "that a hospital is, or should be, a better place for a sick man than his own home however rich that home, and consequently private hospitals and endowed hospitals are preparing to accommodate an ever-increasing and ever more varied demand. . . ."[28] This was a somewhat sanguine, but fundamentally accurate, view; they may not always have been comfortable about it, but increasing numbers of Americans were in fact being treated in hospital wards and private rooms.

The precise reasons for this new willingness remain obscure. It is an obscurity that is a consequence of the seeming inevitability and desirability of this attitudinal change. Until relatively recent years, the growing willingness of prosperous Americans to enter hospitals had seemed to historians and sociologists no more than a natural response to the new technical resources of the medical profession allied with the changed domestic ecology of an increasingly urban population. By 1900, the home seemed no longer the ideal site for diagnosis and treatment of severe illness—as it had still been a quarter century before.[29] In addition, few Americans who sought to treat family members at home possessed the space, servants, and leisure, as well as dollars to hire the private duty nurses demanded by new standards of care. Thus a seemingly more effective technology allied with the intractable logistics of patient care conspired to channel ever-increasing numbers of patients into the early twentieth-century hospital.

This is the traditional and commonsensical view, but it has a number of difficulties. One, as we have implied, is its failure to consider the hospital's positive role in attracting patients, or, on the other hand, its failure to confront the depth of patient resistance. We need to understand more about the factors determining the thousands of separate individual decisions in which that traditional antipathy was overcome. This conventional view rests moreover on an assumed but largely unexamined change in late nineteenth-century lay attitudes toward and expectations of medicine and its technical resources. Middle-class Americans almost certainly did entertain a growing faith in the efficacy of medicine—but how, when, and how widely such attitudes were diffused and how they shaped medical care decisions remains unclear. Attitudes are difficult to evaluate in the present; past attitudes are even more elusive.

The least ambiguous aspect of the private patient question was, in fact, hospital needs and expectations. Most private institutions had consistently sought to maximize the number of private patients they treated. Many provided private rooms and even wings years before a demand for them existed. Again and again, hospitals found such facilities underutilized. From the 1870s on, hospitals had sought to present an inviting and increasingly scientific image to the public. In annual reports and planted newspaper stories, they underlined two themes—first, that their private rooms offered the comfort and convenience of a hotel with the ambience of a home; and second, that professional care and a newly effective technology could only be provided in a hospital. Their private rooms, a North Carolina hospital assured, "are daintily furnished either in oak or white furniture, but every bed is of white enamel or brass with springs and hair mattresses." Any citizen would "find it both pleasant and profitable to pay a visit to this home like systematically managed hospital." Several years later, a new hospital in Richmond was careful to reassure prospective patients that every scientific precaution would be utilized in their treatment. "All the *linen is sterilized* after being laundered, and the *beds are sterilized* after being vacated before other patients are assigned to them. *All germs are destroyed,*" the hospital publicist explained, "by the best and most scientific means—steam heat under pressure." Sterile procedures were, of course, followed with particular scrupulousness in the operating room. "Before operating, the surgeon divests himself of his clothes, takes a shower-bath, dons his sterilized operating suit, sterilizes his hands and arms, puts on rubber gloves and then enters the operating room, where he is enveloped in his sterilized operating cap and gown."[30] Invoking the rituals of science reassured prospective patients, as they justified more generally the social place of America's new temples of healing.

Despite the reiteration of such confident descriptions, however, resistance to hospital care was not easily overcome. No single factor can, in fact, explain the change. The most important were the new promise of surgery, the role of individual physicians, and finally the increasing convenience and economic attractiveness of the hospital as compared with home care.

Urban hospitals soon discovered that private rooms set aside for medical cases remained empty while their surgical counterparts were consistently occupied.[31] Educated Americans were aware by the turn of the century that the elaborate procedures and apparatus required by aseptic surgery were best provided in the hospital's operating and recovery rooms, and that postoperative nursing and medical care were not easily arranged, even in the homes of the very rich. As one hospital spokesman contended at the turn of the century, "The great improvement in the character and management of hospitals which has come about within the last few years through the introduction of antisepsis, a more practical knowledge and application of measures for preventing the spread of disease, and especially through the service of the trained nurse, has almost completely revolutionized public sentiment with regard to these institutions. The prejudices that were so hard to combat only a few years ago have been largely overcome."[32]

This is not to suggest that the change in surgical practice patterns was abrupt or universal. Physicians' memoirs make clear that even major operations were sometimes, and minor procedures often, performed in private homes. Surgical and nursing textbooks of the period provide instructions for the rough-and-ready preparation of ordinary bedrooms or kitchens for surgery. But with each succeeding year it had become clearer that such makeshifts were far from ideal.

From the elite physician's viewpoint, of course, the hospital was a far more convenient as well as safer place to practice than patients' homes scattered about a crowded city or sprawling countryside. The hospital not only possessed the proper tools, it allowed the doctor to see a larger number of patients in a shorter period of time, and it provided (in many cases) a resident physician on call day and night and a supply of trained nurses. No longer would established practitioners have to spend so many of their productive hours in travel; no longer would they have to negotiate arrangements with younger doctors to provide clinical backup in private homes; no longer would they be plagued by the need to find and oversee private duty nurses and worry about their interaction with invalids, their families, and their servants.

As early as the 1890s, at least some eminent surgeons were beginning to limit their practice to the hospital. In 1894, for example, Nicholas Senn, Chicago's most prominent surgeon, explained to his Boston peer J. Collins Warren that he enjoyed "continuous service" at St. Joseph's and Presbyterian hospitals (that is, he did not serve a three- or four-month tour of duty). "It is here I earn my daily bread," he explained, "because I have not the time to operate in private houses."[33] For the urban surgical elite, attending and admitting privileges at large voluntary hospitals allowed them to teach (on the wards) and practice (in private and semiprivate rooms) in the same institution.[34]

Although we naturally think of attitudinal and social change as we try to understand the new willingness of middle-class patients to accept hospital treatment, the key factor in most individual decisions was probably a practitioner's advice. "Excluding accident cases," the superintendent of a small hospital explained in 1914, "over 75 per cent of all patients admitted are sent in by the physician in charge of the case, who generally arranges with us in advance for the patient's admission, states the probable diagnosis, and, when possible, informs us whether the incoming patient is to go into a private room or the ward."[35]

This is not to underestimate the often cramped domestic settings of urban life and the realities of income distribution in shaping these medical care decisions. A comparatively small proportion of late nineteenth- and early twentieth-century urban Americans possessed the combination of space, leisure, and domestic help, the savings to pay for a physician's frequent visits in severe or incapacitating conditions; the hospital could provide all of these with greater convenience and often at lower total cost. "I am going to the New York Hospital at 11 o'clock today," a middle-class woman wrote to her mother in 1909. Her physician had, she explained, told her it was "the finest hospital in New York, & that I will be absolutely comfortable there." The doctor had just let her know "that there was a cheap room vacant that I could get, $25 a week." Her husband had at first opposed her entering the hospital and "wanted to get a nurse & keep me here. But when we talked the matter over seriously last night, we decided the hospital was the best." Our regular servants were ignorant of medical matters while "a nurse is so in the way in this small house. I get absolute rest & freedom from care at the hospital—it [doesn't] cost quite so much as the nurse." Her physician, finally, had reassured her that "he has lots of patients down there—& will see me every day."[36] Just such a calculus of pragmatic consideration in a context of shifting attitude and technical capability must have shaped the decisions of many thousands of families as they reasoned together, seeking the best medical care for family members.

Growth of the Community Hospital

Nowhere was the private patient's role more prominent than in the abundant crop of community hospitals that sprouted in the three decades before America entered the First World War. Some were proprietary, some industrial, a greater number nonprofit, but almost all shared a common dependence on the dollars of private patients and the desire of local physicians to integrate the hospital into their routine of practice. All those factors that convinced elite urban practitioners to embrace the hospital applied to their small-town counterparts, with the intractable reality of longer distances underlining the hospital's appeal.[37] Rural physicians had always spent a substantial proportion of their time in travel, a reality reflected in the way medical society fee bills characteristically specified mileage charges just as they did the fees for particular procedures. The hospital offered the great advantage of bringing the patient or patients to the physician, especially in those severe ills that might have otherwise demanded daily visits to scattered homes. In the majority of towns and small cities, hospitals offered admitting privileges to all "respectable" physicians, avoiding the factionalism that often arose in larger cities.

Small town hospitals were ordinarily community institutions in a very literal—participatory—sense. The opening of a new hospital was the occasion for celebration and proud inspections. The Morton Hospital in Taunton, Massachusetts, opened on January 3, 1889, for example, and on the next two days, thirteen hundred curious townspeople strolled through the novel institution and signed its visitors' books.[38] Fairs, bake sales, theatricals, church collections, and baseball games helped flesh out modest budgets. Most such community hospitals were relatively free from the taint of dependence and pauperism that stigmatized their urban predecessors. The gradient of reluctance among prospective patients could not have been as steep as in many older communities.

Even more than in urban general hospitals, community hospitals were overwhelmingly surgical, a factor that made institutional treatment seem both necessary and proper—a sign of family devotion and not neglect. Of seventy-eight hospitals founded in North Carolina between 1890 and 1910, thirty-seven were proprietary, owned and operated by individual surgeons.[39] Minnesota's Mayo Clinic was only the most famous and atypically successful of small-town enterprises. In hospital after hospital, surgical far outweighed medical admissions. The suspiciously disproportionate prominence of a few procedures—appendectomies most conspicuously—indicates the activist enthusiasm of surgeons and their willingness to solve diagnostic problems with their scalpels.[40]

The surgical domination of community hospitals was a tendency apparent to contemporaries, some of whom still regarded their local practitioners with populist suspicion. A hostile newspaper editor in Waverly, Iowa, for example, bemoaned his original support for the town's hospital. "Before that time," he explained, "a surgical operation in Waverly was so rare that it was always opened with a prayer and the people stood around on tiptoe waiting for the result. Now it is next to impossible to prevent the ambulances and automobiles from running into each other as they bring victims to the hospital to be operated upon." It was a change that had taken place quickly. "At first there was only one doctor who could cut and things were not so bad. But gradually others began returning from Chicago with a post-graduate diploma and a new set of tools, until in one neighborhood there was not a family in which one of the members had not been operated upon."[41] On another occasion the same editor scornfully dismissed the efforts of a Spencer, Iowa medical man ("a physician who seemingly would like to get into the appendicitis game, but is handicapped by lack of hospital facilities") to lobby the state legislature to allow counties to levy a special tax to support hospitals; ". . . it does not seem unreasonable," the caustic newspaperman concluded, "that they should provide their own workshops. The Lord knows that they charge enough for their jobs."[42]

But such sardonic comments expressed a minority opinion. Most communities looked on their local hospitals with pride and hope.

They would have read with pleasure the words of a medical editorialist who contended in 1913 that forty-nine out of fifty patients
would do as well in a competently managed small institution as in
a "million-dollar metropolitan hospital."[43] Although historians
have been little concerned with the phenomenon, there were some
clearly defined patterns in the development of hospitals in small
towns and cities. One was widespread community involvement,
another the growing role of income from private patients, most of
them surgical, another the quiet and rapid integration of hospital
care into medical practice patterns.

Most started with relatively modest aims. "This is not an institution for the exhibition of brilliant surgery and specialties in diseases," the trustees of Durham, North Carolina's Watts Hospital
explained in their first annual report in 1895, "by renowned experts;
it is simply a cottage Hospital,—a home for the care and treatment
of those sick and injured citizens of Durham, who are deprived of
the favorable conditions that are necessary for their comfort, and
the successful management of their maladies." The favorable conditions would have been understood and assumed by educated
Americans a century earlier: ". . . pure air, sunlight, good food and
careful nursing" that could not be provided "under the poorer sanitary conditions of many homes and boarding houses." The Durham
Academy of Medicine had agreed to staff the new facility and six
hundred visitors toured the building during the first two days it was
open. Mr. Watts's benefaction had been designed by a prominent
Boston firm of hospital architects and incorporated electric lights,
telephones, and boasted an interior designed to reduce the accumulation of dust and germs. Nevertheless, the institution's only guaranteed income was the monthly contribution of a hundred dollars
from the town's commissioners.[44]

A quarter century later, the same hospital boasted a half-million
dollar physical plant and an endowment of another half million.
Both city and county contributed to the hospital's current expenses
as did income from its endowment; nevertheless two-thirds of its
costs were covered by private patient fees. The hospital housed a
modern pathology and x-ray department. Thirteen hundred and
sixty-nine operations were performed on 1,094 patients; 286 were
appendectomies! To maintain that volume, the hospital extended
admitting privileges to all Durham county's "white physicians" in
good standing.[45]

The Durham story was typical. The explicitly evangelical Mission

Hospital in Asheville, North Carolina, for example, underwent a similar pattern of growth. The hospital began in 1887 with little more in assets than "earnest prayers for God's merciful protection and guidance." Two years later the hospital remained optimistic, reporting: "The good news that here in our own city the suffering poor can find skillful nursing and medical treatment without money and price, is being passed from mouth to mouth, and the imagined horrors of a hospital are giving place to a pleasing sense of rest against want until health is regained." That year the struggling institution admitted only ninety-three patients and maintained an average census of seven. In 1928, the now flourishing hospital admitted 2,485 patients, while staff physicians performed 1,574 operations on inpatients.[46] Not only had the role of the hospital in medical care increased, but the very definition of that care had changed fundamentally.

As was the case in a good many other communities, Haverhill, Massachusetts's hospital began with the energy and support of a prominent local citizen, E.J.M. Hale. Starting in the late 1870s, Hale had urged his fellow citizens to support a community hospital, bought land for it, and left $50,000 in his will toward its support. Nevertheless, Haverhill's hospital did not open until the very end of 1887. In its first annual report, the fledgling institution repeated what had become accepted wisdom in hospital circles: every community needed one hospital bed for each thousand inhabitants, which meant twenty-five beds for the small industrial city. Each free bed was estimated to cost $300 annually, and since the institution's initial endowment produced only $3,000 each year, the ambitious new institution began operations with a typically inadequate income. Donations, the endowment of free beds, and private patient fees were the sources from which that shortfall had to be made up each year. The trustees planned to reject chronic, incurable, and contagious cases but accept acute and surgical patients—and never exclude patients "because of [their] inability to pay. . . ." Of the 105 patients admitted during the first year, 71 were treated without charge.[47]

The hospital was necessarily dependent on continued local support. In its first year, for example, both the Congregational Church and Catholic Aid Society underwrote free beds, while a gift of $5,000 in honor of a deceased local physician endowed another. In subsequent years, annual solicitations helped meet recurring deficits, while an all-female Hospital Aid Association raised smaller sums for sheets and pillowcases, fruit and ice cream for patients, and operating room equipment. By the early years of the twentieth century, the ladies had developed an annual Donation Day on the hospital grounds. An awning was placed over the reception area and lighted by electricity (the wiring contributed by a local electrician). The ladies poured tea for visitors throughout the afternoon and evening. "A committee to receive contributions has a table near at hand, where all the smaller packages are placed. The barrels of flour, sugar, vegetables, etc., are all carried directly to the basement of the hospital, where they may be seen by anyone who cares to go below." Near the tea table was a desk bearing a placard stating: "Contributions of money received here." A harpist and violinist provided music for those attending.[48]

Such homely stratagems could not well support the growing costs of a twentieth-century hospital. Free beds, for example, had been originally endowed for $5,000; by 1905 the hospital could report that an endowment of $15,000 was in fact needed to meet the real annual cost of supporting a hospital bed. At the same time, the yield on investments had actually decreased; "For obvious reasons," the Haverhill trustees noted laconically in 1906, we "have not been hunting about for patients to occupy beds free of charge, . . ." It is no accident that the hospital at the same time urged any local physician, including the homeopathic, to "place private patients, and obtain the advantages peculiar to a hospital, especially in surgical work." Nor was it surprising that surgical admissions grew most rapidly. In 1905, 384 patients were admitted, and 287 of them were surgical. Almost two-thirds of the hospital's income came from the fees of private patients.[49] Individual histories varied widely, but growth and the struggle for survival forced community hospitals into an increasingly uniform pattern well before any formal agencies sought to regulate them.

Medical Incomes and Hospital Practice

The mid-ninteenth-century physician did not expect to earn his fees in the hospital; hospital patients were, by definition, hospital patients because they could not pay a private practitioner. Nevertheless, as we have seen, attending physicians were anxious to serve on hospital wards and were well aware of the equities associated with such gratuitous service. Professional status, referrals, and student fees constituted benefits that made elite physicians anxious to fill unpaid posts on hospital attending and visiting staffs. For many, of course, a traditional sense of noblesse oblige and pious commitment provided another, less material, form of compensation.

With the increasing plausibility of hospital care for the physician-employing classes this situation changed, as did the place of doctors in and in relation to the hospital. In most communities, there was little conflict at first. Anxious to maximize paying bed occupancy, hospitals typically welcomed the help of the community's "respectable" physicians and offered admitting privileges with a liberal hand.

By the time of the First World War, the problem of relating medical practice to the hospital had already assumed another aspect. So crucial had hospital admitting privileges become that a city's practitioners were sometimes divided between the haves and bitter have-nots, between those with staff privileges and those without. Much older conflicts between the elite of urban hospital physicians and their less privileged professional brethren were inevitably exacerbated as fee-paying private patients found their way into the hospital. Within the many hospitals that had been lavish in extending admitting privileges, problems of discipline and the maintenance of standards emerged. How were incompetent or marginally competent physicians and surgeons to be disciplined? How were their interactions with nursing and housestaff to be overseen? The charging of fees for hospital services posed another set of administrative questions. Were specialist consultations to be billed separately or considered part of the hospital's basic services? How were the costs of the hospital's new technological resources to be underwritten? Were patients to be charged separate fees for x-ray diagnosis and treatment, laboratory tests, anesthesia, and use of the operating room?

Hospital care was being integrated not only into medical practice, but into a complex network of monetary transactions. Like many other social institutions, the hospital was being transformed into an ever-more bureaucratic and market-oriented organism. The author of a recent study of the hospital's political economy in this period chose the apt title *A Once Charitable Enterprise.* Although perhaps exaggerating the sharpness of change, the title underlines a fundamental shift in social function and world view. The early twentieth-century nonprofit hospital, nevertheless, remained clothed with the public interest and insulated from the full impact of market forces by both a lingering sense of noblesse oblige and the sacred aura of sickness, pain, and death. The majority of voluntary hospitals never thought of themselves as being part of a transaction-structured marketplace—even as they conformed themselves increasingly to its dictates.[50]

This was neither an abrupt nor categorical change, and only infrequently did it become the occasion for open debate and conflict. In a few of the nation's older institutions, however, the change was traumatic, and the controversy surrounding it illustrative of more fundamental shifts in the hospital's social role. The most dramatic of such incidents took place in the Massachusetts General Hospital, an institution long shaped by a traditional sense of stewardship. Ever since the 1820s and 1830s, the MGH had treated some private patients, and a larger number had been paid for in part by Massachusetts towns and counties. It was never considered appropriate, however, for a staff physician to charge a patient directly for services rendered in the hospital. The Massachusetts General Hospital's endowment had been accumulated to treat the worthy and dependent—not to underwrite the care of individuals able to employ their own physician. Pennsylvania Hospital, the Massachusetts General's even older Philadelphia counterpart, similarly discouraged staff members from taking fees for treating private patients in its wards and rooms.[51] To do so seemed a betrayal of the function for which the institutions had been created by pious and community-minded Unitarian and Quaker merchants in still small and deferential commercial seaports. "A public hospital is a trust," as a Brahmin physician explained his opposition to hospital fees, "originally set apart as a charity for the sick, and not for the pecuniary benefit of their attendants. Whatever in a charitable institution is practiced for this end, leads to its gradual insidious deterioration." Once physicians were allowed to profit from their hospital work, every aspect of the institution would come to reflect these material ends, and the patients, finally, "who paid their attendants would be not the worst cared for."[52]

But such social assumptions were less and less persuasive in America's thriving cities at the end of the nineteenth century. And they were rejected emphatically by the great majority of a medical profession increasingly confident in its therapeutic skills and ever-more dependent on the hospital for a setting in which to practice them. Physicians resented their being used to attract paying patients to hospital rooms where they would be treated without receiving a separate bill for medical services and thus subsidizing the institution at the expense of potential fees.[53] As early as 1881, the Massachusetts General Hospital trustees felt compelled to print a circular explaining that a physician or surgeon in "accepting an appointment upon the staff, thereby waives all claim for compensation in money, . . ."[54] It was a policy supported moreover by a powerful and traditionally oriented minority among the hospital's attending staff. But controversy continued to build as the great majority of hospitals in the Boston area allowed staff members to charge patients for treatment administered in the hospital. In 1894, the board solicited the opinions of their attending staff. The immediate occasion was a need to make policy in regard to a recently remodeled private ward. A minority of staff members still endorsed an older vision of the MGH as an exclusively benevolent institution; there were many well-regarded private hospitals, they argued, in which the wealthy could be treated and pay their attending physician an appropriate fee. The Massachusetts General Hospital, their argument followed, had a different function and demanded an appropriate dedication from staff members. It became clear, however, that many MGH attending physicians routinely steered private patients to other hospitals in which they enjoyed admitting privileges and in which fees could be charged. (A similar problem plagued the Pennsylvania Hospital, which in fact actively discouraged patients who sought private accommodations as well as forbidding its attendings from charging for hospital services.) Traditionalists, on the other hand, emphasized that physicians were well paid in the coin of status and experience—as well as in the opportunity to support a worthy charity. In the event of conflict, the hospital's interests should take precedence over those of individual practitioners. Pay rooms and fees for service had no place in hospitals originally established to aid the needy working classes and advance medical knowledge.[55]

To physicians outside the elite circles that controlled attending appointments in large cities, such policies seemed to constitute a de facto collusion between the hospital and its wealthy patients that worked to deprive physicians of deserved fees. As the retiring president of the Medical Society of the County of New York ironically expressed such resentment in 1895, "I have seen hospitals stretching out their tentacles so as to include the care of the worthy rich."[56] A 1904 survey of Boston area physicians showed that the great majority (295 as opposed to 22) believed that anyone able to pay for a private room could also pay his or her physician. The great majority of New England hospitals, moreover, were conducted on "sound business principles"—that is, they allowed staff members to collect fees from private-room patients.[57] And even where large hospitals allowed physicians to charge for their services, practitioners without admitting privileges resented their exclusion.[58]

These new economic possibilities implied a host of questions for the hospital and its own medical staff. Some are obvious, such as the shift in power implied by the hospital's growing dependence on the admitting physician's willingness to channel private patients into its rooms. It is not surprising that when faced with underutilized private facilities and rising budgets that hospitals should have added prominent local practitioners to the ranks of physicians with admitting privileges. In 1904, for example, Jacob Solis-Cohen, a well-known Philadelphia specialist, received letters from both Polyclinic and Jewish (now Einstein) hospitals pointing out the virtues of their private facilities and urging him to use them.[59] Even the atypically conservative Pennsylvania Hospital, like its Boston peer the Massachusetts General, could not stand against the tide, and in the first decade of the twentieth century began to allow its surgeons to treat and bill private patients.[60]

Even a hospital so prestigious and well endowed as Johns Hopkins was dependent on the referrals of its internationally known staff and, in particular, gynecological surgeon Howard Kelly. At such institutions, of course, the balance of power was structured rather differently from more marginal enterprises. The medical board and trustees could hold out admitting privileges as a reward for the most successful of its junior staff members, or as inducements to keep them from accepting positions at rival institutions.[61]

Within individual institutions, attending staff members consistently urged the improvement of private room and consultation facilities. In 1909, to cite a typical example, the medical board at New York's Presbyterian Hospital voted to make appropriate "overtures" to the trustees in an effort to increase private patient accommodations. The private service was important for public relations, they argued, and even more significant to staff members. "It . . . concentrates the labors and by doing so increases the devotion of the attending staff which is among the greatest assets of the institution." Perhaps the threat was only implied, but even New York's well-endowed Presbyterian Hospital had become increasingly dependent on the "devotion" of its attending staff.[62] Private practice in the hospital necessitated not only more private and semi-private inpatient facilities, but also the provision of physicians' dressing and consulting rooms, amenities that had not been considered when the hospital had treated only the dependent.

The promise of a potential paying clientele at a time of growing costs implied a wide range of intrahospital adjustments; physical facilities constituted only one aspect of such change. Almost without exception, for example, nineteenth-century hospitals had maintained revolving staff appointments, physicians and surgeons serving three- or four-month shifts attending on the wards. Private practice, on the other hand, was necessarily a year-round commitment—implying a conflict between the needs of practice and conventional staffing arrangements. Should attending physicians have private admitting privileges when they were not "on duty"? (When hospitals had been populated almost entirely by the indigent, no such conflicts existed; the needs of private practice, supplemented by those of teaching, were to make revolving appointments obsolete.) Conflict over specialization and its prerogatives inevitably surfaced as well. If, for example, a neurologist was asked to see a private patient under the care of a general surgeon, could the neurologist submit a separate bill? And was the admitting physician ethically obligated to consult more expert staff members in special areas? Was the hospital in some way responsible for the scale of fees charged private patients? Some institutions decided that fees were to be entirely a private matter, to be settled between doctor and patient; others sought to establish a maximum fee scale.[63]

Allowing community physicians into the hospital was to implicitly endorse their practice, and many institutions were well aware that problems of quality control would emerge. Some hospitals required physicians with admitting privileges but without attending appointments to have the approval of a staff member before they could operate, even on their own patients. And, of course, both ethics and interest dictated that attending staffs maintain exclusive control over the care of ward patients.

Relations with nurses presented another awkward matter. All physicians were accustomed to demanding immediate and unquestioning obedience from nurses, but no hospital's nursing staff could tolerate diverse and inconsistent orders of sometimes scores of physicians, many of them unfamiliar with established procedures (and some of whom treated only occasional patients).[64] None of

these matters was easily worked out; nor was the problem of specifying payment for particular technical services.

Nineteenth-century private patients ordinarily paid a single rate
that included every aspect of their care except possible special nursing or dietary supplements (sherry, for example, or chicken).[65]
Gradually, however, the institution's new technical resources became a source of profit—or at least a mode of amortizing their
original cost. By the beginning of the twentieth century, for example, most hospitals had established fees for use of their operating
rooms, often on a sliding scale, with some institutions imposing an
additional fee for the administration of general anesthesia. The need
to pay for new radiology "outfits" led similarly to the gradual imposition of fees, usually higher for outpatients than inpatients.[66] Almost all demanded payment—usually for a week's minimum stay—
before a patient would be admitted.[67] The American hospital had
evolved a long way from its formative years when the term "board"
and "boarders" had naturally and accurately described the hospital's services and its minority of paying patients. Perhaps most
important, the relationship between hospital and its admitting
physicians had become more intimate and symbiotic, while admitting physicians had come to constitute an increasing proportion of
medical practitioners generally.

Inside the Hospital: Impact of the Private Patient

Private patients had an impact on more than hospital budgets;
within the institution, they helped create a new set of day-to-day
realities. Contemporary assumptions of class-appropriate lifestyles
dictated that private patients should enjoy a very different kind of
environment from that provided ward patients. The hospital's hope
of attracting that elusive minority of Americans able to pay twenty-
five dollars and more a week for private accommodations lent urgency to institutional plans for providing the amenities considered
appropriate to middle-class sensibilities.[68] In many cities, in fact,
hospitals competed actively and self-consciously for the patronage
of a limited pool of wealthy patients. They could neglect the physical comforts that might reassure such patients as little as they could

ignore the desires of those elite practitioners whose referrals could alone keep private rooms filled.

Private patients demanded and were supplied with rugs and draperies, with easy chairs and delicate china; they expected to receive visitors at almost every hour of the day and evening. Nurses, relatives, or companions often occupied adjoining rooms. In most hospitals, private patients would be attended by their regular physicians, perhaps in consultation with attending staff members. (If a resident seemed particularly congenial, a wealthy patient might seek to hire him personally—a recurring embarrassment for hospital administrators.) House officers did not operate on private patients, while contemporaries were unable even to contemplate the possibility that such patients would be used in teaching. Privacy and payment seemed naturally allied.[69]

Not surprisingly, profit margins in private room services were often less than anticipated. Wealthy patients were far more demanding of nurses and house staff, while their presumed necessities (such as a better and more pleasingly served diet, rugs, draperies, and bric-a-brac that needed constant dusting) increased costs. A thriving private service also implied the creation of an extended, and sometimes separate, house staff to deal with their more importunate demands.[70] Private duty nurses created problems of discipline—and frequently of housing, though they were often expected to sleep in the patient's room. Caring for private patients was, moreover, a seasonal business; private rooms and services remained sparsely populated during the summer months when patients as well as their personal physicians fled the hot and unfashionable city.[71] The consequences were obvious—even to contemporaries anxious to increase private services. Between 1905 and 1910, for example, the cost per day of caring for paying patients at New York's Presbyterian Hospital almost doubled, while the cost of ward patients increased only a third.[72] There were in any case, as we have seen, only a limited number of Americans able to pay for private rooms at a rate that promised a comfortable margin above actual costs.

A far greater number of respectable Americans could pay something toward their medical care, but hardly the cost of a private room with its associated clinical and nursing fees. Hospitals soon adjusted, impelled both by experience and deeply felt assumptions in regard to the dignities of class. Since mid-century, older urban hospitals had been concerned by the plight of that anomalous group of "intelligent and sensitive" Americans who could not afford a private room but should not be expected to endure the general ward's "unpleasant associations." One widespread hospital response was to offer ad hoc discounts to "worthy" patients, another to create what would later be called semiprivate accommodations—rooms smaller, less pleasantly located and elaborately furnished than the highest-priced private room, and perhaps shared with one or more patients. Philadelphia's Polyclinic Hospital, for example, established small "pay wards" in 1904 "in which patients can be accommodated who desire somewhat greater privacy than can be obtained in the free and general wards."[73] By the 1890s, moreover, hospitals had also begun to charge even ward patients a modest fee; the intent was to produce some income and at the same time counteract the tendency toward pauperism presumably induced by entirely gratuitous care. Most hospitals assessed ward patients a dollar a day, half or less of most institutions' actual costs. (The widespread policy of not allowing physicians to charge fees to patients other than those occupying private rooms also protected the deserving patient's dignity—if at occasional cost to the practitioner.) Contemporaries argued, moreover, that the mixing of classes in the new-model hospital with its diverse styles of care did not demean the free patients but instead improved their treatment. It is evident, Henry Hurd argued in 1896, "that the mingling of patients of the more prosperous classes with those who formerly resorted to hospitals has improved their dietary, their methods of treatment and especially the nursing and personal care of patients. Now that hospital care of the more prosperous classes of patients has become an imperative necessity, the neglect of the poorer classes in the same hospitals becomes impossible."[74]

Quality of treatment is inevitably difficult to evaluate. What is clear, however, is the fact every private hospital, even the oldest and best endowed, had become increasingly dependent upon patient income and upon its attending physicians and surgeons to attract those patients.[75] Scientific medicine promised unending therapeutic progress—and the hospital had become the place in which those promises of healing were to be redeemed.

The hospital was at the same time becoming a more complex and ambiguous institution. Although it had begun to enter the marketplace of economic relationships, it was still clothed with a peculiar public interest and emotional associations that made it difficult to regard as simply a mechanism for profit making. In the second decade of the twentieth century, however, most of its problems seemed manageable. For the first time, proposals to regulate and evaluate American hospitals were being discussed and tentatively realized. Private patient income allowed smaller institutions to exist and larger ones to continue their traditional role of caring for the poor. Municipalities and localities continued—if in an increasingly bureaucratic fashion—their traditional practice of providing hospital care for the indigent. If some physicians were resentful at their being shut out of hospital staffs and the sometimes lucrative admitting privileges that went with these positions, a larger number benefited from the hospitals' new prominence in medical care.

But the willingness of ordinary Americans to enter a hospital created its own problems. Hospitals were still unable to provide adequate accommodations for the middle class; a contemporary cliché warned that the best medical care could only be purchased by the dollars of the rich or the dignity of the poor. But this still seemed a paradox that could ultimately be resolved through good will and the creation of appropriate semiprivate accommodations. At least for this generation, economic costs seemed containable. Student nurses and house staff provided inexpensive labor—bartered for credentials that were becoming indispensable. Nonprofessional workers were in general paid less than counterparts outside the hospital but were still the beneficiaries of more than ordinary job security. Hospital prospects seemed bright indeed.

The American hospital in the period of World War I had become a vastly different institution from its postbellum predecessor. Just as medical theory and practice had shifted gradually but inexorably away from the holistic, individual, and antireductionist models of the late eighteenth century, so the hospital had ceased to be an institution defined by traditional economic roles and traditional assumptions of stewardship and deference. Medical care was seen increasingly in technical terms, and the hospital population was defined increasingly by physician-diagnosed pathology and not social position. The hospital itself was entering a world of impersonal cash transactions and bureaucratic relationships. It was only to have been expected that human relationships within the hospital would evolve in ways reflecting these new realities.

CHAPTER 11

A Careful Oversight: Reshaping Authority

On the first of July, 1825, "Nathan Gurney Esq. and his wife, took possession" of the Massachusetts General Hospital as superintendent and matron. "The keys of the Building were delivered to them with the inventory of the furniture. The several officers & servants of the institution were introduced to Mr & Mrs Gurney . . . and requested to conform to their orders and directions."[1] The trustees could leave this reassuring scene confident that their house and the "boarders" that filled it were in good hands. Their new superintendent had been a selectman and overseer of the poor and boasted ". . . a judgment naturally sound & discriminating matured by reflection & acquaintance with the world, an active & enterprising disposition, . . . native tenderness & urbanity & an unimpeached moral character."

Character, not special training or certification, defined an appropriate surrogate for the hospital's trustees. Their first superintendent had, after all, been a retired sea captain. A man who had taken the responsibility for valuable cargoes was certainly capable of overseeing a hospital. In any case, the superintendent was no more than the trustee's deputy; he would be observed carefully by board members who regularly visited each room and ward in the hospital. The possibility of appointing a physician as superintendent was not even considered. Nathan Gurney could be expected to place the physical and moral needs of his patients above every other consideration (except balanced accounts); no medical man could be expected to do the same.

By mid-nineteenth century this traditional view of an appropriate hospital authority structure had begun to fracture. It had become clear that at least one experienced practitioner needed to be in residence to make emergency admissions and treat critical cases on the wards. Inevitably such resident physicians began to accumulate day-to-day responsibilities. But the vision of the superintendent as prudent Christian and of the hospital as his home writ large was not easily discarded. Even into the twentieth century it was assumed that the superintendent would live with his wife and children on the hospital grounds. Until late in the nineteenth century, most hospital trustees still felt a personal responsibility for the comfort of workers and patients.

Nevertheless, by 1900 an increasingly bureaucratic reality was beginning to supersede these traditional assumptions. Many of the matron's responsibilities, for example, had been assumed by the training school superintendent, while in many small community hospitals both those positions had been amalgamated in the person of the female nurse-superintendent. Associations of hospital and training school superintendents had come into formal and self-conscious existence. Textbooks and journals for aspiring adminis-trators were available by the time of the First World War. Lay trustees were coming to play an increasingly passive and distant role—concerned with their financial responsibilities but less and less involved with the institution's day-to-day routine.

Physicians and medical values, on the other hand, assumed a central role in shaping those routines. It seemed only a natural response to the ever-more powerful tools at the profession's com-mand and to their increasing demands for bedside teaching oppor-tunities. Staff physicians grew restive at their exclusion from most hospital boards—even as their de facto power on the ward, admis-sions room, and operating theater increased. Admissions, appoint-ments, and control of teaching were all areas of conflict between lay and medical authority—and all areas in which laymen gradually retreated and left the field to their medical staff. The early twen-tieth-century hospital still reflected community attitudes, however, some of a traditional sort (such as the moral dependence of women and the inferiority of blacks) and others of a new sort (such as a respect for professionalism and efficiency). If the patient had been defined by a traditional paternalism at the beginning of the nine-teenth century, he or she had become the object of a rigid and impersonal routine at its end.

An Order of Place and Person: Persisting Stewardship

When New York City's Presbyterian Hospital opened in 1871, its wealthy and socially prominent trustees regularly walked the wards, talking to patients, running their hands over moldings in search of dust. On the eighth of November, for example, they found "everything in good order, except the Kitchen floor, which retains every spot of dirt, and no amount of cleaning can remove it—it must either be laid with marble or covered with some hard surface that has a polish." The next month they noticed a chill draft and advised weather-stripping the windows and doors; this was only one of their suggestions. The gas lantern in front of the building blew out in the mildest breeze; the faucets in some of the ward basins had been improperly attached. They even recorded the need for a new corned beef barrel, since the present one leaked. Two years later they noted that the institution's coal was "poor, dirty & filled with slate." Perhaps the bill should not be paid.[2]

Such personal oversight was only typical, even if performed by atypically wealthy and prominent New Yorkers. Similar procedures were followed in almost every American hospital into the twentieth century. Even the self-consciously efficient and bureaucratic Johns Hopkins began operations with an energetic visiting committee that made regular reports to the full board. In August of 1892, for example, they made three inspections of the hospital and reported with pleasure that it

. . . presented a wonderful aspect of order & cleanliness and ventilation— that the patients seemed to be happy and contented, and that although on one occasion the visit was made at a very early hour in the morning, the wards were in a proper condition to receive a visit of inspection.

Some years later the visiting committee still served as critic of everyday hospital realities. They reported in 1900 that the temperature in the "ironing room" often reached 110 in the summer: "This entails very great suffering upon the women employed there; . . . in an institution intended for the relief of suffering this should not be permitted to continue."[3]

Lay trustees still maintained a sharp sense both of their own responsibilities and of the nature of a truly benevolent institution. To some extent these assumptions accepted an implicit conflict between the interests of physicians and patients, between physicians and lay trustees. It is not hard to find evidence of a tenacious paternalism in American hospitals throughout the nineteenth century. In the generation following the Civil War, the better sort of Americans still entertained firm ideas about the appropriate relationships between the giver and receiver of alms. Not surprisingly, they sought to incorporate these views in the hospital's social fabric. Every aspect of the patient's experience continued, for example, as it had since the beginning of the century to be subject to elaborate rules and regulations. The patients were still inmates—as were the servants, nurses, and house officers. As late as 1898, Cleveland's forward-looking Lakeside Hospital warned that

Patients admitted to the Hospital are forbidden to use profane or indecent language; to express immoral or infidel sentiments; to play at cards or any other game for money; to smoke tobacco in the house, or to procure for themselves or others any intoxicating liquors.

Patients were—almost literally—incarcerated and required to apply for passes should they choose to leave the hospital grounds. The New York Hospital's Executive Committee warned in 1886 that patients ". . . allowed to go out on a pass and remaining beyond the time specified will be regarded as discharged, . . ." Sensitive both to the dangers of improper ventilation and to the costs of heat, the committee warned as well that any patient tampering with windows or registers would also be subject to immediate discharge.[4] Catholic hospitals might have seemed less threatening to immigrant clients than their Protestant peers, but they could be equally paternalistic in their regulations. It was no more than the moral common sense of the matter; wealth, education, and piety implied responsibility— and the forceful exertion of authority.

But it was becoming increasingly difficult for lay trustees to undertake the personal oversight that had characterized the antebellum hospital. Some problems were practical: the increasing scale of many institutions and the growing technical authority of physicians and trained nurses. Another problem was ideological. A growing respect for professionalism as such helped undermine the traditional prerogatives of lay stewardship. The requirements of Christian stewardship were absolute, but so was the condition that it be performed with skill and efficiency. The pastor of Pittsburgh's Third Presbyterian Church expressed this implicitly paradoxical set of

views in 1888 as he commented on the work of his city's homeopathic hospital. Any such institution, he explained, "in its daily
work is simply Christian thought and belief translated into action."
But there were different ways of attaining this goal.

. . . this hospital not only expresses in its work Christian thought and
feeling, and belief, but expresses it effectively—economically, because it
has maintained its patients at a cost per week of less than the average
estimate set down by competent judges to first-class city hospitals—effectively, because, again, out of every hundred treated, the number of those
that have died, as shown by the figures, is not only within, but actually
below the average.[5]

Secular goals and values were quietly and inexorably, if gradually,
replacing older conceptions of social responsibility. Six years later,
at the same hospital, another pastor expressed these shifting imperatives even more unambiguously. The Reverend Courtenay pointed
explicitly to the older style of hospital in which the sick were
admonished and the dying shriven. Now, he explained, "They are
almost exclusively places for the exercise of the healing art." But
this, he explained, was only one example of a more general evolution of authority from the ecclesiastic to the scientific element in
society.

The present relation of the Christian society to the hospital is that of
sympathy and support, with such spiritual ministrations as may be prudent and proper. . . . Even when wearing churchly names they are safely
committed to the charge of men for whom the construction and management of hospitals, and the cure of the sick and hurt is a lifelong study. Of
old, learning was locked up among the priests, and withered like seed corn
long bearded in the granary. . . . Whereas [sic] the dissemination of knowledge and the division of duty has promoted intensive work. So it is well
that hospitals have been given over to specialists.[6]

This up-to-date clergyman then warned of the dangers of shutting
religion out of the hospital entirely. But it was a case of locking the
barn after the horse had strayed. The reverend gentleman's enthusiastic secularism and uncritical acceptance of technical authority and
the laudable division of intellectual labor reflected fundamental
changes that had already overtaken the hospital like so many other
areas of American life. The confident paternalism of an earlier generation could not be restored.

Not surprisingly, such assumptions soon changed the traditionally understood conceptions of lay responsibility that had guided and legitimated trustee behavior since the end of the eighteenth century. Let me refer again to the Johns Hopkins Hospital's Visiting Committee, a group that we have just seen acting out a traditionally intrusive role in the 1890s. In 1902, however, the committee made an explicit and novel statement of policy. They were convinced that their "true object" was to become familiar with the workings of the hospital, "that their interest and supervising care be manifested to those here engaged," but that specific suggestions "should be made with caution, and are rather to be avoided than specially sought."[7] This was a far more modest vision of lay responsibility than philanthropists of an earlier generation would have understood or tolerated. They might well have seen it as an abdication of that proper stewardship enjoined by piety and the responsibilities of class.

Ladies of Charity and Their Erring Sisters

In one area at least, this trend was less apparent. This was the role of women, both as givers and receivers of charity. For women's peculiar social position, affecting both rich and poor if in somewhat different ways, created an at least partially separate sphere of hospital work. Like every aspect of the hospital's internal social world, the place of women within it mirrored precisely the character of women's role outside the hospital's walls. Insofar as a woman was assumed to be a moral minor in need of care and supervision, so would the hospital treat her as such. Insofar as women sought new avenues for social action and autonomy, so would at least some middle- and upper-class women seek to use the hospital for these new purposes.

Before the Civil War, few respectable women would have considered intruding upon the hospital ward and its presumably unsavory denizens, but by the late 1860s and in a few instances even earlier, committees of "lady visitors" had become a standard feature of hospital life. Such pious women would read to patients, pray with them, provide flowers, Christmas trees, and Easter hams. Most important, from the point of view of many such ladies, was the opportunity for alerting the erring to their Master's imminent presence.

Even outpatients were not immune to such earnest efforts. The lady visitors at Philadelphia's Episcopal Hospital, for example, hoped to pay as much attention as possible to the dispensary patients. "This can be done not only by judicious conversation with individual patients, but by reading to them while waiting, such portions of Scripture or other religious reading as shall be deemed best fitted for their use and comfort."[8] (Long hours of waiting on hard benches presumably created appropriate subjects for pious exhortation.) Although such ladies' committees could not well contest the authority of male trustees or medical board members in general hospitals, their presence and the class attitudes and prerogatives they brought with them constituted a concrete extension of middle-class values and authority into the ward's everyday social fabric.

They could, on the other hand, become something of a nuisance if their evangelicalism grew too enthusiastic or if they interfered with nurses or resident physicians. On the whole, however, most hospitals welcomed female help in fund-raising, sponsoring charity beds, or furnishing wards and private rooms.[9] Women seemed, in fact, ideally suited to the maintaining of a watchful eye over hospital housekeeping. "The life-long training of the housewife," a Philadelphia physician explained

of course fits her to see at once in public institutions faults as to cleanliness, cooking, waste, etc., which are only detected with difficulty by the average man, or more often altogether escape his inspection.

But even more important, he explained, were two other female attributes: "a peculiar moral fitness, and in most cases an endless supply of leisure." Leisure was an indispensable prerequisite for the would-be hospital activist; it was a commodity in short supply among men prominent in business. No wonder, he noted, "woman often is to the poor wretches in the hospitals and almshouses as an angel from heaven."[10] There was a little of the ministering angel in every well-bred woman.

In some hospitals, women tended to play an even more prominent role—as trustees and policy makers. These were those institutions that provided medical care for women and children. A handful of such hospitals had come into existence before 1860, but even when ostensibly guided by women, advisory committees of male philanthropists and physicians tended to make key decisions. The New-York Asylum for Lying-In Women was organized in 1823, for example, at the initiative of a group of prominent physicians who called an organizational meeting of wealthy ladies. When they met, one of the medical men "stated to the Ladies the object of the meeting, of such an Institution in our city." The ladies were then presented with a "Constitution previously drafted . . . after which the Gentlemen withdrew, leaving the Ladies to proceed to the consideration of the Constitution submitted."[11]

By the 1850s, another motive had been added to the movement for women and children's hospitals. This was the desire to provide clinical training for the first generation of aspiring women physicians. Women were to play a prominent role in such institutions, both in administration and the provision of care. In these hospitals at least, the presumed special needs of their patient population allowed women to play a more autonomous role than they did in most general hospitals, both as physicians and administrators.

Women patients, and particularly lying-in patients, represented a very special population, at risk both morally and physically. They were patients for whom an all-inclusive paternalism (or in the case of female-dominated hospitals, maternalism) seemed both necessary and proper. Their sex, their class, and their presumed lack of self-control all implied the need for support and guidance. Nineteenth- and early twentieth-century maternity hospitals were relentlessly intrusive in their control of patients. (This was still a period, it will be recalled, when few but the very poor or "abandoned" would enter a lying-in ward.) Hospitals, for example, would typically admit unmarried obstetric patients only once.

It was simply assumed that the hospital and its lady managers and lady visitors would occupy a position in *loco parentis* (in many of the earliest hospitals, assuming the right to find places as wet nurses for women and adoptive homes for their children). "Ordinary routine," the matron of Boston's Lying-In Hospital noted in her journal on February 17, 1873. "Mrs Keeler discharged—her child to be boarded out and the Mother gone as wet nurse to New Bedford." The options for unmarried, widowed, or deserted mothers were few in the late nineteenth century; even had they wanted to keep their children, it was often impossible. "Annie Shattuck who was confined July 2nd '76," the same matron recorded in 1877, "& baby adopted, called to day to ascertain its whereabouts—not to obtain possession of it—only a desire to see it & feel assured it was in a good home with kind people."[12]

Into the early years of the twentieth century, such female oriented institutions presented an atypically and overtly pious, controlling, and sometimes crypto-feminist context for the provision of care. Often smaller in scale, they resisted both the acute care orientation and growing impersonality of the larger general hospitals. The Minnesota Maternity in Minneapolis constitutes a revealing example of such an institution. Its object, when founded in the late 1880s, was to provide for the "confinement of married women who are without means or suitable abode and care at the time of childbirth and may also admit girls who under promise of marriage, have been led astray; and also may care for destitute children born in the institution." Not surprisingly, the hospital's president and lady managers arranged for adoptions and personally inspected prospective foster homes. The board formally voted, moreover, that it "shall be the duty of this association to keep watch over any unmarried girl who is discharged from this hospital—for the space of one year if possible." As part of their program for moral uplift, the ladies invited a city missionary to visit the patients "for the purpose of holding meetings and religious conversation" and were overjoyed to have found a matron able to exert an improving influence through her "Christian example & words of Christian training."[13]

It was natural to move from the moral to the environmental—to question those aspects of society that had made their patients patients. The physician at a lying-in hospital was necessarily sociologist and social worker at the same time she delivered babies and cared for newborns. Dr. Martha Ripley, the hospital's female resident physician, was particularly sensitive to such matters. "As long as there is a double code of morals for men and women, woman must ever find it harder than her brother to regain the right paths. Let the standard of virtue for women not be lowered, but let us insist that the man's be equally high." Dr. Ripley expressed her reactions forthrightly at an 1890 meeting of the hospital's board.

Dr. Ripley could keep still no longer. Said if something was not done soon to improve the morality of the girls of the city she would go crazy. She thought the ladies who employ girls ought to be called together & take some measures to compel girls to be at home as early as ten o'clock. Ought also to have meetings for the girls, especially the Scandinavian, to instruct them in purity.[14]

The hospital provided one of the few contexts in which middle-class women could play a legitimate and, to an extent, autonomous role outside the home. Such hospitals played a similar role for a handful of ambitious women doctors who would never have held positions of authority at large private or municipal hospitals. It is hardly surprising that overtones of feminism and the piety that so often legitimated such activism should have thrived in these institutions.

These were roles that did not always suit male staff members. In many hospitals, attending physicians fought an endemic guerrilla war against female board members and committees of lady visitors; in only a handful of hospitals did women exert an unquestioned authority. Women had certainly planned and raised funds for many new hospitals, but this worthy contribution did not mean they were regarded as capable of managing those institutions once established. Few women, as an authority on hospital management explained in 1906, "have any opportunity for becoming acquainted with business principles and their application. As a rule the husband bears 'the white man's burden' . . ." Some men took an even more categorical position; women were simply not "fitted by nature" for decision-making positions.[15] The very social activism of many women implied a continuing personal involvement in the hospital—but it was an involvement that many male staff members found difficult to tolerate. Male trustees might be occupied elsewhere during business hours, while their wives and sisters could be an annoying presence in wards and corridors. It was an especially irritating presence at a time when medical men were becoming more and more resentful of any lay intrusions into hospital management.

A Physician's Workshop

Physicians felt increasingly constrained just as they attained an unprecedented influence within the hospital. Their growing technical skills and clinical dependence on the hospital made a lingering subordination to lay boards and administrators more and more intolerable.

No one could deny that the scale of the hospital enterprise had increased, but this did not justify the businessman's easy assumption that practical matters were beyond their capacity. The traditional policy of excluding physicians from hospital governing boards seemed indefensible to most doctors, especially when allied with an often explicit policy of appointing only lay superintendents. Medical training could at least help an able superintendent bridge the gap between the realities of ward and operating room and those financial realities that confronted board members. "The ability to make cheap bargains," as an argumentative commentator put it, "should not be compared to the ability to restore to health the sick and injured." Clinical and scientific skills were ultimately more central both to the treatment of individual patients and the making of hospital policy. "One who has the knowledge and wisdom to direct the treatment and bring about the restoration of a patient must not be classed with one who attends only to the physical needs of an institution."[16]

It was a conflict both of power and legitimacy. Physicians, of course, preferred to see it as simply a recognition of the necessary autonomy of medical skill and knowledge. Was the hospital to be a curative institution organized around scientific procedures and capabilities or was it simply a species of welfare home? Once one conceded that the hospital was a curative institution, the argument followed, it was obvious that no interference by laymen should be tolerated.[17]

The hospital's very centrality to medical careers seemed, ironically, to have maximized the power of laymen—or so at least physicians complained. There were always more than enough physicians willing to volunteer their services on attending staffs. "The hospital managers with patronizing smile tell the poor doctor that he is no business man;" a medical editorialist put it in 1896, "the doctor admits it, and with hat in hand begs for an opportunity to give his services free."[18] So long as there were far more physicians anxious to fill staff positions than there were positions to fill, lay managers would have the leverage to back up their traditional sense of prerogative.

In some hospitals, the grasp of lay authority was particularly tenacious. The nursing orders that administered Catholic hospitals were accustomed to managing every aspect of the institutions they staffed—and could dominate both lay and medical boards. Municipal hospitals represented a rather different problem. For here the prerogatives and imperatives of electoral politics often imposed themselves on the institution's internal order. The "audacity" of Philadelphia General Hospital's Board in settling medical questions was, for example, characterized by a prominent clinician as exhibiting the "complacency of a hog in his wash." In such cases, another critic urged, it was the physician's duty to take part in politics so as to oust the "political henchmen" who filled too many hospital offices.[19]

Most physicians, of course, accepted an implicit division of labor; the doctor was presumed to be master of the ward in which he or she practiced. "When the physician is authorized to cross the threshold of the ward," as one medical writer articulated this particular vision of clinical transcendence,

he is vested with authority, which must be recognized, and can not be gainsaid, until that right is withdrawn. He has been placed at the helm, and has the right to command, and to expect an immediate response to his guiding touch. The resources of the hospital are at his disposal, . . . He has been assigned his own province, and is bound to defend it, even from the intrusion of his own colleagues.[20]

But the transferring of that authority from the ward—from the legitimating context of clinical decision making—was no easy matter. It could be accomplished only gradually. In larger and older hospitals, especially, lay managers did not easily abandon their traditional sense of power and prerogative. Physicians in community and specialty hospitals, of course, often found themselves de facto administrators as well as clinicians. And in hospitals generally, as I have argued in a previous chapter, the gradual introduction of private patients meant that physicians would have an important role in filling paid beds and thus in balancing the institution's books. But even while this development was taking place, most American hospitals had already seen a gradual shift in the day-to-day structure of decision making and medical autonomy, a shift reflecting and incorporating the growing authority of medicine.

A Contested Terrain: Negotiating Power

Conflict did not ordinarily manifest itself in dramatic incidents or categorical statements of principle. Power did not pass convulsively from lay to medical hands. Instead, the sum of day-to-day decisions became increasingly medical; lay authority gradually withdrew from the admitting process, the ward, and the autopsy room. The demands of staff members for teaching privileges became gradually more insistent and plausible.

Hospital policies begin with admission. Here lay authorities had traditionally exerted a firm hand; morality, stewardship, and chronically shaky budgets dictated a careful attention to admissions. Chronic and incurable patients, like the venereal and alcoholic, were ordinarily excluded from free beds at private hospitals. The popular nineteenth-century practice of raising funds for endowed beds ordinarily brought with it power to name occupants of that bed. (A typical arrangement at midcentury might confer the title of life trustee to the donor of a thousand dollars and with it control of a particular bed, although even with the endorsement of such benefactors a medical certification of need was ordinarily required for admission.)

Physicians had obviously to play a coordinate role; even when an individual appeared bearing a trustee's letter authorizing admission, the prospective patient was still required to be examined by a physician to determine whether he or she were a "proper subject" for hospital care. By midcentury, as we have seen, admissions procedures were becoming increasingly medical. Trustees and wealthy donors were less and less likely to be accessible—and to be able to treat the hospital as part of a network of patronage and deference. The admitting power of physicians was constrained only by the occasional ad hoc intrusions of the superintendent or particular trustees and—more systematically and indirectly—by frugal budgets that limited the number of available free beds.

At New York's newly founded Roosevelt Hospital, for example, the "number of vacant beds, both free and pay," was posted each day for the "information of the examining physician." Thus medical men could make clinical decisions—but within boundaries defined by budgetary necessity.[21] Many hospitals indeed sought to place these decisions firmly in medical hands and discourage lingering patient assumptions that influence was an inextricable part of the admission process. "No paper of admission is needed," the steward of Philadelphia's Pennsylvania Hospital explained to a prospective patient in 1885: "Let the man present himself at the Hospital and he will be examined."[22]

Trustees, of course, maintained some role in admissions into the twentieth century. In many institutions this was limited to the casual endorsement of a particular patient. Cleveland's Lakeside

Hospital allowed any trustee or member of the visiting medical staff to admit patients by "written permit"; Massachusetts General Hospital's Board required individual justifications for any patient retained more than ninety days.[23] At city hospitals, of course, both party politics and welfare administrators continued to play a role in individual hospital admissions. But it was clear to most contemporaries that the role of laymen was being gradually eroded; most had come to accept it as inevitable, if not laudable.

A few, however, continued to mistrust medical men and motives. In a minority report to the New York's Hospital's Executive Committee, Elbridge Gerry warned in 1887 that patient care and dignity might suffer at the hands of medical staff concerned more with their professional interests than the needs of particular patients. "Unless the case is what is termed an 'interesting one'," he contended, "the patient is soon discharged from the Hospital, oftentimes half-cured, and sometimes without any benefit at all." Gerry objected as well to a suggestion that the hospital's staff shift from rotating to continuous service; it recalled the professional domination of European hospitals where patients received shabby care. "The patient whether living or dead being handed over to the physicians without any right of appeal, and the government maintaining the hospital for the improvement of medical science."[24]

The words "living or dead" were hardly accidental. The patient's experience started with admission; it could end with death. Thus another area of endemic—and revealing—conflict surrounded the question of autopsies. It was a particularly sensitive area, mobilizing religious, class, and cultural anxieties and inevitably reflecting differences between lay and medical values. Most of us, as a Jewish leader explained, are naturally revolted by such "an outrage on the body of the dead." There could be no doubt but that it is a "shocking practice in public institutions to degrade the remains of the poor into mere *subjects,* to teach young physicians the structure of the human frame and the diseases to which it is subject." No matter how loud the claims of science they could hardly excuse the "profanation of the helpless dead."[25] This was 1867, but the attitudes expressed were still widely accepted a half century later—and exacerbated by the grim reality that only the poor were ordinarily subjects for postmortems. No matter what their personal views, trustees had to be conscious that such anxieties simmered in the community; every hospital was dogged by the fear that sensationalistic newspapermen might exploit legitimate autopsy policies.

Physicians regarded the subject in a different light. Ambition and intellect conspired to make staff members at leading hospitals advocates of routine postmortems, certainly in those cases of clinical interest. This was a generation in which American medicine looked to Europe for intellectual leadership and matters were handled very differently there. At Vienna's sprawling General Hospital, for example, all cases were autopsied as a matter of routine. Most staff physicians were impatient with the traditional contention that the hospital's mission was the effective treatment of those patients who happened to fill its beds. The demands of clinical investigation could be as absolute and all-encompassing as those of traditional benevolence, and the authority of science could be as transcendent as that of a more conventional piety.

The living as well as dead could evoke conflicts between the imperatives of medicine and those of morality. Alcoholism and venereal disease, for example, implied occasions for conflict at every private hospital. By the last quarter of the century, most clinicians—and particularly specialists in dermatology and syphilology—felt that venereal patients should be admitted, especially syphilitics in the later, noncontagious stages in which neurological and cardiovascular symptoms demanded treatment. But trustees were hostile or hesitant to accept such undesirable and unworthy patients; as late as 1894, the Massachusetts General Hospital trustees pondered the appropriateness of accepting a bequest underwriting the treatment of venereal disease.[26] Alcohol created an even more pervasive and ambiguous problem. It might be easy to write a bylaw excluding alcoholics from hospital admission, but difficult to administer it humanely. Physicians were well aware that the symptoms of other, sometimes critical, ailments might mimic those of drunkenness. Or what of cases in which patients suffered from ills that resulted from the ingestion of alcohol, ranging from fractures and lacerations to liver disease? Did a failure of will in the past mean that an individual should be denied treatment in the present? Physicians were well aware that delirium tremens, "immediate alcoholic poisoning," often required medical treatment and not the cold floor of a police cell. A realistic understanding of clinical realities underlined the inadequacy of rules flatly denying admission to cases of "pure and simple inebriety."[27] Most hospitals tried to formulate compromise procedures reflecting both lay and medical points of view. Particularly embarrassing were incidents in which gravely injured patients were refused ambulance service and hospital admission because they appeared to have drunk too much.[28] Mundane issues perhaps, but such recurring instances illustrate the never-ending process of negotiation between lay and medical authority.

Conflict could arise over the staff physician's behavior as well as his values. Discipline was not limited to patients and servants. Physicians too might need to be prodded into a due respect for their obligations. Senior attending physicians often slighted the hospital wards. Outpatient physicians were often late; house and attending physicians sometimes ignored calls to critically ill or dying patients; junior house officers might become drunken and unruly, harass nurses, or protest the quality of food provided. In all such cases, lay boards and superintendents had to step in and impose an appropriate order.[29] Senior medical staff had their problems as well maintaining control over their own assistants and interns in wards they visited only a few hours each week.[30]

Although holders of the medical degree were still a minority on private hospital governing boards, separate boards representing the attending medical staff began to play an increasingly prominent role in everyday hospital routine. They were advocates for new programs and facilities, and adjudicated the career demands that often led to undignified strife among physicians. They spoke in a formal way for the corporate needs of medicine and the individual ambitions of particular practitioners. How were promotions from junior to senior positions to be made? Was seniority or some other standard to be used in making such promotions? How were cases to be divided between medical and surgical services? How were the new specialties to be integrated into the institution's clinical services? Only when the medical staff could not make amicable decisions or when they lacked the financial resources to enforce the decision they desired, did they turn to the trustees.

In such negotiations the hospital superintendent often served as intermediary, exerting a power based not only on newly proclaimed professional skills but on his or her strategic position in the hospital. No one else could plausibly mediate between the claims of lay and medical authority. No one else could make a plausible claim to understanding the hospital in both its care giving and financial aspects.

A Third Force: Emergence of the Superintendent

Lay boards removed themselves only gradually from the hospital's wards, kitchens, and corridors. But that distancing was as inexorable as it was gradual; delegation of authority was a natural response by men and women of affairs who found hospital affairs time consuming and even intimidating. Appointing a strong executive was increasingly seen as a key duty. At the Hartford Hospital, for example, the board's executive committee had at first overseen much of the institution's routine management. In 1877, its members embarked upon a new course, deciding that their most important duty was to appoint well-qualified executive officers ". . . who have purity of character, equable temper, and the power of self-control. They should also possess faculties adapted to their position. When this is accomplished it is not necessary for committees to spend much time in details. Their principal duty is to keep these appointments as perfect as possible."[31]

The superintendent was the most important of such appointments, although his key attributes were still personal: honesty, common sense, financial prudence. The superintendent still had no special training and claimed none. In this sense, hospital governance had changed little since the first half of the century. But with growing size and diversity, the demands made on the hospital's executive officer increased steadily. His was an almost impossible task.[32] One of the answers to this dilemma was a gradual diffusion of executive responsibility. By the end of the century, and at larger hospitals even earlier, the functions performed by the superintendent and his wife had devolved into the hands of three separate officers: a superintendent, matron, and head nurse. The matron, no longer assumed to be part of the superintendent's family, remained in charge of cooking, cleaning, and laundry, the traditionally female part of the hospital.[33] A trained nurse ordinarily supervised the nursing and nurse training school. At the same time, most institutions relied on the decisions of a chief resident physician in day-to-day hospital routine and disciplining junior house officers. This was a far more elaborate administrative structure than anything that could have been anticipated by antebellum hospital advocates.

To some extent it was simply an inevitable response to increases in scale coupled with the growing professional authority of medical and nursing staff. But it was also a response to a more complex set of responsibilities—a physical plant that included elevators and steam boilers, telephones and electric generators, a training program that included student nurses and interns, an enormously more complex and demanding financial structure, a patient population divided among pay, part-pay, and charity accommodations. By the first decade of the twentieth century, the superintendent could not realistically expect to visit each ward or room—and even less could members of the institution's governing board.

There were exceptions to this rule. One, of course, was many of the Catholic hospitals, even the larger ones, where nursing orders still maintained administrative control. A sister could still provide strong executive leadership while remaining in contact with everyday ward routine. Community hospitals constituted another exception, for in such smaller institutions a trained nurse often occupied the role of superintendent as well as supervisor of nurses. But this was not true of all community hospitals. In some, the superintendent and resident physician roles were fused so that one salaried practitioner could admit patients, treat emergencies, supervise nurses, and bill patients.[34] In either case, an able man or woman could maintain a firm and knowing hold on an institution.

Superintendents of large hospitals, on the other hand, soon began to conceive of their complex tasks as demanding a special kind of experience and training. A proper ordering of administrative roles, routines, and authority had become a necessity. Florence Nightingale and other mid-century hospital reformers had emphasized this principle, and subsequent increases in hospital scale only underlined its continuing relevance. The hospital's "usefulness," as one aggressive superintendent explained it, "depends upon a proper organization, in which certain fundamental principles should be supreme which form the natural laws of such institutions."[35]

Natural law implied systematic investigation and a new kind of superintendent well versed in the application of this new understanding. But most superintendents of American hospitals had, as one authority put it in 1912, been "pitchforked into their positions without special training," although the demands of the position were extraordinarily diverse and consuming.[36] "He requires the strength of Samson, the meekness (at times) of Moses and the patience of Job. He ought to be a good beggar, a good business man, a physician, a bit of a lawyer, and have enough piety to admit him to the pulpit."[37] Despite such requirements, there were still no formal training programs for hospital administration at the time of the First World War; successful superintendents learned on the job—whether they were laymen or physicians. Visits to prominent hospitals and the availability of handbooks supplemented but could not replace that experience.[38]

No technical understanding was more important than the political acumen that allowed a skillful superintendent to define his authority in opposition to and in cooperation with medical men and lay trustees (and with a glance over his shoulder at a public and press still suspicious of the hospital). The most important of a superintendent's management skills was that which allowed him to manage his trustees. In this diplomatic task, an alert superintendent had a number of advantages. One was the fact that no trustee lived in the hospital and could only rarely be familiar with the details of a particular problem; second was the widely held assumption that authority must be unified—that like a military unit the hospital must have a clear chain of command.[39]

The superintendent must be supreme in relation to every aspect of the hospital, the argument followed. It is not surprising that superintendents were fond of invoking military and mercantile metaphors in explaining their sense of prerogative. "The work of running a hospital is made unnecessarily hard oftentimes," the Pennsylvania Hospital's superintendent contended in 1908, "by conflicting ideas of the board of managers, and the sooner people having hospitals in charge realize the nearer a hospital organization is to military discipline, the more perfect the organization is going to be." It was not that the managers should remain ignorant of hospital affairs, but after they have chosen an executive officer, "it is absolutely undermining of all discipline for individual managers or committees to go about with an attitude of expecting that something is wrong."[40] Equally important was the need to maintain exclusive access to the trustees; matron and supervisor of nurses were to report to the superintendent. "It is just as impossible," the shrewd administrator explained, "to run a hospital successfully and smoothly with two heads, as it is to run a business enterprise with antagonistic forces at its head."[41]

Lines of authority were not always as clear in reality as they were in the rhetoric of administrators. Few superintendents before the 1920s actually exerted the unfettered authority they sought. Too many trustees, as one superintendent put it, treated their executive officer like a "sort of hired man . . . for fear that something may be done without the initiative of the board."[42] Board members were potentially and often in reality antagonists to be placated or openly opposed. In 1906, for example, when it was proposed that lay trustees be allowed to join the American Hospital Association (until that year the Association of Hospital Superintendents), the measure was opposed on the ground that candid discussions could not be held if they were present.[43] Many superintendents continued to resent the paternalistic and arbitrarily intrusive policies of governing boards. Would the owners "of a great commercial house," as one spokesman put it, ask their manager to sleep on the premises? Or would the editor of a great metropolitan daily be asked to sleep in the publisher's office? Yet trustees in 1913, when those rhetorical questions were posed, still assumed that the hospital superintendent must live on the grounds of the institution he managed. Another habitual grievance lay in the habit of individual trustees bypassing their superintendent and dealing directly with subordinates. "Boards are disposed to do this without realizing that the first result of it will be subversion of all discipline," followed necessarily by the superintendent's inability "to control people and things." Resignation was the superintendent's only recourse if board members persisted in such subversive behavior.[44]

Conflict with medical men and medical needs was a more frequent reality; every aspect of hospital routine implied differences in priority and perception. One constant irritant was the need to discipline house staff. When surgeons abused patients or failed to answer emergency calls, it was the superintendent's responsibility to punish the offender (especially when the incident had become public).[45] Less dramatic but more frequent was the need to fit junior house officers into a bureaucratic routine.[46] The superintendent, on the other hand, could be a pivotal mediator between medical staff and lay trustees. When, for example, the Boston City Hospital surgical staff sought a reorganization, they voted that the superintendent "should do whatever was possible, in personal interviews with these gentlemen, to secure the requests."[47]

Medical men often contended that friction between staff and administration could be reduced by the simple expedient of appointing physician superintendents, ideally medical men with both clinical and administrative experience. The more optimistic could even contend by the time of the First World War that "there has grown up a school of hospital administration in which the graduates are medical specialists, just as other medical men are specialists in other branches of the profession." Such experts had not only mastered the financial and technical aspects of administration, "but know enough about medicine to deal with the medical men and furnish them with the facilities they need."[48]

Lay superintendents often failed to share this bland view. They saw the medical profession as faction-ridden and sometimes exploitative in its relationship to the hospital.[49] And as might have been expected, even when administrators were physicians, their altered responsibilities often implied conflict with their sometime colleagues; it was a result not simply of training and allegiance but of social location.[50]

From another perspective, of course, both medical staff and administrators benefited from the hospital's growth; there were abundant perquisites to be divided in a period of expansion and the feudalization of authority. One group, however, benefited very little: the men and women who worked in the hospital's wards, laundries, and kitchens, drove its ambulances and shoveled coal into its furnaces.

Forgotten Men and Women: Workers and Bureaucracy

If the hospital relationships of doctors, nurses, and administrators can be seen in terms of the accumulation and negotiation of authority, the experience of lay workers must be seen rather differently. They adjusted to authority rather than exerted it. Work conditions often deteriorated as the paternalism that had traditionally tempered bleak realities was gradually transformed into a self-conscious and impersonally bureaucratic style of management. Wages had always been lower than in comparative jobs outside the hospital, but greater security and a casual tempo of work had seemed sufficient compensation to some.

With each decade after the 1870s, however, hospital managers sought to impose a firmer order upon their work force. Since the great majority of hospital workers lived in the institution itself, every aspect and moment of their lives could be subjected to an increasingly vigilant oversight. To hospital reformers, the energy and relentlessness of that oversight was an index to the hospital's efficiency. In 1877, for example, the New York State Charities Aid Association—dominated by a handful of ladies who sought to rationalize benevolence—published a guide to *Hospital Housekeeping*. It warned hospital matrons to be rigid and methodical; casual discipline guaranteed disaster. "This sort of lax rule," they warned, "may sometimes earn a cheap popularity with the lower quality of attendants and the weaker sort of officers, but it is a mistake to believe that conscientious and intelligent persons like it. This class prefer order and system and respect those officers most who steadily and kindly enforce them." And enforcement meant a total and unrelenting vigilance. "The matron should not fail to look into every attendant's dormitory, under the beds, behind the doors, and into the closets, at least once a day, and occasionally at other and unexpected times."[51]

Imposing order meant in practice rooting out the areas in which nonprofessionals controlled the pace and quality of their own work. At the beginning of the nineteenth century, the relations between hospitals and their employees were typical of those in a more traditional economic world; like other employers, for example, hospitals still provided liquor rations to male nurses, laborers, and washerwomen, who as we have seen largely controlled the day-to-day fabric of life and work in wards, kitchens, and laundries.[52] Hospital reform implied that these domains of manual labor had to be controlled just as nursing had; they could not be allowed to exist as autonomous enclaves of power and value.

A minor but illuminating incident at the Massachusetts General Hospital in 1893 suggests these tensions. The hospital's resident physician, Dr. John Pratt, sought to ease the reins of power in the kitchen away from Grace McLeod, who had been a loyal MGH employee for more than thirty years. Although Dr. Pratt conceded that he respected McLeod, she was not "progressive. Under her supervision things run in a rut." She did not guard the stores carefully, and he hoped to hire an assistant cook and storage clerk to increase administrative control and to "begin with these changes and to gradually lessen the rule and authority of Grace." A few months later—almost too neatly—the hospital trustees hired scientific nutritionist Ellen Richards. The resident physician, not surprisingly, approved fully of Miss Richards' attempt to bring science and cost-cutting to the hospital in place of the traditional practices that still shaped many aspects of the institution's everyday life; it was a tradition he could not understand and only partially control. "An important part of Miss Richards' work," a trustee committee shrewdly observed, "has been to secure throughout the kitchen department capable and honest people working loyally in accordance with her wishes."[53] Ellen Richards with her academic training and professional aspirations is in many ways an admirable figure— an inspiration to women seeking careers in the sciences. She must have appeared in a rather different light to the cooks and kitchen workers at the Massachusetts General Hospital.

Coupled with substandard wages and poor living conditions, such intrusive policies made it hard for hospitals to attract and hold a stable workforce.[54] It is hardly surprising that a "labor problem" plagued hospital superintendents in the first decades of the present century. Orderlies were a particular worry, because they played a vital role in care and came into contact with patients and visitors. The situation at New York Hospital became so awkward that the trustees appointed a committee to investigate the problem in 1907. The report suggested that the much-criticized orderlies would provide much better service "provided in turn better recognition is given to them."[55] In most hospitals it was assumed that orderlies were recruited from "a class which is shiftless"; the pay was so poor and the work so menial that everyone connected with the institution simply assumed and acted as though they were an inferior class—a perception underlined by the fact that "everyone gives them orders & they give orders to no one." Nevertheless, the report continued optimistically, the hospital did have a number of hardworking and self-respecting orderlies who were in fact appreciated by the hospital's officers. The problem was to increase the number of such workers. One method was raising salaries; the report suggested that salaries be adjusted gradually until they reached forty dollars a month after five years of service; pride could also be instilled by providing service stripes reflecting years employed.[56] Orderlies should be given uniforms and not required to do manual work when they might be called at any time to assist with patient care. "They of all persons come closer to the patients and should be cleaner in a sanitary sense than almost any of the other employees of the hospital." Bathrooms should be provided and the hospital insist that "they take baths at regular intervals and . . . change their underclothes at certain times." Finally the report urged that orderlies be given instruction before they began to work on the wards. Class was still a tangible element in the hospital's social structure; pay, prerogatives, dress, even smell distinguished those members of the working class who were to be subdued to a bureaucratic discipline—and whose underpaid work still subsidized the hospital's benevolence.[57]

A final group ignored in the hospital's redistribution of power and prerogative were the patients who filled its wards and rooms. Unwilling participants, perhaps, they were necessarily affected by all of those changes we have described.

CHAPTER 12

Life on the Ward

In the spring of 1874, the Board of Managers of Philadelphia's Pennsylvania Hospital appointed an Officer of Hygiene—a young physician whose task it would be to inspect the building from basement to attic and report his findings. This delegation of authority might well be seen as the forerunner of more bureaucratic ways of controlling a still traditional institution, a significant break with the personal oversight that the hospital's lay managers had always exerted.

But this incident is more significant in retrospect than it was in substance; the building through which the Officer of Hygiene walked in 1874 had in many ways changed little since the beginning of the century. Nurses were often absent from assigned wards and servants insolent or evasive. Chamber pots remained unemptied for hours under wooden bedsteads, and mattresses were still made of coarse straw packed tightly inside rough ticking. Vermin continued to be almost a condition of life among the poor and working people who populated the hospital's beds, and lice, bedbugs, flies, and even rats were tenacious realities of hospital life.

The patients were still largely recruited from a culture very different from that which had socialized staff physicians and lay administrators. They used the hot air flues for spittoons and emptied their urinals into the sink instead of the water closet.[1] Patients hoped and expected to find relatives and friends a source of emotional support in strange and threatening surroundings; visitors not only smuggled in forbidden food and drink but milled about in large numbers and with casual disregard for stated visiting hours. On one occasion, the harried Officer of Hygiene reported eleven visitors at a bedside and another day, four men and a dog sitting on a bed. Clothing provided another test of will. Patients were often unwilling to give up their own garments and insisted on wearing them—even in bed. The Pennsylvania Hospital's problems were no more than typical; the ward was inevitably a battlefield of values in postbellum American hospitals.

The same year that the Pennsylvania Hospital's earnest young Officer of Hygiene surveyed its wards, the bylaws of the New Haven Hospital specified that patients take off their hats in the wards and their boots or shoes before lying down. "All patients able to leave their beds will wash themselves in the ward bath-rooms," the Connecticut hospital's regulations continued, "and comb their hair, immediately upon getting up in the morning. Every patient is expected to bathe the whole person once a week, . . ." Philadelphia's Jewish Hospital similarly warned its patients in 1874 that they had to remove all their outer clothing before getting into bed and refrain from "Using tobacco . . . spitting or throwing anything upon the floors or steps, and throwing or hanging anything whatever from the windows, balconies, or verandahs."[2]

In every hospital, both private and municipal, ambulatory patients would, as they had since the eighteenth century, be expected to help with the cleaning, serving, and mending. The superintendent of one large city hospital suggested in 1883 that recovered patients be made to work for two weeks after they would normally have been discharged.[3] It was only right that they pay with their labor for the care that had helped them recuperate. Social position, not sickness, was still the primary determinant of a patient's hospital identity.

An enormous gap separated the hospital's normal patient population from the genteel presumptions and comfortable styles of life assumed by those who administered the hospital and practiced in it. Nothing symbolizes this distance more aptly than the lice that seemed an almost inevitable part of slum life—and thus a problem for hospital authorities. "Vermin," as one attending physician put it in 1876, "are constantly introduced with the patients brought from places alive with these pests, and nothing can protect the wards from their disgusting prevalence but the want of harboring places, vigilance and care."[4] The hospital in the mid-1870s seemed always to be on the defensive—always grappling with fresh onslaughts of dirt, insolence, swearing, and alcoholism, as well as the lice and bedbugs that symbolized and embodied the distance between hospital inmates and their social superiors. A resident physician, as one who served in Philadelphia's municipal hospital warned in 1877, would have to "be wary if he wants to have control of his wards, for the vicious and often criminal characters therein will stop short of nothing to circumvent him."[5]

Imposing a New Order: Sources of Change

By the first decade of the twentieth century, the average patient's experience had become something very different from that which had been the lot of his predecessor a half century before. One source of change grew out of scientific and technological innovation. The germ theory and related public health practices reshaped not only the incidence of infectious disease, but the status and prerogatives of the medical profession as well. Therapeutics too had changed, particularly the increasing prominence of surgery in the hospital. Lengths of stay decreased during the same period, necessarily altering the texture of ward life. And every aspect of hospital life was, finally, affected by those multifaceted economic and technological changes that were reshaping Western society generally—from telephones and electric lights to elevators and inexpensive textiles.

Changes in the hospital's social organization were also important in reshaping the patient's experience. The larger institutions had been internally restructured by the prerogatives and perspectives of the developing professions of nursing and hospital administration, and the elaborate specialization that had come to characterize urban medicine. The gradually increasing presence of bedside teaching and beginnings of clinical investigation on the ward guaranteed that its occupants would in all likelihood be exposed to more frequent and intense contacts with house officers and medical students.

Patients were also likely to be victims of different sorts of ailments. Although the relationship between changing morbidity and mortality patterns and the acceptance of the germ theory does not seem as unambiguous as it did a generation ago, there are some direct interconnections, especially in regard to infectious disease. Typhoid fever provides an instructive example. By the 1920s, the typhoid cases that had proved so labor-intensive in the nineteenth century had ceased to be a significant element in hospital admissions. A combination of progress in civil engineering, allied with bacteriological and serological screening along with the establishment of isolation procedures, had worked to vastly decrease typhoid incidence. Diphtheria, to cite another instance, was still a menacing presence in the 1870s; by the 1920s it had become far less common in most parts of the United States. Similar, though hardly identical, circumstances had changed the incidence of other infectious ailments—and helped create the familiar picture of late twentieth-century disease and death: an increasing life expectancy and the consequently growing role of degenerative disease and cancer in medical care.

Knowledge of pathogenic microorganisms had an even more direct impact on the American hospital; this was the stimulus it provided for the enormous growth of surgery in the four decades between 1875 and the First World War. It had a number of important consequences. One, as we have seen, was in convincing middle- and upper-class patients that a hospital was an appropriate place in which to be treated. As a result of the growing amount of surgery allied with a desire to cut costs, the average length of patient stays, both free and pay, decreased steadily between 1870 and 1900, from an average of roughly six weeks to one closer to three.[6] The ward's social order necessarily reflected this changing pattern of morbidity, therapeutics, and length of stay. Patients were less likely to be ambulatory and thus less likely to develop a supportive network of fellow patients on the ward.

And these wards—as well as the increasing number of private and semiprivate rooms—were likely to be quite different from their predecessors in the 1860s. Electric lights, elevators, metal bedframes, and easy to clean composition floors had become a part of every well-run institution. Cheaper textiles meant more frequent changes of linen and gowns, gauze that could be discarded and need not be washed for reuse. A more varied and inexpensive food supply implied a more adequate hospital diet, as it did for Americans outside the hospital. More effective modes of heating and ventilation also affected the patient's experience; no more could patients complain that beds near a central stove were too hot, those in remote corners of the ward too cold. None of these developments were strictly medical, but all were the product of scientific and technological change considered broadly. All altered patient experience directly—and indirectly as well by conspiring to make the hospital an inexorably more capital-intensive enterprise.

The architectural and organizational aspect of the Nightingale reforms had profoundly affected the hospital. The uniform arrangement of wards and fanatical attention to ventilation had become omnipresent realities by the 1880s. They were not always welcomed by ward inmates (as when patients complained of the cold drafts engendered by an aggressive commitment to cross-ventilation no matter what the season). By the turn of the century, however, the original Nightingale doctrines were being modified; ward sizes, for example, had become somewhat smaller (twenty instead of over thirty beds in each) and the supervising ward nurse was no longer ordinarily housed in an adjacent room.[7]

Other technical changes were related more directly to the physician's ability to diagnose and treat. The routine use of the thermometer, the clinical laboratory's armamentarium of blood, urine, and tissue tests, and the x-ray at the very end of the century all helped reshape the traditional interaction between doctor and patient. Although it has perhaps been overstated, there is a core of truth in the notion that the patient was becoming more and more an object— "clinical material," the kidney in H or appendicitis in G—rather than an individual whose class and style of life were his or her most distinguishing characteristics.[8]

Diagnosis was decreasingly dependent on the patient's own words and the physician's immediate sense perceptions. Hospital practice had, of course, always been more impersonal and routine than its private counterpart—so that the change in institutional practice was in some ways from that of casual neglect to an impersonal, intrusive, and highly structured routinism. For the first time, physicians could call upon a set of procedures and techniques that subsumed the individual sick person to the increasingly lesion-oriented and disease-specific notions of pathology that had become gradually dominant in the profession's world view during the course of the nineteenth century. Allied with the increasing ratio of house staff to patients and the presence of student and graduate nurses on the ward, this new technology could monitor—and thus control—patients more likely to be seriously ill and less able to call upon the social and emotional resources offered by his or her wardmates. The inmate was becoming a patient—and the patient a diagnosis.

Administrative as well as cognitive and technological change impinged directly on ward life. Most important was the advent of trained and student nurses, for they constituted the mechanism through which the period's drive for order and system was articulated throughout the hospital. The desire of this fledgling group for professional acceptance meant that every routine procedure nurses learned and administered would serve to act out and legitimate their status. The very sacredness of impersonal routine erected an increasingly rigid barrier between nurses—already distanced by social origins and aspirations—and their still predominately lower-class patients.

Bureaucracy and efficiency meant the pious and unrelenting invocation of numbers just as they demanded an unbending routine. By the mid-1870s, hospitals were already beginning to impose a statistical order on their operations just as they had always sought to impose a suitable decorum on their patients, servants, and junior house officers. The clock and the time-clock became important tools in regulating the hospital; they had played almost no role in its prebellum predecessor. When New York's Presbyterian Hospital opened in 1873, its visiting committee found only one clock in the entire building—and that in the kitchen.[9] As the clock and time-specific work schedules began to control the work of aides, nurses, and house staff, the chart and clinical case record came increasingly to define the patient's ward identity.[10] These developments brought a host of everyday consequences. Temperature curves meant patients being awakened at night or disturbed during the day to have their temperatures taken; rigid work schedules meant that ward patients could be awakened as early as four in the morning so that prescribed cleaning tasks might be completed.[11] Such petty but by no means trivial annoyances soon became a part of accepted hospital experience.

The well-managed institution sought to impose a segregated order of place as well as of time. Uniforms, for example, were seen as important not only for instilling morale, but could set individuals apart from one another and place them immediately in the hospital's social hierarchy. By 1900, a visitor could tell house from attending staff, graduate nurse from student, and student from probationer or servant by their dress. In the older municipal or almshouse hospitals, physicians and administrators sought to separate the sick from the merely dependent; dress was an invaluable signifier.[12]

Just as the late nineteenth-century hospital hoped to identify individuals and place them in functional categories, so it sought to physically separate the institution's several functions. At the beginning of the century, admittance, diagnosis, surgery, and even death were not segregated; all took place in the ward. By the end of the century, all had been (or were being) defined and physically separated. Even at midnineteenth century few institutions had proper receiving and admitting rooms or separate entrances for emergencies.[13] Diagnostic workups, like much surgery, the dressing of wounds, and finally death, took place in the ward among presumably calloused onlookers. Individual patients could do little to ensure their privacy even during the most intimate or painful examinations and treatments. (By the 1870s, curtains were sometimes available on the ward, but in at least some, only for "naturally modest women.")[14]

By the end of the century, admission had become a routinized, physically segregated procedure. A standard physical examination preceded admission to a bed, as did a compulsory bath and, in many institutions, delousing. The patient's street clothes were removed, locked away, and replaced with a hospital gown. Hospital rules no longer forbade patients from wearing shoes and hats in beds; all of an individual's personal effects would have been systematically removed before they reached the ward. The admissions process might be thought of as a ritual separating the patient from his or her previous identity—and especially those class-specific attitudes, behaviors, and possessions administrators sought to exclude from the wards. This depersonalization was carried out as well in the fashionable practice of referring to each new admission by the number of his or her bed; this not only symbolized the efficiency sought by superintendents and trustees since the 1870s, but discouraged the "inappropriate" familiarity that sometimes developed between nurses and patients. Such impersonality was not only uncomfortable for many patients but could on occasion contribute to embarrassing mistakes in therapy. When a Hahnemann Hospital surgeon, for example, discovered that the wrong patient's head had been shaved preparatory to an operation, he urged that orders for surgery or other therapies mention patients by name as well as bed number.[15]

Death too was removed from the ward. Moribund patients were systematically transferred to special rooms. "Such cases," New York's Presbyterian Hospital explained in its annual report for 1891, "however guarded, are depressing to other patients in the ward, as is also the removal of the body afterward; nor is the ward, however well managed, so fitting a place for the last hours as a room where the patient is separated from all but the necessary attendant or friends." Presbyterian was actually a bit in advance of some other institutions. It was not until 1906, for example, that the Board of Managers of Philadelphia's Episcopal Hospital decided that "for humane reasons towards co-inmates" patients "shall not be allowed to die in the wards of the Hospital unless from sudden or unforseen causes; . . ."[16] Decades earlier, administrators had sought to remove surgical procedures (other than emergencies or routine dressings) from the ward; even with the availability of anesthesia, surgery on the ward could be emotionally traumatic for onlookers. The advent of aseptic surgery added prophylatic to humanitarian reasons for limiting surgery to special operating rooms.[17] It will be recalled as well that in the first half of the century, even some laundry and food preparation remained the ward nurse's responsibility and took place in the ward or nearby. The well-administered hospital in 1900 boasted a separate laundry and kitchen (though small pantries for the preparation of special diets were still considered necessary for individual floors or wards).

This segregation of function affected patients differentially according to class. The gradual entrance of paying patients into the hospital was significant for the institution's budget, but also created new social realities in the hospital. The comparative minority of well-to-do patients could be catered to in their "hotel-like" rooms: they were never subjected to the prying eyes, hands, and instruments of students; they might have relatives in the same or adjacent rooms; they could call upon the services of a special private nurse; they ate "dainty and taste tempting" food from fine china. Marketplace considerations as well as social assumptions demanded such genteel amenities. When accommodations were less than appropriate, the urban hospital could find itself at a competitive disadvantage. "This is necessary," a concerned member of New York's Presbyterian Hospital inspecting committee warned in 1896, "from a purely business motive, as well as for the reputation of the hospital." The committee had been dismayed to discover that despite their institution's none-too-modest fee schedule, private room meals were poor in quality.

. . . there is a noticeable failure, and I am sorry to say, this reputation prevails outside of the Hospital. Persons accustomed to good living, on entering the Hospital, must first provide for having a part of their food sent to them from outside, or satisfy themselves with a poor meal. The Bouillon and Soups are not delicate and free from grease, and are not served in that inviting condition they should be for private patients.

On the other hand, the same committee concluded, "the table for the Wards is excellent. Bouillon and Soups, possibly, could be clearer and freer from grease."[18]

Food quality was only one of the distinctions between free and paying patients. Private patients, for example, had the privilege of receiving visitors at almost any time of the day (though many hospitals did try to discourage all visitors before noon), while ward visiting hours were sharply limited.[19] Every detail of a hospital's accommodations reflected both the need to attract paying patients and contemporary assumptions concerning differences in class sensibilities. Heat might be more abundant and easily adjusted in private rooms than in wards. Floors on free wards, like those of kitchen or utility areas, an authority explained in 1912, should ordinarily be made of tile or terrazzo. For private wards, on the other hand, wood was appropriate. "The traffic on such floors is comparatively small, they can be kept polished fairly steadily, and they give the home touch, a point the psychological importance of which is worth remembering."[20] Curtains, window boxes, and individually designed rooms were all recommended as useful in reproducing that homelike atmosphere considered indispensable to an ideally curative atmosphere.

Care as well as decor reflected such assumptions. Women and private patients, for example, were more likely to receive anesthesia for the same procedure. Surgical house staff rarely operated on private patients, except in dire emergency. The superintendent of Pennsylvania Hospital urged attending surgeons to leave private patients in bed in their own rooms until the surgeon actually arrived on the scene; with free cases, the practice had been to prepare patients and place them on stretchers before the surgeon entered the building. In some institutions, the patient might be brought into the operating theater and anesthetized before the surgeon was actually in the hospital. The presumed dignities of class did not end with consciousness; even under anesthesia, it was assumed that private patients would be spared the inquiring eyes and presence of medical students.[21]

If the wealthy could hope to reconstitute a version of their accustomed domestic style while in hospital, the reality was far grimmer for the "intelligent" and "cultivated" of limited means. Although they might need the specialized care (often surgical) that only a hospital could provide, they feared the ward's demeaning associations. The lower middle class might share the social values and preconceptions of their wealthier fellow citizens, but not the resources to pay for private or semiprivate rooms. Yet the mixing of classes (and sensibilities) was something most administrators regarded with instinctive distaste; both empathy and equity dictated that respectable Americans be spared the free ward's polluting contacts.

By the turn of the century, hospital administrators were well aware of such problems. They could hardly avoid them as they made individual decisions in regard to admission and billing. "My means are very limited," Anna Baird of Staunton, Virginia wrote to the superintendent of the Johns Hopkins Hospital, "my father being an invalid Presbyterian minister & I a music teacher—& I cannot afford the luxury of a room to myself. Please let me know what would be the least that I could have the advantages of the Hospital for, without going into the free ward."[22] Self-respect demanded that one do everything possible to keep family members—especially wives, daughters, and sisters—out of the "charity ward." The small minority of the relatively well-to-do could be catered to in hotellike accommodations, but the far greater number of less financially secure Americans who thought of themselves as middle class needed private or semiprivate arrangements that might spare them the double humiliation of accepting alms and being forced to mingle with those beneath them in the social scale.

The gradual transformation of the hospital into a potential site of medical care for Americans of every social and geographic location inevitably altered the experience of all; the rich had to adjust to hospital life—no matter how slavishly the hospital sought to recreate their accustomed comforts. The middle class had to face a difficult choice between borrowing or using limited savings to avoid the free ward, while also facing the fear and anxiety that confronted all hospital patients regardless of social origin. The experience of working men and women may have changed least of all; hospital amenities did improve steadily throughout the period but at the cost of a parallel depersonalization.

The problem of treating contagious disease provides another example of the tenacity of class assumptions as well as the creation of a new class of potential hospital patients. Once medical men and

boards of health accepted the idea that certain infectious ills needed
to be isolated, they accepted the practical necessity of sequestering
individuals suffering from such ills—and thus created the dilemma
implicit in the mandatory mixing of classes in municipal contagious
disease facilities. Administrators were particularly sympathetic
with the plight of respectable fellow citizens forced to share class-
blind isolation wards. In describing their Branch (contagious disease) hospital, authorities at the Cincinnati General Hospital complained in 1904 that among their patients had been many

. . . from the better walks in life and most respectable and prominent
citizens, and many were from the lowest of the low; but owing to inadequate facilities for complete isolation and separation, we have not been
able to separate as completely as should be done, the better class of people
from the depraved and criminal class.[23]

A solution depended on the city providing facilities in which individuals could be segregated by class as well as sex. In other communities similar experiences led to calls for the creation of pay
hospitals for the treatment of contagious disease; such ailments
were no respecters of persons. Mandatory co-existence with the
poor and uncouth seemed an unjustified punishment for individuals
whose only crime lay in having fallen ill.[24]

Another characteristic aspect of the two-track system within voluntary hospitals lay, as we have seen, in the immunity of pay
patients from the hands, eyes, and stethoscopes of students and
teachers. When clinical teaching became more routine and more
frequently took place in small groups at the bedside, individual
patients were correspondingly more likely to be subjected to such
indignities. For sensitive patients, even being in a room where such
instruction took place could be humiliating. Outpatient clinics
could be particularly brutal in their impersonal and episodic way;
"she was poor," as one lady clinic patient complained, "but had not
always been so, and could not sit there with others present and
listen to what she had to."[25] It is not surprising that medical schools,
hospitals, and dispensaries sought to control the casual affronts of
students and house officers. "Students are required," as one faculty
committee expressed it, "in the interest of their own education and
in deference to the dictates of humanity, to examine the patients
with the consideration due to sick people."[26]

It is clear that patients did not always welcome the teaching hospital's ministrations. New York's Sloane Maternity Hospital, for example, discovered that its occupancy rate plunged during the academic year and increased when classes were not in session. The hospital's medical director scrawled in exasperation in 1901, that "if we *could*, we would shut up the hospital when we closed the doors of the College in June."[27]

In the great majority of early twentieth-century hospitals little clinical research was undertaken—even in institutions where a good deal of bedside teaching was accepted. But clinical investigation was already well established in a handful of the more academically oriented hospitals.[28] Systematic clinical research provided another context in which conflict might arise between the immediate interests of the individual patient and the ultimate accumulation of knowledge—knowledge that might, as research advocates claimed, serve in the long run to benefit humanity, but which might be garnered in studies conceived with little thought to the comfort of a particular patient who happened to find him or herself serving as an involuntary datum. Even if it meant no more than frequent blood tests and temperature readings, clinical research could still increase the patient's anxiety and discomfort. By the turn of the century, in fact, contemporaries were well aware that conflict between patient welfare and the compulsions of medical science could and did arise. "No man should be a member of a hospital staff," a prominent Cleveland physician warned in 1898, "whose zeal for the advancement of science or the promotion of his own ambition will sacrifice the interests of his poorest patient."[29] The implicit dilemma has in the past four generations been restated but hardly resolved.

The Intractable Institution

In the last third of the nineteenth century and first decade of the twentieth, the hospital had been transformed. Every aspect of change affected the individual patient's experience, but in a context in which continuity was also strikingly marked, especially for those poor and working-class Americans who had always been its natural and earliest constituency. The hospital remained, as it had necessarily to be, a microcosm of the social relationships and values that

prevailed outside the institution. Social values could not be transformed as easily as the physician's diagnostic tools.

Fundamental aspects of the sick role were perhaps even more
tenacious. Sick people tended to become patients, infantilized
whether treated at home or in the hospital. "Men under such conditions," as a prominent surgeon expressed what seemed only a
truism, "are mentally speaking, reduced to the condition of children; they can not be chastised with the rod; they can hardly be
reasoned with; they must and will have their own way." A more
than ordinary endowment of patience and understanding was demanded of those who cared for such difficult charges. "We must
always remember," readers of a nursing journal were warned in
1888, "that the sick are selfish, that it is their right to be so, and that
to the strong their little whims often appear rediculous [sic]; yet we
must always treat them with thoughtful consideration and kindness." It was only to be expected that they would be "exacting and,
in some cases, querulous"; the problem was in imposing an appropriate discipline. Unending demands could not be tolerated in an
efficient ward. "It is then the staff's privilege to control the patient,
by the highest of all forces, the love and respect the patient bears
them."

If the patient continues willful, designedly, or from impulse, from weakness, or, as often happens, from having been spoiled, the staff may still be
able to control her by talking to her—by taking away her little privileges
she has been enjoying—by passing her with a curt "Good morning" and
so on, until she realizes she must obey the general law.

A patient, like any emotional dependent, needed to be treated with
a mixture of kindness and authority; as with children, only a "tight
hand" would keep them from becoming "absolutely unmanage-
able."[30]

The urban hospital was still not the primary locus of medical care
for most Americans. Special domestic circumstances or the need for
major surgery might bring the wealthy and respectable into urban
hospitals—but they remained a predominately working-class institution before the First World War. Men far outnumbered women,
and among males, the single and widower were disproportionately
prominent. The hospital still constituted for most of its potential
clients a feared and stigmatizing institution. "Among the very poor
people," as social worker Jane Addams explained in 1907, "there is

a deep-seated prejudice against hospitals as such. I have heard," she elaborated, "the absurd stories they tell—that if you go to a hospital they will cut you up, if you go there they will find out what is the matter with you in all sorts of queer ways."[31] Even more starkly, the hospital remained for many among the poor a place to die—a deeply internalized fear that no recitation of cure rates could easily counteract. At least as general as such visceral fears were those of being humiliated in the acceptance of free care. Many working people were anxious, for example, to pay the dollar a day that became standard in the "part-pay wards"—thus distinguishing themselves from the even less affluent who were treated without charge.

Not surprisingly, there remained an enormous social distance between medical men (and the comparative handful of women physicians) and patients. The growing number of new immigrants from Southern and Eastern Europe (Jews, Slavs, and Italians) with their jarring languages and behaviors only exacerbated the situation. The Irish had seemed sufficiently alien and disquieting at midcentury; ethnic stereotypes only intensified the structured misunderstanding and hostility that often characterized doctor-patient interactions in hospitals and clinics. In 1896, a Boston physician recalled how the Irish had seemed to represent a step down from native-born patients whose self-respect demanded that they consult a private physician if they possibly could. The situation had only worsened as the century drew to a close. "Since the Slav and Latin nations have come in, they always expect to be hospital patients; they never mean to employ a doctor in any other way." The Irish were alcoholic, Italians filthy and garlic-smelling, Jews timid and intolerant of pain. "Sam, a young Polish Jew," had had his right foot crushed under a streetcar wheel, an observer of "hospital life" reported in 1888:

A very good boy he is, only he has not been gifted with the amount of courage most American boys have. An approach of the visiting physician to his bed-side is a signal for a blanched face, panting breath, and dilated eyes; the announcement that he will do his dressing now, call forth a cry of protest which is increased to a yell like that of a young savage, when he is carried to the dressing room and the cutting of the bandage is commenced.

The lack of communication between doctor and patient was often literal as well as figurative. A prominent dermatologist, for example, recalled that in his clinical work among Italian patients at the New York Dispensary, he accumulated a working vocabulary consisting in its entirety of the Italian phrases for "undress," "rub it in," and "three times a day."[32]

Although an increasing proportion of medical men spent time as house officers, they still represented a group disproportionately well-off and ambitious when compared with the population generally—and certainly with the urban hospital population. (And this is not to consider the absence of women, blacks, and recent immigrants among the ranks of interns and residents at America's "best" hospitals.) Physicians and nurses seem in retrospect to have often been insensitive to the needs and perceptions of their institutional charges—beings alien to the social expectations of the more genteel house officers. Some medical men sometimes noted and recorded, for example, the "quaint" sayings of their charges (routinely an aspect of the institution's oral tradition and a practice hardly unknown today). W. Gilman Thompson, a house officer at New York's Roosevelt Hospital in the 1880s, made note of "Odd remarks of Dispensary and Hospital Patients."[33] Such "odd remarks" included those of an Irishman who exclaimed "I'm the father o 4 poor childhren & the mother of em gone, & if I be laid up, God help us." Several years later, he recorded the plea of another Irishman who begged: "Docther, I don' want to lose this one, for I buried 7 out o' 9 with bronchitis!" His four-year-old was being treated for the same ailment.

Patients were assumed to be uncouth in language and filthy in their habits. A hospital authority rejected the possibility of using commercial dishwashing machines for ward dishes, as was done in hotels and restaurants, partially because of breakage, but partially because of the condition of ward dishes, "left by a patient, who is of a very different breeding from the epicure at an hotel."[34] It is hardly surprising that hospital boards should have had to discipline nurses and house staff for occasionally striking and cursing intractable patients. "I have heard say," a young woman physician complained in 1902, "it is unwise to try to explain the cause of disease to patients, that it is throwing pearls before swine." She herself rejected the notion, but it was clearly a common attitude.[35] It was only consistent that convalescent and ambulatory free patients should still have been expected to help with cleaning and sewing; both class attitudes and chronically straitened budgets guaranteed that the practice would maintain a tenacious hold on ward life into the twentieth century.[36]

The impact of professional nursing was also related to class. In their embodiment of bureaucracy and enforcement of an increasing medical authority, trained nurses helped bring social change into the ward. On the other hand, the makeup of this new nursing force reaffirmed the social distance that had always characterized the institution. The older nursing corps had been recruited largely from among the sort of people who populated the wards and then "trained" informally on those same wards; the new model nurse, especially those who wielded administrative responsibility, had been recruited from a rather different class. (And training schools worked hard to instill "proper" styles of behavior even in students drawn from working-class families.) The nurse's own social and professional insecurities only heightened the emotional distance that separated her from her hospital patient.[37]

Class was not the only social relationship that reenacted itself within the hospital. As might be expected, race and conventional moral categories were also powerful realities. Black patients continued to occupy the least desirable locations in nonsegregated hospitals; in some cases they remained in older wings when new wings or buildings were constructed. In others, they were shunted into basements or attics. When white wards were refurbished, black patients might receive the cast-off furniture to replace their even less presentable ward furnishings. (And the fact that a particular institution admitted both blacks and whites did not mean they occupied the same wards or rooms; locational segregation remained standard within nominally unsegregated institutions.) A 1907 authority on the "race question" in hospitals explained the prevailing wisdom:

. . . the negro department must always be as far from the white and executive department as possible. . . . The equipments in all departments are practically the same; however, the linen, gowns and every individual article of the different departments must be kept as separate as if in a different part of the city. Say, for instance, at a glance you can note where each article belongs, as all are marked in large letters—cream and white blankets for private rooms and white wards; slate-colored blankets for colored wards, and red blankets for ambulance service.[38]

Hospitals varied of course according to the mechanisms with which they turned racial assumptions into everyday routine. Most older Northern hospitals were discreet about their policies, but even if their bylaws remained silent on the subject, actual practice reflected prevailing attitudes. At the New York Hospital, for example, even the plea of an attending physician failed to move the institution's superintendent as the medical man sought to have a middle-class black patient admitted to the "intermediate ward" of the hospital's private building. "The patient is of light complexion," the administrator explained to the chairman of the hospital's visiting committee:

(probably quadroon) is eminently respectable, quiet and dignified in bearing and has means, is able and willing to pay and was sent to Dr. Johnson by General James Wilson, who is greatly interested in her . . . Without prejudicing the decision in any way, I may say that the question of admission of colored patients came up early in the history of our Private Patient's Building. The Committee decided that they preferred not to put on record any legislation on the subject. They thought, however, that the admission of such patients would be unwise and instructed me, in the event of there being an application to seek to evade it, rather than quote any Hospital rule against it.[39]

Private white patients would hardly patronize an institution in which they might be expected to share rooms (or even floors) with blacks.

Ironically, however, black poverty and the general lack of black-sponsored and staffed hospitals made blacks all the more dependent on available hospital facilities—no matter how undesirable the terms on which those facilities might be made available. Sex ratios among black patients were not so sharply skewed toward males as they were in white admissions. In some general hospitals, "colored wards" were filled to overflowing, while white wards were partially occupied. At Atlanta's Grady Hospital, for example, the superintendent reported in 1899 a sufficient number of beds for white patients, but a waiting list for "colored beds." Two years later, the situation was even worse; there was still a waiting list in the colored wards—while facilities for whites remained more than adequate.[40] Although there were occasional problems in finding staff for black hospital units, the presence of black patients was in fact often welcomed by attendings at the largest hospitals: "the negro," as one contemporary put it, "is more docile and does not object to being used in clinic for teaching purposes and is one of the most prolific sources in the study of medicine."[41] (Black nurses and doctors did not, of course, benefit from this source of teaching "material," since they almost never gained access to student or staff positions at white hospitals. It is not surprising that black physicians should have been leaders in founding the first hospitals supported by and for the "race.")

Children played an even more ambiguous role. Romanticized as victims of ills they could not understand and often appealing as individuals, they were almost always representatives of a social class far lower than that of their nurses and physicians. They were minors in more than one sense. Doctors could take real pleasure from the affection children might provide. "The only endurable hour in the day," a Hopkins house staff member wrote to his fiancée, "is the one outside of G. with all the poor crippled up little beggars climbing over me—why I feel really pleased & proud to have them remember me overnight, & set up a shout of 'Good mornin', Doctor Billy' when I come into the ward for the visit."[42]

But these eager little faces presented a peculiar discipline problem; it lay in the need to avoid spoiling them so that they could return happily to their tenement apartments. The hospital should seek to restore children "to their homes unspoiled by the necessary comforts its fostering care has given them."

The soft bed, the warm clothes, the comfortable bath, the abundant food, and constant unremitting care give place to the bare walls, the scanty table and crowded room of the poor man's home. The luxuries of the nursery have no proper place in the ward of the hospital and the most discriminating care should be exercised lest the "pet" of the ward return, cured it may be in body, but ill at ease and dissatisfied, to its place by the hearth from which it has been so greatly missed.[43]

The contrast seemed all too stark. Children often arrived at hospitals in rags and covered with lice. "They are thoroughly washed," as a newspaperman visiting New York's Babies' Hospital explained in 1886, "dressed in clean, comfortable clothes and put to bed, for the first time in their wretched little lives experiencing the sense of comfort." If such ambivalence and condescension were unavoidable, attitudes toward the little sufferer's parents ordinarily lacked even ambivalence. "The greatest obstacle," as a Philadelphia General Hospital physician explained his work in the infant ward, "to contend with in these cases is the vicious stupidity of many of the mothers, the dreadful condition in which many of the children are brought to us."[44]

Moralism and the paternalistic assumptions of a more traditional society remained alive in hospital routine well into the twentieth century. Hospital patients were still moral agents, responsible in some sense for their sickness as well as their poverty. Contemporaries felt no difficulty in making such associations. It was not the diminution of tuberculosis in their city that reduced their admissions, a Cincinnati General Hospital physician explained in 1906, but rather "an effort to limit our admissions to worthy patients; those who would not lend their personal aid in curing or bettering their condition, where possible, being discouraged from admission."[45]

The connection between traditional moralism and the paternalistic framework of social relationships in which it was articulated was maintained with particular tenacity in regard to childbirth—and especially the large proportion of unwed mothers who filled maternity hospital beds at the end of the century. This was certainly a category of patient in which volition was related to the necessity for hospital admission. Hospital boards were both protective and punitive. One evidence of these mixed motives was the age-honored practice of limiting admission to "first-time losers." An innocent girl might be forgiven one mistake, but hardly a second. Control over the erring young mother's child also seemed an appropriate responsibility for her social betters: many maternity hospital administrators felt no hesitance in placing these products of untoward alliances in respectable homes. Even in a self-consciously modern and scientific institution like Johns Hopkins, maternity patients filled a particularly passive and sentimentalized niche, "a portion of the community, which either from poverty or disgrace demands the pity of an institution founded for purposes of beneficence and education."[46]

The punitive component of these attitudes was even more prominent in regard to another class of patient—those suffering from venereal disease. Such ailments, as one widely read clinician put it, "are the result generally, not of misfortunes, as other inflictions are, but of imprudence, and are self-inflicted. And for this reason," he explained, "venereal patients have not the usual claim upon your sympathy."[47] Voluntary hospitals still rejected such patients (although attending physicians often urged that only patients with primary lesions be excluded and that those suffering from the neurological or cardiovascular symptoms of more advanced syphilis be treated).[48] Throughout the period, however, such patients were admitted if they paid; it was not simply a question of economics—but of class, for the great majority of female venereal patients were prostitutes and the men, common laborers or sailors.

Even when admitted to municipal hospitals, venereal patients were, as we have seen, still treated as pariahs. A resident at PGH, for example, noted that the venereal patients had

nothing in common with anybody else in the house. Their dress is of a peculiar color and make, the ugliest that ever could have been devised by man. They are not allowed to associate with any but their own class, nor allowed to use anything except what is set aside for the use of their own floor. Instruments used in these floors cannot be used in any part of the house.[49]

This particular description was written in 1880, but the segregation and stigmatization of venereal patients and their treatment as less-than-equal continued into the twentieth century. They might be forbidden to take books out of the library or provided a diet less abundant and of worse quality than that enjoyed by other patients. Even outpatient clinics represented a problem to conscientious administrators; male and female venereal patients had to be carefully segregated and both classes kept as separate as possible from other outpatients. It was a never-ending problem to find space "enabling us to better segregate the most objectionable people we are called upon to treat, viz—those suffering from genito-urinary or venereal diseases."[50]

Alcoholic patients too were treated with disdain. The solution for dealing with such patients was well established by the end of the century: transfer them to a city hospital. Private hospitals could to some extent choose their clientele; city and county hospitals could not. This policy, however, could lead to embarrassment when hospitals failed to treat gravely ill patients exhibiting symptoms that mimicked the drunkard's erratic behavior. On occasion such unfortunates might die in transit between voluntary and municipal facilities; now and then such examples of seeming callousness provoked newspaper exposés.

Such incidents had little in the way of lasting impact. The fundamental relationship between the public and private sector continued—and affected the experience of patients at both voluntary and municipal hospitals. Aged and chronic patients were, like the alcoholic, consigned in the great majority of cases to stigmatizing public care. The willingness of some religious hospitals in the 1870s and 1880s to make room for such patients sometimes failed to survive into the twentieth century.[51] Even though individual hospitals might continue to treat the aged and chronic (or support a division that did), newer hospitals oriented themselves as much as possible toward acute care. Most were unwilling to admit tuberculosis cases, for example, or even cancer. As late as 1909, none of New York City's general hospitals would accept cancer patients; ". . . aside from the Almshouse Hospital," a prominent New York surgeon observed, "the number of places where the poor can go and spend their days in comparative peace are sadly inadequate."[52]

Although change also came to chronic and municipal hospitals, it always arrived slowly in such institutions, plagued as they were by constrained budgets, an almshouse heritage, and the dispiriting awareness that the brave new weapons of medical science were of little use in treating the victims of degenerative ills. The ward experience changed slowly indeed for aged and chronic patients consigned to beds in city and county hospitals.[53] Both social and biological realities remained intractable; and, not surprisingly, chronic facilities were operated more as custodial than curative institutions—on an inevitably lowest-cost-per-day basis. In small cities and counties, even general and acute care hospitals were sometimes far less imposing than the glass and marble "palaces" that foreign visitors admired in New York, Boston, and Chicago. Wyndham Blanton, a practitioner and historian of medicine in Virginia, described Richmond's Old Dominion Hospital, for example, "as a sort of reconditioned barn, poorly equipped and redolent of odors compounded of feces, food and ether."[54] The nineteenth-century heritage died hard.

Even in the most avowedly scientific hospitals an older paternalism continued to remain very much alive. Patients still had to be disciplined to the use of combs and toothbrushes; friends still had to be stopped from providing companionship, food, and bracing—if forbidden—drinks; rules still enjoined the use of profanity and the expression of infidel sentiments. Sponsorship by individual board or attending staff members could still affect admission and treatment. At the Massachusetts General Hospital, the resident physician had to report individually on the moral worth of applicants for wooden legs. He recommended one boy, the son of a widow, for he had "looked up his record and we find that he is a good little boy." A laborer was approved because he had "a family to support and has never had aid from town or city." The superintendent of another hospital routinely informed the employers of patients diagnosed as suffering from gonorrhea—"as diseases of this kind are often transferred to innocent persons while using the same toilet utensils etc."[55] Although the hospital's technical underpinnings and economic logic had changed dramatically in the generations since the Civil War, the free patient remained a moral minor subject to the decisions and condescension of administrators, nurses, and medical men.

Most of those who inhabited the turn-of-the-century hospital were not the sort who kept journals or diaries. Few wrote to concerned family members, who then carefully preserved their letters. Many physicians and nurses did publish recollections of their hospital experiences, but their accounts are in most cases so wooden and stylized that they tell us more about the writer's attitudes than about the patient's experience. A few personal accounts do escape these strictures, and I would like to use one to provide a somewhat more textured insight into life on the ward as it was experienced by Katherine Hammond, a student nurse at Johns Hopkins Hospital in 1893–1894 who described her everyday routine in regular letters to her mother.[56] This particular hospital may have been in some ways atypical; it was a leader in the avant garde of medical care and teaching. But by the same token, Johns Hopkins provided a foretaste of the future—to be observed and emulated by hospitals throughout the country.

Every aspect of the institution seemed shaped by a relentless drive for internal order. "There was never anything so monotonous & clock like as our work here," she complained, "its exact regularity."[57] At the same time, she was well aware of the advantages provided by the hospital's bureaucratic structure. "I find my cap and uniform," she explained after graduating from probationer status, "a great help in managing the patients—now that I work in this dress they cant tell how little I know but will obey almost unquestioningly."[58]

It was easy to feel an instinctive sympathy with the patients. The physicians seemed often to care more about refining their skills than they did about the helpless men and women on whom they practiced. "I was quietly letting my man die," Hammond complained on another occasion in describing a terminally ill patient, "only keeping him as comfortable as possible—when the Dr. came in and began to torture him. I would never come here to be nursed if I were ill."[59] The hospital's all-pervading regimentation was an even more depressing reality. On another occasion, the student nurse was upset when her graduate ward supervisor confiscated pictures drawn by a youthful patient, "because they littered up his bed. He looked at me in such an injured way, he cant understand a word of english, so I could not make him know why I did it. She made me stop him from whistling. I felt very bad about it."[60]

In keeping with the institution's desire for order and impersonality, patients were never to be referred to by name, but only by bed number. "Another hard thing about these numbers," the anxious young woman wrote,

is that they are so unfeeling—to address a dying man as No 8—and ask if you can help him seems very heartless—and yet it's often the case. I will do everything for a man for a week or more without knowing his name—and always in speaking to the Dr. or other nurses you speak of them in that way . . . I wonder if it is because these people are sick—that they seem so different from many of the people I have ever seen before. You know a lot of them are immigrants from all parts of Europe, but laying aside this fact, there is a curious sort of phlegm and indifference about them, very different from what I consider now, the excitability of the people I have been accustomed to.[61]

Hammond was not alone in this observation; other nurses and medical men noted that even hospitalized young children soon learned not to cry for attention that rarely materialized.[62]

Just as these passages illustrate Hammond's sympathy with the plight of her ward charges, they also illustrate the emotional and social distance that separated them. When she worked in the male medical ward, for example, Hammond complained that it was difficult for her "to make a man put on clean shirt and to see that his finger nails are clean."[63] She was surprised that her patients seemed not to notice the economic slump that had caused so much concern among her parents and their friends. Her charges were, as she put it, "absolutely poverty-stricken" and their economic prospects so chronically hopeless that the depression seemed not even perceptible to them.[64] In this situation, class lines were exacerbated by ethnic difference. One day she referred to a "Russian girl—as wild & untamed as a young animal," while the Irish served, as they had throughout the century, as a convenient occasion for whimsy.[65] A particularly poignant instance of such cultural misunderstanding arose when a young Italian was admitted with a fractured skull.

At first he did nothing but sleep—but now he is getting better—and sits up in bed and talks the wildest lingo to us all. . . . If you do anything that pleases him he will catch your hand and kiss it—and makes violent efforts to embrace you. He is filthy like all Italians—and sly too. He steals the peaches out of the other men's table . . . eats them and hides the stones under his mattress.[66]

"My Dago boy," she wrote two days later, has gotten out of bed and walks around "in the funniest way you ever saw. When any of the men speak kindly to him he stops and kisses their hands—much to their confusion." Some months later the exhausted student nurse wrote in summation that "the patients in this ward are now an awful common lot—you don't care what a person is when they are very ill—but when they begin to get well you feel utterly disgusted with them."[67]

The Johns Hopkins Hospital embodied and symbolized a new scientific medicine, but it still replicated in microcosm the social realities that shaped the larger society outside its reassuring red brick walls. And it was an environment in which patients still paid a price in dignity and discomfort for the new clinical skills and efficiency that they hoped would restore them to health.

CHAPTER 13

The New-Model
Hospital and Its Critics

In the summer of 1911, Joan Smith's ninety-year-old father died at the Massachusetts General Hospital. His treatment and hers had left her with bitter feelings toward the hospital and its "uncivil and apparently inefficient" employees. Questions were answered with rudeness, often with a clerk not even looking up from his desk. "While the majority of the people calling at the hospital are poor and ignorant," she contended, "that is no reason why they should not be treated like human beings and not like cattle."

Family members could only speak with physicians at three o'clock and then the brief exchange of words had to be held in a "common entrance way" with the doctor "who is also standing . . ." Might not the families of gravely ill and dying patients be "allowed the privacy of an office, where, if only for a few minutes, they might receive the attention and courtesy due them." The nursing too was inadequate; several times she had found her father's ward entirely unattended. After he died, she and an undertaker were kept waiting for some time until an official appeared to receive payment for two days' charges. Only then was she allowed to claim the body. Even though her father was a ward patient, she concluded, "he and those interested in him, should receive common courtesy." He had been born in Massachusetts, "and his father and mother before him, and he lived a useful and respected life for nearly ninety-one years, but it will never cease to be a regret to me that he died in the Massachusetts General Hospital."[1]

The bereaved and indignant Brookline resident was hardly alone in her feelings. Although the early twentieth-century hospital was in general an enormous source of pride and optimism, it had already provoked a variety of critics. Even many of the self-consciously professional leaders in the new field of hospital administration were aware of imperfections in their proud new temples of healing and sought to make them as humane as they were scientific and efficient. At the beginning of the twentieth century, thoughtful hospital executives such as George Rowe of Boston City, George P. Ludlam of the New York Hospital, and S.S. Goldwater of New York's Mt. Sinai, were aware of flaws even in their prestigious institutions. They feared the emergence of a hospital that would, as one such critic put it, become a "great machine" reducing to cogs those unfortunate enough to find themselves within it or, in the words of another contemporary, an "experiment station" of interest chiefly to a small clique of ambitious publishing physicians.[2]

By 1910, in fact, almost all of the criticisms that were to become so familiar in the late twentieth century were already being directed toward American hospitals. From the patient's perspective, the hospital seemed impersonal and bureaucratic. Staff physicians infrequently treated the whole patient, the critique followed, certainly not as part of a specific family and specific community; specialists addressed themselves to a focus narrowed by their training. Paralleling this structured myopia was a disproportionate concern with acute ailments, especially those in which the hospital's technical capabilities might be employed, and a corresponding lack of interest in convalescence and chronic illness.

The urban general hospital was, finally, coming to seem a facility for the very rich and the indigent alone. As we have seen, the great mass of middle-income Americans would not willingly enter a hospital as ward patients but could not afford private room rates. Something had to be done to make the hospital an available choice for these neglected families. Thoughtful critics of the early twentieth-century hospital also sought to moderate the already-alarming escalation of costs that seemed inevitably associated with an emphasis on acute care; the hospital needed to become a more flexible institution. Both economics and humanity underlined the need for regional planning, for improving, and even expanding outpatient facilities, for better convalescent and long-term care, for the provision of socially appropriate yet economically viable facilities for middle-income patients.

Meanwhile, the municipal hospital had still to escape its alms-

house heritage and the constraints of an always mundane and sometimes corrupt political process. No matter what their class, sick
people deserved competent and nonstigmatizing care; reformers
hoped to make the municipal hospital humane, efficient, and scientific—clearly differentiated from its almshouse roots and as much as
possible a mirror image of its not-for-profit peers.

In this progressive generation, the desire to make urban social
institutions both rational and responsive flourished among hospital
spokesmen as it did among social workers, socially minded educators, and municipal reformers. Yet the impact of their shared convictions was necessarily limited. Efficiency, science, and planning,
the tools that legitimated and would presumably implement reform
efforts, were to prove in some ways antagonistic and in others
irrelevant to those efforts. The forces that had already shaped the
the hospital were bound too deeply into its fabric.

A Social Vision

Disease was more than a pathological process, and the hospital's
role more than that of a repair shop. The reform program emphasized the arbitrariness of the barriers separating hospitals from the
communities that surrounded and supported them. "Many medical
and social workers," a prominent advocate of hospital social work
contended, "who are thoughtfully searching for the causes and
treatment of human misery ask whether the hospital is ready for a
broadening of its functions; whether or not it should now look
. . . beyond its walls to the community which it more or less consciously serves."[3] Truly effective medical care and a more humane
society were inextricably related.

Traditional medical thought had never questioned the significance of the relationship among environment, style of life, and
illness. Environmentalist assumptions persisted among public
health reformers in the late nineteenth and early decades of the
twentieth century, despite the increasing influence of the germ theory. Even in the world of academic medicine, the reductionist view
of disease had not swept all before it; work, diet, stress, individual
habits, and dwelling-places all might play a role in predisposing to
illness. The incidence and severity of disease was determined by

more than a chance likelihood of exposure to specific disease agents. Such assumptions pointed compellingly toward the need for a medicine with roots in the family and community.

And a vocal minority of socially oriented doctors did advocate an increased intervention in the hospital patient's social milieu. Richard Cabot, for example, a Harvard professor and Massachusetts General staff member, was probably the most outspoken and articulate of these activists. He pictured each patient in hospital or clinic as a kind of sampling device (like the bacteriologist's sample of a water supply) reflecting in his or her sickness aspects of the society that helped produce such disability.

As a bucket let down into an artesian well or into the ocean brings up from the bottom a sample of what is widely distributed there, so a patient with lead poisoning, with tuberculosis, with a court record, brings us into touch with conditions which we should not ignore.[4]

It was entirely consistent that Cabot should have been instrumental in establishing America's first hospital social work department (at the Massachusetts General), and that he should have condemned the disjunction between patient as citizen and family member and the same patient as hospital case; the two dimensions of experience could not be disassociated without reducing the quality of care. "Beyond the special disease," Cabot argued, "of a special child or adult who comes to us in the dispensary, stands a family problem, ultimately a community problem, poverty, bad housing, bad food, bad habits and associations, ignorance of the ways and means of making a clean and healthy life on scanty means."[5] Such arguments paralleled the motivations and assumptions of contemporary social welfare advocates, many of whom, like the nurse and settlement house leader Lillian Wald or industrial toxicologist Alice Hamilton, had a professional interest in medical care.[6]

Although historians have found it difficult to agree on the distinguishing characteristics and social roots of progressivism, there is no doubt that the first two decades of the twentieth century witnessed a broadly conceived attempt to expand the traditional responsibilities of urban social services. Health played a prominent role in that more general program of social renewal; hospitals could hardly remain immune from the critical attentions of would-be reformers. The responsibilities of the hospital did not stop with perceived sickness, they contended, nor were its boundaries defined by admission and discharge. Outpatient clinics could be a place for educational lectures and instruction, the moment of discharge a signal for shifting attention to the home and away from the hospital bed. Attention to such "medical prophylaxis" would aid the hospital as well—relieving crowding by attacking disease at its source: the homes and workshops of the poor.[7]

Within the hospital, outreach centered on public health nursing and social service. Both were predicated on the need to follow the patient into his or her home; both presumed a need for flexible modes of delivering care. Visiting nursing had the older history, reflecting pioneer mid-century English efforts.[8] By the 1880s, a number of American hospitals and dispensaries were already employing nurses to visit convalescent patients after discharge. Their primary duties were therapeutic, to oversee the changing of dressings, for example, or the proper use of orthopedic appliances, but they were to have an educational function as well, bringing knowledge of proper diet and hygiene to the presumably benighted tenement home. At roughly the same time, the first of the autonomous (and often female directed and funded) visiting nurse associations began their work in urban tenement districts.[9] Although structured around the delivery of care, the visiting nurse associations also saw themselves as providing education and enlightenment.

It was not until the first decade of the twentieth century that a hospital social service emerged.[10] Led by the example of Massachusetts General Hospital's pioneer program, other institutions began to appoint social workers whose task it was to follow discharged patients, provide hygienic advice, monitor the patient's compliance with instructions and, perhaps most importantly, evaluate his or her social and economic as well as physical health. A patient could hardly remain healthy while unsure of his or her livelihood; hospital social workers were thus expected to cooperate with public and private welfare agencies.

Despite such energetic beginnings, however, some aspects of the early twentieth-century hospital seemed fundamentally antagonistic to a social understanding of health and disease, even to a sensitive treatment of the particular men and women who occupied its beds. The hospital had organized itself to provide the most advanced technical services in an efficient bureaucratic setting, but in doing so, its critics charged, had lost sight of the individual patient. Jane Addams, for example, dramatized such organizational inhumanity to a group of hospital administrators by citing the case of a woman suffering from a ruptured appendix who had been admitted and in conformity with regulations had been bathed and had had her hair braided before being seen by a physician. She died during surgery.[11] The problem was worst in the largest hospitals and especially in those with active teaching programs. We do not want the patient, as the superintendent of New York Hospital argued, to think of himself as an object of charity, nor do we "want to allow a patient to become a 'case;' we do not want to have him simply amalgamated with the mass of clinical material; we want to preserve his individuality." The great majority of patients entered the hospital in fear and only as a consequence of unavoidable necessity; the patient had a right to expect ". . . 'environmental treatment,' and consideration for himself as an individual, not a mere unit lost in routine."[12]

Some of the reasons for the trend deplored in these already commonplace arguments seemed bound up with fundamental aspects of twentieth-century medicine. Specialization was one such factor. With too much specialization, as Mt. Sinai's Goldwater warned in 1906, the hospital "ceases to be a satisfactory or even a safe instrument for the relief of its patients." Treatment might well be determined not by the patient's needs but "by the special aims and practice of the department in which he happens to be placed." Research-oriented surgeons might, for example, consciously or unconsciously discharge patients who were of no "interest" prematurely; gynecologists might dismiss ailing patients simply because a surgical procedure did not figure in their care.[13]

The patient had become, so the already-familiar argument ran, not a person but a configuration of organs and potential syndromes. Richard Cabot expressed and dismissed these attitudes with whimsical acidity as he quoted the words of his clinic assistant. The young man greeted him one morning with the enthusiastic report that there awaited: "a pretty good lot of material. There's a couple of good hearts, a big liver with jaundice, a floating kidney, three pernicious anemias, and a flat-foot." Understanding the patient was a prerequisite to understanding his or her disease, yet, Cabot lamented, "the average practitioner is used to seeing his patients flash by him like shooting stars. . . . He has been trained to focus upon a single suspected organ till he thinks of his patients almost like disembodied diseases."[14]

Cabot was hardly alone in entertaining reservations about the reductionist tendencies of an increasingly technical hospital medicine. Many ordinary practitioners shared a lingering hostility to specialism and suspicion of the laboratory. Test results might obscure as much as they revealed, and the findings of test tube and microscope were, in any case, no substitute for the experienced clinician's understanding of the whole patient.[15] As one ironic practitioner put it, private practice forces us, "the possibly prejudiced and misled practitioners—to treat the patient as well as the disease or diseases he is suffering from, and here sentiment helps as well as science and art."[16] To some physicians at least, hospital care was not always and inevitably the best care.

Of course, most contemporaries did not see the achievements of the hospital and laboratory as necessarily antagonistic to the hopes of social medicine. To the great majority of able and idealistic physicians the laboratory and hospital ward seemed, in fact, the appropriate places to seek means for ameliorating man's physical lot. Older and more inclusive views seemed in comparison vague and diffuse. Questions of resistance, of predisposition, of family situation and individual idiosyncrasy, of the relation between social environment and health seemed less and less relevant, or more accurately, less amenable to controlled investigation. Moreover, implementation of the social program implicit in environmental views demanded the difficult and unsettling consideration of political and social action— the reform of industrial and housing conditions, for example, or the establishment of national health insurance.[17] Intellect, professionalism, and prudence all conspired to center the energies of medicine's elite on the hospital's inpatient beds.

Inpatient and Outpatient in the Culture of Medicine

But as contemporaries were well aware, far more Americans were treated outside than inside the hospital. Only 13 percent of the sick were admitted to hospitals, a prominent authority on hospital management emphasized in 1913. We did not need and could not provide a bed for every sick person. The dispensary and social service department were the appropriate response.[18] It was the urban hospital's duty, in the words of another administrator, "to give its help in the earliest stage of the disease, . . . and keep the wage-earner from being obliged to leave his work and become an inmate of a hospital ward."[19]

Free outpatient treatment had always been an important aspect of health care in American cities—even though its provision had never enjoyed high status among physicians. Originating in the late eighteenth century, dispensaries and hospital outpatient clinics had by mid-nineteenth century become the principal form of institutional care for the working poor and the indigent. In terms of case loads, they were to remain so well into the twentieth century. Antebellum hospitals and independent dispensaries had always offered "walk-in" treatment to those unable to afford their own physicians. In many, staff physicians paid house calls on the more seriously ill.[20] The policy was effective, in keeping with both the career patterns of physicians and the social perceptions of those benevolent stewards of society's wealth who supported the dispensary's work. At minimum cost, the laboring poor could be kept out of the hospital's pauperizing wards and returned to work.[21] Physicians, at the same time, found volunteer work at a dispensary or hospital outpatient facility an attractive way of accumulating clinical experience.

In the hierarchy of professional achievement, however, outpatient appointments were, as we have seen, always less desirable than their inpatient parallels. Control of beds, the opportunity to monitor "interesting" cases, the opportunity for surgeons to perform "important" operations, and, equally important, the prestige traditionally attached to the position itself guaranteed that the inpatient attending physician would enjoy more status than his outpatient colleague. Details might have changed between 1800 and 1920, but the distinction between inpatient and outpatient care remained fundamental.

The status gap between inpatient and outpatient appointments could hardly have narrowed as medicine's technical capacities increased over time. Equally significant was the fact that institutional outpatient services remained essentially gratuitous, not related directly to the economic relations that shaped private practice. The treatment of hospital inpatients, on the other hand, had become a promising, and to some physicians significant, source of patient fees by the early twentieth century. (When they did not need hospitalization, private patients were still seen in their homes or, less frequently, the physician's office and only in unusual circumstances in an institutional setting.)

Outpatient work, on the other hand, remained a formative stage in the physician's professional evolution, a stage decreasingly central as hospitals increased in number and opportunities for clinical training expanded. At the turn of the century, however, outpatient and clinic appointments still constituted an important phase in medical careers and would until more elaborate residence and fellowship programs reshaped outpatient staffing. Some specialties, moreover, such as ophthalmology, dermatology, and otology were particularly well adapted to clinic contexts.

Although undoubtedly important to such budding specialists and their students, early twentieth-century outpatient medicine was marked by a number of persistent problems. One was the frequently poor quality of care. Clinic hours were short and waiting rooms crowded and lacking in privacy, records casually kept, and attendance by senior physicians sometimes equally casual. Enormous caseloads made examinations perfunctory and long waits routine. Therapeutics was limited to minor surgery and the dispensing of prescriptions—in many institutions limited to a list of approved (and inexpensive) formulas, sometimes kept in a row of bottles labeled one through ten or twelve.[22] A second problem was organizational. How was the outpatient staff and its functions to be related to the hospital and its senior attending staff? Such institutionally powerful physicians saw outpatient clinics as useful in serving to "feed clinical material" to their hospital's inpatient beds and as an important site for training medical students and nurses. Friction developed when these goals were not met. Inpatient and outpatient physicians could also squabble over facilities and privileges. A third problem developed at the very end of the nineteenth and beginning of the twentieth centuries: it became increasingly difficult to interest "first-class" young men in routine outpatient work.[23] Such positions, as a New York Hospital report explained in 1906, had become progressively more undesirable as clinical instruction became an integral part of medical education. "The acquirements of recent graduates of our medical school[s] have been so greatly increased," they explained, "that the men no longer feel the need of doing dispensary work for self-improvement."[24]

Although it may seem judgmental, it must be understood that patient care as such was not ordinarily a consideration in these discussions—beyond the institutional and moral inertia implicit in the traditional assumption that medical care should be supplied to the working poor temporarily in need and to the unambiguously deserving among the permanently indigent (the crippled, blind, aged, and widowed).[25] Certainly few if any physicians categorically opposed the need for gratuitous outpatient care or the responsibility of the medical profession to provide it. But the provision of such care was rewarded neither with material goods in the form of fees nor the opportunity for intellectual achievement (for few outpatient services were conducted in a way that would allow the systematic accumulation of data by even the most energetic young physician).[26]

No one within the hospital world opposed outpatient care, but neither did more than a few care greatly about it as such. The significance of outpatient work to the medical profession, as I have argued, lay in the opportunity it provided junior physicians for acquiring clinical experience and hospital seniority.[27] To attending physicians, an outpatient service was a source of challenging and instructive cases for admission to their wards. In some ways, such pragmatic considerations pervaded all decision making within the hospital. Institutional policies were determined, that is, only partially by the needs of a specific population: they responded far more sensitively to some institutional dilemma, such as financial stringency, or some professional imperative, such as access to patients for teaching purposes. If optimum care for the working poor had been an explicit priority in shaping the delivery of outpatient care, clinic hours, to cite only the most mundane of examples, would hardly have been limited to the working day.[28]

Ordinarily such matters remained hidden from the public—if not from clinic patrons—and often from trustees as well. In the public mind, and in the thoughts of the great majority of rank-and-file medical practitioners, the central dilemma of outpatient care was subsumed under the rubric of "charity abuse." And unlike quality of care or the relationship between a hospital's inpatient and outpatient services, this issue stimulated a persistent and egregiously public debate. Even those administrators and staff physicians convinced of the need for a vigorous outpatient effort had become increasingly defensive by the late 1890s. Critics of an unsystematic and promiscuous benevolence emphasized not only the drain of unjustified demands on hospital budgets, but also reiterated the already traditional fear of instilling a pauper mentality in the recipients of unearned and thus unappreciated benefits. By the turn of the century, most hospitals and dispensaries had found ways to respond to such criticisms. Some institutions arranged with professional social work organizations to check the truthfulness of patient avowals that they could not pay a regular physician. Others conducted their own financial investigations or began to make small charges for clinic registration or for individual prescriptions. Inpatients were less subject to charges of misrepresentation; men and women occupying an acute hospital bed seemed truly in need, a need demonstrated both by the admitting physician's diagnosis and a willingness to enter the institution's forbidding walls. Traditional assumptions that the medical profession was morally responsible for the provision of gratuitous medical care to the needy had faded by the beginning of the twentieth century. Only a minority of doctors still felt it preferable that a few dissimulators receive undeserved care rather than the genuinely needy being either discouraged or humiliated by probing questions.[29] Some medical staff members opposed outpatient fees and financial inquiries for more pragmatic reasons, particularly the way such policies could inhibit clinic attendance and thus inpatient admissions.[30]

In reading between the lines of this debate, it becomes apparent that a good many patients—especially at the outpatient departments of the largest and best-known hospitals—did have some small ability to pay, but came to specialty clinics seeking more definitive diagnoses than their regular practitioners were capable of providing. Many indeed were referred informally by family physicians who recommended a consultation their patients could not have afforded as private patients. "The patients come very largely for diagnosis," as one contemporary explained it, "and care little for the prescriptions. They will be treated at home, but wish to know if the Doctor is right."[31]

Despite much opposition to existing programs, a minority of early twentieth-century physicians and administrators did articulate a positive defense of the outpatient clinic and dispensary as necessary parts of an effective medical care system and not simply an adjunct to teaching and the need to recruit inpatients. Outpatient services should not be constrained, they argued, but made more accessible and upgraded in quality. The rapidly increasing costs of acute hospital care only underlined the need for such measures. Michael Davis, administrator of the Boston Dispensary in the years before the First World War, was perhaps the most inventive among his contemporaries in shaping plans for improved outpatient medicine. Davis sought to turn the staid Boston Dispensary into something resembling a health maintenance organization, not for the indigent alone, but for any Bostonian who could not afford the most advanced and specialized care.[32] He emphasized both the need to reach into patients' homes and the unsettling fact that many even among the city's skilled workers, middle-class clerks, and managers could not afford the fees of an array of specialized consultants in the event of illness. He contended that such services should not be limited to the treatment of acute ills, but utilized in prevention as well; the Dispensary should disseminate the truths of cleanliness and proper diet.[33] The dispensary and outpatient clinics of major hospitals could thus fill logical gaps in the prevailing system of urban health care. Davis was hardly alone in expressing such views. Yet just as his ideas and pilot programs were being elaborated, changes in medical ideas, institutional practices, and related medical career patterns were making the independent dispensary (such as his Boston Dispensary) well-nigh obsolete, and even the thriving hospital outpatient department became less and less important to the plans of most aspiring physicians. Twentieth-century outpatient clinics continued and continue to treat vast numbers, but this had little to do with their limited status in a medical culture increasingly dominated by inpatient care.[34]

Dispensaries and outpatient clinics were left with the residual function of providing casual and largely gratuitous medical care. The hospital's increasing technical capacities seemed only to justify the clinic's marginal status. A hospital bed was the proper place for treating severe ills; even childbirth and death were moving into the hospital by the 1920s. Both intellect and material interest pointed toward an increasing concentration on the hospital's inpatient role. That energetic minority of ambitious young physicians unwilling to remain content with the mere accumulation of fees and a local clinical reputation were, as the twentieth century advanced, ordinarily attracted not by social medicine, but increasingly by the "higher" and seemingly less ambiguous demands of research. The hospital was inevitably the locus for those kinds of clinical investigation that garnered the highest status. The reward systems of medicine and the expectations and values of society reinforced each other, offering their highest inducements to those physicians controlling hospital access and hospital practice. The hopes of those who sought to make the hospital a more flexible and less costly institution by expanding outpatient services were doomed to failure.

Despite some foundation and government support in the 1920s

and 1930s, outreach programs continued to suffer from the stigma
of welfare medicine and the antagonism of many ordinary physicians who saw in them a portent of "medical socialism"—and potential competition for a still-slender supply of paying patients.
During the 1920s organized medicine even opposed government
support of clinics for venereal disease control and for maternal and
child health, areas in which the special circumstances of target
populations might have been expected to imply a certain tolerance.

Almshouse or Hospital: Reforming the Public Hospital

Throughout the nineteenth century, much of inpatient medical
care was provided in almshouses and county poorhouses. Yet concerned physicians and laymen had always felt that treatment in
such surroundings would be inferior and demeaning. Insofar as
residence in an almshouse was a punishment for past economic
inadequacy and a deterrent to future imprudence, it seemed unfair
to subject hard-working men and women or the elderly to such
conditions simply because they had fallen ill. So long as laymen
were aware that admission to a municipal hospital was determined
primarily by dependence, they would regard it with fear and hostility. To be treated in Bellevue or Cook County or Philadelphia General Hospital was to confess a culpable lack of options.

The nineteenth-century almshouse hospital was often unsatisfactory in terms of medical staff members' needs as well. Its wards
filled with chronic patients, its budget both chronically emaciated
and controlled by political appointees, the municipal hospital offered a less than ideal niche for ambitious practitioners. But positions
in such hospitals were a good deal better than nothing, for physicianships in the most desirable voluntary hospitals were scarce and
highly competitive. Unlike the vast majority of educated and well-
to-do Americans, medical staff members actually came in contact
with the grim life inside almshouse or municipal hospital walls—
humanity allied with professionalism in motivating their calls for
reform. Since the second quarter of the nineteenth century in fact,
staff physicians had taken the lead in urging that municipal hospitals admit only the remediable and worthy poor, that they be

defined as healing institutions exclusively, physically and administratively distinct from their almshouse predecessors.

The attempt to reform municipal hospitals had a long history. As early as 1835, for example, when Philadelphia moved its almshouse to a new location, its medical staff urged that the medical wards be referred to as the Philadelphia Hospital—thus demarcating it from the institution's other functions.[35] When Boston physicians urged the establishment of a city hospital in the late 1850s and early 1860s, they marshaled similar arguments. It was important to segregate the healing aspect of the municipal hospital function from the sediment of incapacity, age, and illness that more properly constituted an almshouse population.

Central to the logic of such reform pleas was a faith in medicine's healing powers and the egalitarian corollary that every individual had a right of access to therapeutic resources. This assumption of technological entitlement implied an increasing gap between the hospital's welfare and curative functions. Insofar as human problems could be defined in medical—and in practice episodic—terms, they made a strong appeal for public sympathy and support. The reform program promised a community's taxpayers practical benefits as well. Effective medical care could help decrease welfare rolls. "It is certain," a Minnesota physician defended the municipal hospital in 1889, "that the better the surroundings, the more complete the facilities, the more skillful the care and the treatment furnished the sick or injured, the greater are their chances for recovery from disability, the more likely they are to be restored to a life of usefulness and self-support."[36]

Therapeutic and welfare functions should be separated; an almshouse and a hospital should and must be separate institutions. The movement to achieve this goal is illustrated perhaps most dramatically in Philadelphia, the American city in which the physical entanglement of hospital and almshouse persisted longest. In 1873, for example, Isaac Ray, a prominent psychiatrist and expert on institutional care, addressed the reformist Philadelphia Social Science Association, and reaffirmed the already half-century-old demand that almshouse and hospital be disassociated. It was a necessary step toward providing adequate medical care for the city's working poor. Minor improvements, Ray emphasized, "will fall far short of the end in view, if the hospital is to be managed in the spirit of a pauper establishment. The paramount consideration must be, not how cheaply the patients can be kept, but how speedily they can be cured, and how far their sufferings can be alleviated."[37]

Ray's reform contentions rested in good measure on the widespread assumption that there was a real and categorical distinction between the worthy and unworthy poor, between the demoralized pauper and the hard-working but unfortunate ailing laborer. The essential issue did not change in the course of the century, even as Philadelphia's municipal hospital grew ever larger and more prominent. In 1900, for example, its medical staff again formulated the now commonplace demand. The hospital "being a part of the Almshouse," they warned, "there is a strenuous objection on the part of many people to take advantage of the treatment therein accorded patients, because of the stigma of pauperism . . ." The only solution was a physical removal of the almshouse to another part of the city, "and to make the present location a hospital in every sense of the term, one from which the stigma is removed, and that no citizen would hesitate to enter when in need of treatment." Significantly, this plea was made as part of an effort to "promote, encourage and enlarge the clinical teaching at the Philadelphia Hospital" so as to "make it one of the best medical and dental schools in the world."

And as a matter of fact, Philadelphia physicians allied with elements in the city administration were able to bring about a great deal of change in their city's hospital. By the First World War, it could compete in most respects with facilities at local voluntary hospitals—and because it had almost no paying patients offered diverse and increasingly unfettered teaching opportunities. Wards had been reorganized in terms of diagnosis, and a respected nursing school flourished. Clinical pathology and radiology were available for routine patient care; in such technical matters, Philadelphia General Hospital had grown increasingly similar to its prestigious voluntary neighbor, the Hospital of the University of Pennsylvania. By the First World War, at least a dozen specialties had established themselves in the hospital's wards and teaching routine; it had become an institution that felt itself to be a hospital and prided itself on the quality of its teaching, care, and the opportunity it offered the pathologist and clinical investigator. In 1890, *Philadelphia Hospital Reports* was begun as a vehicle for clinical studies conducted at the institution. In 1904, annual reports began to include a bibliography of articles in which PGH "materials" had been used. Philadelphia's municipal hospital had been gradually integrated into the world of medical status and teaching.

By 1910, the year of the Flexner Report and its call for a closer integration of hospital, medical science, and medical education, Philadelphia General had become in some ways a hospital like any of its large, metropolitan, voluntary sisters. Indeed it was far larger than most and boasted an enviable reputation as a place to teach and study clinical medicine.[38] Its 13,000 admissions demanded the attention of 73 visiting staff members (10 surgeons, 12 physicians, 8 each of obstetricians and neurologists). A majority held teaching positions in the city's medical schools. The hospital also boasted a house staff of 27 interns directed by a chief resident, an assistant chief resident, and a resident pathologist. Philadelphia General had become part of the twentieth-century medical world, articulated into both its intellectual and social structure.

On the other hand, it was still an almshouse. The hospital's death rate remained at 12 percent, and a large proportion of its patients were chronically ill. The average stay at PGH was thirty-five days in 1910, and nineteen at the Pennsylvania Hospital. The more things changed, the more they had remained the same. PGH was still residuary legatee for those cases desired least by Philadelphia's voluntary hospitals. It was still physically part of the almshouse complex—one known and feared by the city's working people. It was not until 1920 that Philadelphia opened a physically separate "Home for the Indigent," and not until the years between 1919 and 1926 that the "insane hospital" was moved to a separate location in a then still-rural section of the city. Philadelphia's social problems were not as amenable to a seeming technical solution, or even redefinition, as its medical ones. The chasm in status between the public and private sector remained. Social location was still the primary determinant in deciding who would occupy Philadelphia's municipal hospital beds, and the problems of class, age, race, and chronic disease loomed if anything more prominently as the twentieth century progressed.

Philadelphia was by no means atypical. Other cities followed parallel paths. New York's larger scale made for an earlier physical differentiation of function, but Bellevue and Kings County hospitals, the city's largest and most prominent acute care facilities, shared many of Philadelphia General's characteristics.[39] In Boston, the founding of the City Hospital in 1864 created another variant of the municipal hospital dilemma. Boston City emerged as an acute care-oriented institution much earlier than its Philadelphia peer. But even more significantly, Boston's creation of a self-consciously medical institution did not address the city's burden of age and chronic disease. Long Island Hospital became the refuge for Boston's dependent and chronically ill, who were in fact often sent from Boston City Hospital where they had originally been admitted, but which would treat patients for only a limited number of days.[40] In Charleston, South Carolina, a very different sort of community from either Philadelphia or Boston, a new city hospital organized in 1880 experienced very similar problems as it sought to define a sphere of responsibility distinct from that of the almshouse. The mere act of a city council could not well approximate the problems of human beings who groped their way through the community's welfare system. The chronic sick "found their way" into the almshouse and some of the aged drifted into the hospital, which complained that it was not a home for incurables. Like Philadelphia, Charleston had sought to rationalize and separate its welfare functions, but it too found little success in placing particular people in discrete categories.[41]

The differences between New York, Boston, Charleston, and Philadelphia were more circumstantial than fundamental. In each case muncipal authorities were left with an intractable burden of age, dependence, and chronic illness. In one city, they were treated at separate sites, in another at a single location, but if one thinks of the municipality's health and welfare function, the differences tend to dissolve. Within each system of municipal and county care, it was difficult to make definitive distinctions between disease and dependence, between dependence and disability. In every city, private voluntary hospitals exercised their ability to select among an available patient population, avoiding chronic and contagious ills—just as they had in the first half of the nineteenth century. "Voluntary hospitals," as Henry Hurd, the superintendent of Johns Hopkins candidly argued in 1912, "cannot receive these patients without detriment to the interests of their own special patients."[42]

The rationale for municipal hospital reform called upon a consensus of reference and expectation that transcended the peculiarities of history and scale that set one community's institutional development apart from another. Concerned physicians and laymen invoked the prestige of scientific medicine and coupled it with a humanitarianism that decried the stigma traditionally associated with publicly funded inpatient care. Both the community's economic interest and humanity urged that working men and women have access to potentially healing hospital services.

Such arguments worked to preserve the distinction between the hospital's therapeutic and welfare functions, between the legitimate and the stigmatizing, between the worthy and unworthy poor. The technical rationale underpinning this argument made it largely irrelevant to the intractable problems that had been aggregated in the antebellum almshouse. The plausibility and legitimacy of reform contentions were in fact based on the rejection of precisely those problems. The argument for municipal hospital reform necessarily obscured the magnitude of chronic illness and helped skew priorities toward acute interventionist care. The allure of what I have called technological entitlement helped earnest and well-meaning Americans to ignore that inevitable burden of age and chronic illness built into the imperfect human body. Reformers at the beginning of the twentieth century were well aware of the problems that resided in the municipal hospital but ill equipped to find a lasting solution.

Organizing Benevolence

The hospital system's linked burden of chronic disease, age, and indigence was only one aspect of a more general problem. Even the best run hospitals seemed often inefficient and poorly managed, while local resources were dissipated in the duplication of increasingly costly services. There were a number of seemingly useful responses. One was the invocation of something called efficiency. Second, and seemingly related, was a faith in the potential of medical science; and the methods of science could point to the rational management of limited resources as well as to a more effective therapeutics. Related to both the efficiency movement and a faith in the problem-solving capacities of the scientific method was a small but promising commitment to regional health care planning.

Efficiency was a term invoked so frequently and with so little precise content that one must approach it with appropriate caution. In the first two decades of the century, it offered a varied assortment of equities to administrators of schools, corporations, municipal governments, and factories. The prestige of "scientific management" influenced hospital managers as well. American hospitals spent $250,000,000 a year, one influential committee report argued in 1913; they were "a large business undertaking and should be managed in accordance with sound business principles." But that was by no means a reality. At least 20 percent of that quarter-billion dollars was wasted each year.[43] Efficiency and scientific management had revolutionized profit making in business and industry; it must revolutionize philanthropy as well. If business enterprise could band together and cooperate to reduce costs, why not "institutions established for humanitarian purposes," a prominent administrator contended a few years earlier: "Let us not illustrate in our own little sphere the truth that children of the world are wiser than the children of light."[44]

Within the hospital, efficiency had a number of distinct meanings. One centered on the mastery of an intrinsically forbidding task: reducing the complex internal life and external relationships of the hospital to an at least minimal order. It is only to have been expected that the meetings of hospital superintendents should often have concerned themselves with such matters as the best forms for maintaining patient records, for submitting bills, and for controlling accounts payable.[45] Efficiency meant as well the creation of a hospital routine, one that would simplify medical care and avoid waste. If every aspect of the patient's treatment, from admission through discharge, were carefully specified, nurses, attendants, and house officers could provide an optimum level of care. Mistakes could never be eliminated, nor could accidents be entirely avoided, but a carefully monitored routine could minimize such mishaps. This ordering of tasks would not only shape an irreproachable level of care, but applied to purchasing, cleaning, and cooking, allow the hospital to make the most effective use of its limited financial resources.

Efficiency meant discipline as well as routine; it implied centralized control over an increasingly diverse and specialized work force. The desire to impose an ordered discipline upon the hospital was not limited to the sphere of rhetoric, nor did it originate with the vogue of scientific management at the beginning of the twentieth century. It had begun in the 1870s with an effort by most large hospitals to control costs, as well as their sometimes intractable patients, employees, and house officers. Even the word efficiency itself was used in its modern sense during these postbellum years; any competent administrator sought to run his institution with "the perfection of a machine."[46] Like the military metaphors equally fashionable at the turn of the century, images of the factory and machine production promised rationality, discipline, and economy.

Few contemporaries questioned such goals—even when they conceded that the hospital could not and should not be operated like a factory. Efficiency advocates contended in fact that the visible signs of an unbending bureaucratic order did not intimidate but in fact contributed to the hospital's psychological resources by reassuring patients that they were in capable hands. "It is a great inspiration to the patient," as one hospital administrator contended in 1911, "when entering a hospital, be he the most intelligent or the most ignorant, to note the system and regularity of the institution; that there is no confusion, no criticism of the orderlies and nurses by each other."[47]

The avowal of efficiency played a legitimating role, in addition, implying devotion to a mode of decision making untainted by self-interest. E. A. Codman, for example, a Boston surgeon and perhaps the most fanatically dedicated among American advocates of hospital efficiency, was well aware that the "efficiency ideal" might play this valuable role. Without such a selfless goal, he warned the President of the American College of Surgeons, the organization could offer little to differentiate it from a trade union.[48] Codman was famous within the world of Boston medicine for his indiscreet attacks on the Massachusetts General Hospital's venerable seniority system and, nationally, for his advocacy of the "end result" system for evaluating the long-term effects of surgery. In Codman's thinking, efficiency meant the objective evaluation of a procedure's efficacy; at one level, scientific management constituted an attack on arbitrary and ill-considered aspects of contemporary practice, on another it reaffirmed the system's already agreed-upon technical goals.

But the rhetoric of efficiency was not easily fashioned into a corresponding reality. Critics at the time were well aware that scientific management would not easily reshape the American hospital.[49] As Codman himself emphasized, for example, uncompromising efficiency implied the evaluation of medical men, medical procedures, even medical fees; this was not easily achieved. The expensive treatment that a physician might see as necessary and appropriate might be construed as mere luxury by a hard-pressed administrator; the administrator's efficiency might seem like power-grabbing or mere penny-pinching to the dedicated clinician. And, as many contemporaries were aware, improved efficiency—if related to quality of services provided—more often increased than decreased hospital costs.[50] Second, even those administrators most committed to scientific management realized that a hospital could not be run with the relentless discipline of a factory or army barracks; it had also to be a family writ large, providing sympathy and concern as well as economy and clinical virtuosity. The hospital, as one influential executive put it before the turn of the century, ". . . has a peculiarity not commonly recognized: while it conducts a *business,* it is the *home* of those who live in it." Henry Hurd, the much respected superintendent of the Johns Hopkins Hospital, agreed. Although discipline was necessary, he conceded, "it is unwise to establish and enforce a semi-military discipline or even one which would be practicable or advisable in a railway, a large factory, a corporation, or other business enterprise."[51] The substance of the debate had not altered since the 1880s; little more than terminology had changed. "Efficiency" in the hands of many early twentieth-century administrators was simply an intensely fashionable term dramatizing long familiar policies.

In practice it often meant old-fashioned penny-pinching. An efficient hospital, for example, was one that discouraged waste, and the zealous systematizer might enforce considerable savings. Butter could be salvaged from trays and made into soap; gauze could be carefully sterilized and used again; linen darned rather than discarded. Waste baskets could be spot checked to detect the discarding of usable food or rags. Generations of contending with skimpy budgets had made such tactics acceptable, if not in fact commendable, while the administrator's search for a legitimating body of knowledge lent system and enthusiasm to this traditional repertoire of mundane household stratagems.

At a level beyond the individual hospital, "efficiency" might logically have been expected to imply regional planning, but this was no realistic goal in a decentralized and uncoordinated medical care system. Within every city, individual hospitals duplicated services and multiplied costs as they competed for both status and paying patients. As early as the 1870s, New York City hospitals had sought to cooperate, dividing the city up so that ambulance and outpatient services would have clearly demarcated responsibilities. It was even suggested that hospitals might specialize in particular ailments.[52] By the turn of the century, hospital administrators complained routinely of the local maldistribution of beds and services.[53] However, little came of such often-repeated criticisms or of attempts to form regional hospital associations early in the twentieth century. New York and Philadelphia did establish long-lived agencies (now the

United Hospital Fund in New York and Delaware Valley Hospital Council in Philadelphia), but they were to exert comparatively little influence on the internal policies of their constituent institutions. Even efforts to impose uniform disease classifications and modes of cost accounting struggled to gain general acceptance.[54] The American Hospital Association (founded in 1899) provided a forum for tactical debate among would-be professional administrators, but it too had little impact on policy before the 1920s.[55] Institutions continued to compete, not only for funds and private patients, but for medical reputation as well. Such rivalries in a decentralized system meant, in the words of a well-informed contemporary in 1911, that cooperation between hospitals would remain at the level of rhetoric.[56] The frequent repetition of similar criticisms in the succeeding half century only underlines the tenacity of these decentralized yet fundamental patterns and the motivations they reflected.

Perhaps the most important subject of concern for would-be planners was the problem of care for middle income Americans. Surveys of available beds and occupancy rates could not deal with the problem of potential patients: men and women who might have benefited from inpatient care but who would not enter a ward and could not afford private rooms. Well-informed administrators and physicians feared that large urban hospitals would become a refuge for the rich and poor alone. The municipal hospital would serve the poor, the voluntary hospital would serve both rich and poor, but in a fashion calculated to provide very different accommodations and privileges. Hospitals thus began, naturally enough, to create facilities for the middle class. This had been a goal at the Massachusetts General Hospital, for example, since the turn of the century. At first, an informal system of graduated rates was instituted, and MGH attending physicians might at their discretion waive or reduce room charges for the appropriately worthy and genteel. Finally, the hospital was able (in 1930) to open a pavilion designed to serve this middle income constituency.[57]

Ultimately this trend was to become a general pattern, one instance at least in which conscious planning seemed to correlate with subsequent policies. But such middle income accommodations came into being not because some collective decision had been made and enforced, but because it was so clearly consistent with the well-established interests of hospitals (which sought increased patient income) and physicians (many of whom would now be able to treat and bill private patients in hospital settings). It was consistent as well with ever increasing lay expectations and the medical profession's intellectual emphasis on acute care. Other efforts at planning, especially those calling for improved outpatient services or the public provision of care, had rather less impact. Technically legitimated services for the morally deserving were easy to support—for hospitals, for physicians, for foundations. Care for the indigent or the chronically ill presented an altogether different public image. The ideology of medicine as science coexisted peacefully and naturally with far older American attitudes toward welfare and the unworthy dependent.

Science as Arbiter

If the invoking of efficiency served in part as a means of avoiding a serious critique of the hospital as a social institution, a parallel faith in scientific medicine played a similar and perhaps even more fundamental role. A late eighteenth-century understanding of the hospital's social mission had been rooted in the assumptions of Christian stewardship allied with a perhaps less strongly felt commitment to medical education. The late nineteenth-century hospital and its leaders found their justifications increasingly in the claims of science and a scientifically oriented clinical education.

To the generation that came of age at the end of the nineteenth century, these claims were compelling indeed. Aseptic surgery, the x-ray, applied immunology all seemed to provide objective evidence of the promise offered by continued investigation. A decade later, even more fundamental investigations beckoned: to an aspiring physician in 1910, the promise of biochemistry, of bacteriology, of physiology seemed limitless, their application in clinical medicine no more than a matter of time. "The hospitals," S.S. Goldwater contended, "which have been, and are doing, most for hospital patients and for humanity, are those which provide liberally for clinical and laboratory research and for the education of the medical student." Traditional attitudes toward the hospital's proper sphere only impeded the liberating accumulation of healing knowledge.

In wet-blanketing the ardor of scientific enthusiasm, in shutting their doors in the face of the research worker and its medical students, hospitals have abandoned their claims to distinction and have stunted their own growth. Sentimentality has commanded them to lock up their priceless storehouses of knowledge, and medical science in America has been half starved in consequence.[58]

In the uncompromising light of science, older concerns for the patient and his or her views had become mere "sentimentality"—even to an administrator atypically concerned with the social dimensions of a patient's experience.

Not surprisingly, early twentieth-century hospitals sought to capitalize on their image as temples of science. Administrators emphasized the sophisticated equipment in operating rooms and laboratories as they appealed for funds, reassured private patients, and impressed visiting committees. European physicians often commented on the opulent appearance of American operating rooms— the use of glass and marble, for example, where less expensive materials would have sufficed. Annual reports of the period refer again and again to sophisticated machines and instruments; the photographs that adorned such reports were routinely posed in front of gleaming apparatus, physicians and nurses solemnly regarding these inanimate icons of technology that occupied emotional center stage. Such photographs often contained no human figures at all.

Private patients and their visitors were suitably awed by displays of technical capacity. The hospital with an irreproachable scientific reputation could hope to enjoy a similarly elevated standing in the community. It had become apparent by the 1890s, moreover, that scientific reputation would serve as an advantage in attracting the brightest and most ambitious young medical men—and, it soon developed, the support of individual and corporate benevolence. The promise of scientific achievement rapidly became a cliché of administrators, fundraisers, and an influential group of foundation advisors. "While the field of research in medicine does not yield direct profit in dollars and cents," as one enthusiast put it, "the world can and does draw from the laboratory of the research worker knowledge which, passing almost duty free into the possession of the community, can actually be estimated in *terms of millions* of dollars."[59] By the era of the First World War, the arguments of a late nineteenth-century professional elite had become a reassuring formula relevant to a much broader constituency. It is hardly surprising that reformers who urged the accreditation of hospitals should have emphasized technical facilities in setting standards. "In constructing a true hospital," as one prominent advocate of standardization argued, "certain scientific departments should first be provided for; the balance of the hospital should be built around these departments."[60]

But as we have come to understand, the relationship between scientific capacity and its application in clinical medicine is hardly simple or unambiguous. Real achievements can obscure real shortcomings. New capabilities reinforced an interest in ills amenable to medical intervention, while insuring a continued lack of interest in ailments for which therapeutics could do little. Second, the increasing faith in medicine as science inevitably magnified the physician's authority, if not always his or her efficacy. Medicine was becoming both more technical and more inaccessible to laymen, and this reality also undergirded the decentralized quality of hospital organization. The esoteric knowledge a physician brought to bear in treating a particular patient loomed ever more important and became in fact a symbol of the hospital's social legitimacy. Within the tightly focused interaction between doctor and patient, social variables could seem insignificant and diffuse. The locus of clinical decision making—and responsibility—had to be concentrated in professional hands. With an increasing technical capacity, each hospital and its managers sought to make that interaction as successful as possible and to provide the physician with as many tools as might—in the worst case—prove necessary. The acute care hospital was becoming a more rigid and capital-intensive institution.

In the face of such powerful trends, well-meaning attempts to shape new social programs within the hospital had comparatively little impact. Chronic and convalescent patients remained a low priority as did outpatient clinics. Reform of municipal hospitals was, as we have seen, predicated on the desirability of turning them into high quality medical facilities—an implicit rejection of the hospital's welfare function and, most specifically, of chronic and geriatric care. Medical social work, so enthusiastically advocated by Richard Cabot and a good many of his contemporaries, did make a permanent, but in sum marginal, place for itself in the hospital. The attitude of most administrators was similar to that of the medical superintendent at the Massachusetts General Hospital who after several years finally visited the social service office, somewhat bemused at this bustling nest of earnest ladies, but unable to understand their relevance to his more central concerns. Ida Cannon, the guiding spirit in the social service department, reported in 1908 that the superintendent had actually come in "and sat down to see what was going on. I am glad he is becoming more interested or curious or whatever it is—but you can imagine there is little inspiration in it for us—except to make him feel some of our enthusiasm."[61] If the hospital is likened to the kitchen of a busy restaurant, social service workers might be likened in hospital priorities to the cleaners and scourers who removed the debris left by the chef after the day's inspired efforts and prepared the pots, pans, and utensils for the next day of skilled creativity. Outpatient and dispensary care (like social service) were never to escape the stigma of poverty medicine; never a part of the economic structure of medical practice and generally occupying an area of minor technical interest, they remained a marginal concern for the profession.

In retrospect, the deeply felt and often acute observations and meliorist programs of early twentieth-century critics of the hospital's social role had little impact, their commitment a mere glance outward of little significance in comparison to the compulsion exerted by the forces that shaped the hospital in its inward vision. The social mission of the hospital seemed to most physicians not so much indefensible as secondary—diffuse and politically unsettling, while the most prestigious scientific insights (a word chosen advisedly) looked inward to the realms of bacteriology, biochemistry, and pathology. Even that concerned and socially committed minority who spearheaded the reform efforts of the Progressive period shared a liberating faith in science and efficiency. Richard Cabot, to whom we have referred as a zealous advocate of social medicine, was perhaps even better known for his role in making the individual case method a central part of medical education.[62] It is certainly possible to see an individual patient as the site of a lesion and at the same time an idiosyncratic member of a family and community, but it has not proven an easy task. Cabot's remedy for slipshod outpatient services was "more science and more Christianity."[63] But these particular oxen were more easily yoked in Cabot's Brahmin sensibility than in America's system of medical care.

Scientific medicine offered a powerful vision of an increasingly effective therapeutics. It promised to liberate men and women from pain and premature death. To the great majority of reformers in the period before World War II, the shortcomings of American medical care lay not in any tendencies within scientific medicine, but in the inequitable distribution of an unambiguous good. It was a necessary part of the solution, only social injustice made it part of the problem. But not every aspect of medicine has proven itself amenable to technical solutions—and even progress has its costs.

CHAPTER 14

Conclusion:
The Past in the Present

When Thomas Jefferson was inaugurated as president in 1800, there were only two American hospitals—one in Philadelphia and the other in New York. And these novel institutions played only a minor role in the provision of medical care; the great majority of inpatient beds were provided in almshouse wards, and even these were comparatively few in number. Most Americans still lived on farms and in rural villages.

Although in this demographic sense marginal, the hospital was nevertheless a characteristic product of the society that nurtured it. The hospital could not help but reproduce fundamental social relationships and values in microcosm. Early national America was a society in which relationships of class and status prescribed demeanors and specified the responsibilities of individuals and the community. It was a society in which bureaucracy and credentials meant little—bearing and social origin much. Even in America's largest cities, traditional views of Christian stewardship shaped assumptions of a proper reciprocity between rich and poor. It was an urban world in which benevolence could still be imagined—if not always realized—in a context of face-to-face interaction between the giver and receiver of charity.

Allied with medicine's limited technical resources, these demographic and attitudinal realities produced a medical system minimally dependent on institutional care and in which dependence and social location, not diagnosis, determined the makeup of institutional populations. Sickness in itself did not imply hospitalization—

only sickness or incapacity in those without a stable home or family members to provide care.

Late eighteenth-and early nineteenth-century hospital advocates felt two kinds of motivation. One was the imperative of traditional Christian benevolence in urban communities already burdened with large numbers of "unsettled" individuals needing care. The other sort of motivation grew out of the clinical and educational goals of an elite in the medical profession. Both lay and medical supporters of private hospitals contended that there could be no conflict between the hospital goals of laymen and physicians, for citizens of every class would ultimately benefit from the clinical instruction that could be most effectively organized around the aggregated bodies of the poor.

But such bland assurance of a necessary consistency between the professional needs of physicians and the benevolent goals of lay trustees were not enough to banish conflict. From its earliest years, the American hospital was marked by a structured divergence of interest between those of the pious laymen who bore the moral and legal responsibility for the institution and the doctors who practiced and taught within it. Drawn largely from the same social circles, attending physicians and lay authorities shared most values and assumptions, but in regard to professional matters such as autopsies, for example, or admission policies they could and did differ. Where they did not, however, was in their assumption of stewardship and the mingled authority and responsibility that constituted it; wealth, gender, and social position implied both the right and duty to direct the lives of dependent fellow citizens.

And the hospital was—insofar as its trustees and attending physicians could manage—a reflection of such relationships and responsibilities. Patients, nurses, attendants, and to an extent the junior house officers were considered moral minors in need of direction and guidance. Trustees felt a personal responsibility for every aspect of the institution and regularly inspected its wards and interviewed patients just as they personally oversaw admissions and settled accounts.

Poverty and dependence were the operational prerequisites for hospital admission. Sickness was a necessary but insufficient condition; aside from the occasional trauma victim, even the laborer or artisan preferred to be cared for at home—if he had a home and family to provide that care. It was only to have been expected that men should have far outnumbered women among nineteenth-century hospital patients. Urban America's abundant supply of single laboring men provided the bulk of admissions.[1] If age and sex justified the father's authority in an ordinary home, so gender and class identity legitimated that authority in the hospital and implied the unquestioned deference that patients were supposed to show toward superintendent, attending physicians, and trustees.

The intimate scale of early nineteenth-century hospitals provided a context in which these more general social realities could reproduce themselves. It was expected that the superintendent would see every patient every day, that he would know all their names and be aware of their personal situations, just as he knew the cook and laundress and coachman, all of course resident in the hospital. Not surprisingly, many of these employees worked for long years at their jobs and were paid on a quarterly or semiannual basis. Like the patients they cared for, the hospital's workers bartered independence for security. This harsh quid pro quo provided nevertheless a measure of stability in a world that offered few such choices for the great majority of Americans who worked with their hands.

The hospital was part of an institutional world that minimized cash transactions, subsisting instead through a network of less tangible interactions. Physicians were paid in prestige and clinical access; trustees in deference and the opportunity for spiritual accomplishment; nurses and patients were compensated with creature comforts: food, heat, and a place to sleep. Patients offered deference and their bodies as teaching material. Few dollars changed hands, but the system worked in its limited way for those who participated in it.

In part this was possible because the antebellum hospital was not burdened by a capital-intensive technology. There was little that could be done for a patient in the hospital that could not and, in practice, was not provided equally well at home—at least if that home could provide food, warmth, and care. Just as medical treatment was not segregated in the hands of a licensed and trained corps of practitioners, so the provision of acute care was not limited to a specific institutional setting. The domain of antebellum medicine was ill defined. Domestic and irregular practice were a significant part of medical care—a vital reality even in families well able to employ trained physicians.

Boundaries between hospital and home were similarly indistinct. A limited technology as well as traditional attitudes blurred the practical distinctions between home and hospital. In architecture as well as in terms of their social organization, America's early hospitals differed little from any large home or welfare institution. As late as the Civil War, much surgery was still done on the wards—laboratories, x-ray units, and sterile operating theaters were far in the future. The rationale for construction of early nineteenth-century surgical amphitheaters was primarily pedagogic.[2] Many antebellum hospitals did not even have specific spaces adapted to the treatment of emergencies or the evaluation of individuals for admission. A limited technology demanded little in the way of functionally differentiated space. A socially undifferentiated patient population similarly implied no need for class-distinct accommodations. Most nineteenth-century hospitals did have a few private rooms, but they were generally insignificant in terms of space or numbers of occupants. The large open ward seemed appropriate to the presumably blunted sensibilities of those sort of individuals who became hospital patients—and to the hospital's own need to minimize costs. Until the twentieth century, hospital current expense budgets were dominated by the cost of food, heat, light, and labor—costs little different from those of an orphanage, boarding school, or rich man's mansion.

Medical ideas and skills were widely disseminated in the community as well and not segregated in the profession, justifying in part the hospital's marginality and paralleling its lack of internal differentiation. Every educated gentleman was presumed to know something about medicine; every woman was something of a general practitioner. Medicine provided a striking example of a still-traditional society's more general lack of specialized roles. In terms of authority, class relations, technology, administration, and even architecture, the hospital was very much a microcosm of the community that produced it. The boundaries, in fact, between community and hospital, between medicine and its clients, remained indistinct in American cities until mid-nineteenth century—and in rural areas until much later. Even ideas of disease causation reflected, incorporated, and legitimated social values generally; this was an era in which disease was still a holistic and nonspecific phenomenon. It could be caused by poor diet, stress, alcoholism, constitutional weakness, or more frequently, some plausible combination of several such factors. Laymen could understand as well as manipulate these ideas—medicine was still practiced in the home in terms mutually understandable to medical men and their patients.

A New Kind of Hospital

All of this had changed drastically by 1920. The hospital had become a national institution, no longer a refuge for the urban poor alone. On January 1, 1923, there were 4,978 hospitals in the United States, 70 percent of them general hospitals. (In 1873, the first American hospital survey had located only 178 hospitals.)[3] By the early 1920s, few enterprising towns of any size had failed to establish a community hospital; it had become an accepted part of medical and especially surgical care for most small town Americans as well as their urban contemporaries. Diagnosis and therapeutic capacity as well as an individual's social location had begun to determine hospital admission. Technology had provided new tools and, equally important, a new rationale for centering acute care in the hospital. Medical men and medical skills were playing an increasingly important part in the institution—gradually supplanting older norms of lay control. Bureaucracy had reshaped the institution's internal order: a trained and disciplined nursing corps, a professionalizing hospital administration, as well as an increasingly specialized medical profession had all played a role in transforming the nineteenth-century hospital.

But certain older aspects of the hospital remained tenaciously intact. One was the stigmatizing distinction between public and private sectors. Municipal or county hospital care—like its almshouse predecessor—was clearly the less desirable, less adequately funded sibling of the private sector. In some ways, however, the formal boundary between public and private remained indistinct; all hospitals were clothed with the public interest, yet not easily subjected to the control of public authority. Decentralized funding and decision making continued to characterize the hospital. The lack of formal planning did not deter long-term trends from acting themselves out in parallel ways in institution after institution and locality after locality. But collective decision making was not easily imposed on an array of institutions that jealously guarded their autonomy and often associated independence with the prestige of localities, of ethnic and religious groups. This competitiveness was, in fact, one of those trends that manifested itself in parallel fashion in city after city; planners could deplore but do little to moderate its effects.

A first generation of hospital reformers had already discovered the structural rigidities beneath the seemingly inconsistent assortment of autonomous institutions that constituted the universe of early twentieth-century American hospitals. Regional planning for the most effective use of available resources was sought after as early as the first decade of the present century. Yet, despite polite words of support, few individual institutions were willing to change their normal priorities or concede any meaningful aspect of their operational independence to some larger group. By 1910, the hospital had already begun to appear to some of its critics as a monolithic and impersonal medical factory.[4]

Many social functions were moving from the home and neighborhood to institutional sites in late nineteenth- and early twentieth-century America—but none more categorically than medical care. And in no other case was the technical rationale more compelling. From a late twentieth-century perspective, the resources of hospital medicine in the period of the First World War may seem primitive, but they were impressive to contemporaries. Antiseptic surgery, the x-ray, and the clinical laboratory seemed to represent a newly scientific and efficacious medicine—a medicine necessarily based in the hospital. Few practitioners could duplicate these resources in their offices or make them easily available in the homes of even their wealthiest patients. Successful physicians had come to assume, and had convinced their patients, that the hospital was the best place to undergo surgery and in fact to treat any acute ailment.

But none of these events could have taken place without changed expectations—on the part of both physicians and their patients. Each decision by a middle-class American to enter a hospital reflected the attitudes and needs of both, even if it was the physician who ultimately referred his case to a hospital bed. Although attitudinal changes are difficult to document, respectable Americans would not have begun to enter hospitals had their perceptions of the institution not changed.

Not only the hospital, but the image of medicine itself had changed radically in the last third of the nineteenth century. The establishment of the germ theory, the advances in diagnosis and therapeutics made possible by immunology and serology, and the x-ray provided a dramatic series of highly visible events that cumulatively recast traditional attitudes toward the physician. It not only raised patient expectations, but also identified medicine's newfound efficacy with the laboratory and the image of science. Few would or could have agreed on what that science might be, but such assumptions nevertheless invested medical men with a new identity, one that based its legitimacy and claims to authority on something called science.[5]

Physicians were hardly immune to the attractions of scientific medicine. A cadre of bright young men had begun in the 1880s and 1890s to orient their careers in terms of the exciting new possibilities in surgery and the specialties. Reputations would be won or lost in these areas—reputations for hospitals as well as their staff members. The stakes were high for ambitious clinicians. Technical virtuosity was being inextricably related to status for institutions as well as individuals.

By the 1920s, surgery had become the acknowledged key to hospital growth and status. Although most patients still saw physicians in their own homes or the practitioner's office, major surgical procedures had shifted to the hospital. Not surprisingly, costs rose steadily; although simple and technologically unadorned by contemporary standards, the hospital of the 1920s was a capital-intensive institution, certainly by comparison with its mid-nineteenth-century predecessors. An increasingly sophisticated technology, both medical and nonmedical, implied higher capital and operating costs and thus a ceaseless quest for reliable sources of income and endowment. Yet only a minority of proprietary hospitals could entirely dispense with the institution's traditional mission of caring for the needy. And treating the poor and lower middle class threatened unending deficits. Administrators of nonprofit hospitals thus energetically sought to maximize private patient income. Competition in terms of elegant rooms and restaurant quality food began in the 1890s, but few institutions filled enough of these private rooms to provide a comfortable cash flow—let alone underwrite costs of treating the indigent. There were simply not enough well-to-do patients.[6]

A far greater number of Americans found themselves unable to afford private rates, yet were unwilling to enter charity wards in voluntary hospitals or their even more stigmatizing counterparts in municipal institutions. America's first generation of hospital planners had, as we have seen, grown acutely aware of this group—shut off by income or place of residence from private hospitals, consultants and specialists. The hospital had become an indispensable element in American health care, yet just as it achieved that status experts decried its failure to provide optimum care at reasonable cost.

Within the hospital itself, physicians and medical values had become increasingly important in decision making. Although there was no abrupt or categorical shift, the general trend was clear enough; even where lay authorities still controlled public or private governing boards, they deferred to doctors in a way that would hardly have been approved by their self-confidently intrusive predecessors a century earlier. The growing complexity and presumed efficacy of medicine's tools seemed to make the centrality of physicians in hospital decision making both inevitable and appropriate. More than technical judgments were relevant. Once hospitals became dependent on patient income, they became dependent as well on the doctors who could fill their private beds. Similarly, increasing scale and an ever larger and more specialized house and nursing staff also distanced laymen from the institutions they formally—and formerly—controlled.[7]

In most hospitals, the influence of attending staffs did not go uncontested, however. Like many other institutions in this period, the hospital was becoming increasingly bureaucratic, governed by a new kind of chief executive officer with the aid of a middle management of nursing superintendent, senior residents, and comptroller. Authority was negotiated as well as imposed.

No single change transformed the hospital's day-to-day workings more than the acceptance of trained nurses and nurse training schools, which brought a disciplined corps of would-be professionals into wards previously dominated by the values and attitudes of working-class patients (and attendants originally recruited from the same strata of society). In a period when few careers were open to women, trained nursing attracted a far greater variety of women, many of them rural and only a minority from the urban working class. Professional ambition and social origin set these first generations of credentialed nurses apart from the ward's accustomed occupants as much as any specific aspect of their schooling.

The status of trained nurses reflected but could not rival the growing influence of a male-dominated medical profession. In the hospital, as in the world outside its walls, female-identified occupations tended to become exclusively female and subordinate to male authority. Central to the professional identity of trained nursing was a relentless emphasis on discipline and efficiency, paralleling medicine's newly scientific self-image. This emphasis and the trained nurses who embodied and enforced it helped impose a new social order in the wards and rooms of the hospital. Nursing added an additional layer to hospital management—yet on balance enhanced rather than undermined the growing power of medicine within the hospital.[8]

The increasing prominence of technology and the physicians who employed these impressive new tools expressed itself in another and particularly tenacious way. This was the prominent role of acute care in the nonprofit hospital, and a parallel lack of interest in the chronically ill, who tended to pile up in county, municipal, and state institutions. In a good many rural areas in the 1920s, the county almshouse continued to serve as the community's repository for "chronics and incurables." Such patients were expensive and fit uncomfortably into the priorities of an increasingly self-confident medical profession. Most chronic facilities, for example, found it difficult to attract housestaff; the duties were depressing and the cases "uninteresting."[9]

Surgery in particular had helped shorten voluntary hospital stays, attracted a new mix of patients and reinforced an already well-established emphasis on acute care. Diagnosis had become self-consciously scientific, determined increasingly by medical men and medical categories. By the 1920s, diagnosis had replaced dependency as the key to hospital admission (although *which* hospital one was admitted to still reflected class and ethnic factors). Socially oriented critics of the early twentieth-century hospital were already contending that the patient was in danger of being reduced to his or her diagnosis—to a biopathological phenomenon.

The hospital had been transformed not only socially and technically, but physically as well. New medical tools coupled with a new industrial and building technology had made the early twentieth-century hospital a physical artifact very different from its forerunners a century earlier. The needs of radiology and clinical pathology, of hydrotherapy and electrotherapy, and, most importantly, of antiseptic surgery demanded reorganization of the hospital's interior so as to minimize steps for its medical and nursing staff. The growth of fee-for-service practice in the hospital implied examining and consulting rooms more private than facilities previously available in ward and outpatient departments. The presumed needs and desires of valued pay patients led to the creation of more and more private and semiprivate accommodations.[10] And like every other large institutional structure at the time, hospitals were being built with electric lights, dynamos, elevators, partially mechanized kitchens and laundries. Added to the cumulative impact of a mid-century reform movement that had underlined the need for improved modes of heating and ventilation, these technological necessities were turning the early twentieth-century American hospital into a capital-intensive and internally differentiated physical entity—mirroring in a different sphere the changes in professional organization and the distribution of knowledge that were reshaping medical care more generally.

Medical knowledge, like medical practice, was gradually but inexorably being segregated in professionally accredited hands. No longer was it assumed that an educated man would understand something of medicine (or law, classics, and theology). No longer was it assumed that midwives would provide the bulk of care during childbirth and early infancy. Drugs were purchased not gathered—and even in rural areas, most Americans turned sooner to physicians than they would have several generations earlier.[11] Within the medical profession too, knowledge was gradually being segregated so that ordinary practitioners were no longer presumed to be omnicompetent (even if they might have to ignore such limitations in rural areas or choose to ignore them in cities). Practitioners as well as educated laymen assumed that the hospital was and must be the site for medicine's most advanced and specialized care.

Although laymen were certainly impressed by the scientific style and seeming efficacy of medicine, it was physicians who in fact determined the content of that medicine. The medical community shaped professional expectations and defined career patterns. And if the optimum relationship between science and its clinical applications remained unclear, the place of the hospital did not. It was central to every aspect of medicine by 1920. The hospital's wards and rooms were the place to learn clinical skills, to master a specialty, often a place to practice, and, for an increasingly influential academic minority, a place to pursue research.

If the hospital had been medicalized, the medical profession had been hospitalized in the years between 1800 and 1920. This intraprofessional development has attracted far less attention from contemporary historians than the hospital's social and economic evolution—but it is no less significant. They are in fact inseparable; the structure of medical careers and changing medical perceptions and priorities are fundamental elements of hospital history.

Hospital service had always been central to the ambitions and careers of America's medical elite. By the First World War, it had become central to the education and practice of a much larger proportion of the profession, which was itself becoming more tightly organized, uniformly trained, and systematically licensed. Since the eighteenth century, hospitals had played a key role in disseminating as well as accumulating medical knowledge, helping to communicate ideas and techniques from a metropolitan elite to a new generation of practitioners. With an ever-larger proportion of physicians serving as interns and residents, the twentieth-century hospital became an increasingly effective tool for the diffusion of ideas and skills. By the 1920s, hospital experience had become an accepted part of medical training. With the national accreditation of hospitals and internship programs and the integration of residency and fellowship programs into board certification, the hospital had become with each passing decade more tightly integrated into the career choices and aspirations of the medical profession.[12]

With consulting and surgical practice moving increasingly into the hospital in the 1920s, interest as well as intellect united in emphasizing its importance to the practitioner. Cash transactions had become increasingly important, not only to the individual physician, but to the hospital as it sought to maximize income in the face of growing demands and rising costs. Older commitments to the provision of gratuitous care allied with institutional rivalries implied that most hospitals would not tolerate falling too far behind in their efforts to provide first-rate staff and facilities. Costs would inevitably increase.

The American hospital can be seen as having moved by the 1920s into a marketplace of discrete and impersonal cash transactions—to a style of benevolence that would have seemed inappropriate to the sort of men who managed hospitals in the first third of the nineteenth century. Efficiency, not stewardship, threatened to dominate the early twentieth-century hospital—as it did the school, state, government, and factory.

But the hospital never assumed the guise of rational and rationalized economic actor during the first three-quarters of the twentieth century. It was never managed as a factory or department store. The hospital continued into the twentieth century, as it had begun in the eighteenth, to be clothed with the public interest in a way that challenged categorical distinctions between public and private. Private hospitals had always been assumed to serve the community at large—treating the needy, training a new generation of medical practitioners, and attracting a varied and eclectic assortment of subventions from city, county, and state authorities.[13] The late eighteenth and early nineteenth centuries had in any case never been comfortable with absolute distinctions between the public and private sphere; the idea of commonwealth subsumed collective responsibility for that community's health. It was natural for most hospital authorities to assume that they should continue to receive public funds, just as they assumed they should be free of local taxes and the constraints of tort law.

The hospital's transactions involved pain, sickness, and death, as well as the public good. An insulating sacredness surrounded the activities of the twentieth-century hospital; its "products" were, in a literal sense, beyond material accounting. The newly intensified expectations of scientific medicine were, that is, both material and transcendent. A growing number of Americans hoped and expected that this new institution could provide a refuge from the sickness and premature death that had always seemed immanent in man's corporeal body. It is not surprising that (except for a minority of proprietary, for-profit institutions) the private hospital's operations have never been entirely disciplined by the logic of profit maximization or easily bent to communally determined demands for planning and cost control. A deficit could be construed as a sign of worthiness and not culpable administrative failure.

Nor is it surprising that transactions within the hospital continued until the Second World War to be structured in part around the exchange of labor and status. The hospital was in but not of the marketplace. Nurses and house staff still exchanged labor for credentials; attending physicians bartered their ward services for prestige and admission privileges in private services. Nonprofessional workers traded a measure of autonomy and the higher wages they might have received on the commercial labor market for the security and paternalism that, presumably, characterized the hospital. Thus, even as it was being transformed into an increasingly technical and seemingly indispensable institution, the hospital remained clothed with a special and sacred quality that removed it from both normal social scrutiny and the market's discipline.

Even if the hospital could not turn itself into an income-maximizing marketplace actor, it did serve as an equity-maximizing vehicle for many of those connected with it. I use the word equity advisedly, for the hospital provided rewards in several forms. To private practitioners, it could provide income; to attending physicians, income and status; to lay trustees, it offered prestige and, in many cases, affirmation of individual or group status; to hospital suppliers, it constituted an increasingly voracious customer; to academic physicians, it provided "clinical material" for teaching and research; to nurses, workers, and attendants, it offered security; and to some, a measure of status. Even the Depression-era hospital reflected and incorporated all these, sometimes conflicting, motives as it struggled with limited budgets.

The late twentieth-century hospital already existed in embryo, waiting only the nutrients of third-party payment, government involvement, technological change, and general economic growth to stimulate a rapid and in some ways hypertrophied development. New and abundant sources of support after the Second World War only intensified well-established patterns. They provided funds on the provider's terms without fundamentally changing the provider's orientation; cost-plus contracts and outright grants are hardly ideal mechanisms for the enforcement of external control.[14]

The Past in the Present

If the hospital in Thomas Jefferson's or Andrew Jackson's America had been a microcosm of the community that nurtured it, so is the hospital of the 1980s. Although we live in a very different sort of world, the hospital remains both product and prisoner of its own history and of the more general trends that have characterized our society. Class, ethnicity, and gender have, for example, all shaped and continue to shape medical care, and the hospital has become a specialized, bureaucratic entity of a kind that has come to dominate so many other aspects of contemporary life. National policies and priorities have come to play a significant role in affairs that had been long thought of as entirely and appropriately local. The origins of America's hospitals are hardly recognizable in their quaint forerunners in a handful of early nineteenth-century port cities.

The hospital is a necessary community institution strangely insulated from the community; it is instead a symbiotically allied group of subcommunities bound together by social location and the logic of history. This insulated character is typical of a good number of social institutions: the schools, the federal civil service, the large corporations. But there are some special aspects of the hospital that have facilitated its ability to look inward, to pursue its own vision of social good. This institutional solipsism developed place in ironic if logical conjunction with the hospital's defining function of dealing with the most intimate and fundamental of human realities.

Like the U.S. Defense Department, the hospital system has grown in response to perceived social need—in comparison with which normal budgetary constraints and compromises have come to seem niggling and inappropriate. Security, like any absolute and immeasurable good, legitimates enormous demands on society's resources. Both health and defense have, moreover, become captives of high technology and worst-case justifications. In both instances, the gradient of technical feasibility becomes a moral imperative.[15] That which might be done, should be done. In both cases, cost-cutting could be equated with penny-pinching—inappropriate to the gravity of the social goals involved. Absolute ends do not lend themselves to compromise, and the bottom line is that there has been no bottom line.

In both areas, material interests obviously play a role; hospitals, doctors, and medical suppliers like defense contractors and the military have interests expressed in and through the political process. But ideas are significant as well. It is impossible to understand our defense budget without factoring in the power of ideology; it is impossible to understand the scale and style of America's health care expenditures without an understanding of the allure of scientific medicine and the promise of healing. Both the Massachusetts General Hospital and the General Dynamics Corporation operate in the market, but they are not entirely bound by its discipline; both also mock the categorical distinction between public and private that indiscriminately places each in the private domain.

This analogy can, of course, be carried too far. The hospital has, as we have emphasized, a special history incorporating and reflecting the evolution of medicine and nursing, and the parallel development of our social welfare system. The high status of medicine has been built into the hospital, not only in the form of an undifferentiated social authority, but in the shape of particular, historically determined techniques and career choices. The ideas that rule the world-view of medicine and its system of education and research have very practical connections with the pragmatic world of medical care and medical costs.

An increasingly subdifferentiated specialization, an emphasis on laboratory research and acute care, for example, have all played an important role in the profession and thus, in the hospital. So complex and intertwined are these interrelationships that changes in any one sphere inevitably impinge on other areas. Some aspects of modern medicine seemed at first unrelated to the marketplace. One, for example, was the increasing ability of physicians to disentangle specific disease entities. This was an intellectual achievement of the first magnitude and not unrelated to the increasingly scientific and prestigious public image of the medical profession. Yet, we have seen a complex and inexorably bureaucratic reimbursement system grow up around these diagnostic entities; disease does not exist if it cannot be coded. It was equally inevitable that efforts to control medical costs should have turned on these same diagnostic categories. Thus the 1980s controversy surrounding Diagnosis Related Groups can be seen in part as a natural outcome of the intellectual and institutional history of the medical profession—and of the hospital as well.

To most contemporary Americans, rising costs have been the key element in transforming the hospital into a highly visible social problem. And it is true that an apparent crisis in hospital finance may well be creating the conditions for fundamental changes. After all, it was not until after the Second World War that the hospital gradually emerged from the world of paternalism. Unions and a more assertive nursing profession, ever-increasing capital costs, a growing dependence on federal support, and rising insurance rates, even the need to pay house staff in dollars have moved the hospital system into the market—and exposed hospitals to the prospect of increasing external control.[16] Still clothed with the public interest and promising immeasurable equities, the hospital remains a rigid and intractable institution.

As we contemplate its contentious present and problematic future, we remain prisoners of its past. The economic and organizational problems that loom so prominently today should not make us lose sight of fundamental contradictions in the hospital's history, contradictions that have fueled two decades of critical debate.

Scientific medicine has raised expectations and costs, but has failed to confront the social consequences of its own success. We are still wedded to acute care and episodic, specialized contacts with physicians. There is a great deal of evidence that indicates widespread dissatisfaction with the quality of care as it is experienced by Americans. Changes in reimbursement mechanisms will not necessarily alter that felt reality. Chronic and geriatric care still constitute a problem—as they always did. We cannot seem to live without high-technology medicine; we cannot seem to live amicably with it. Yet, for the great majority of Americans, divorce is unthinkable. Medical perceptions and careers still proscribe or reward behaviors that may or may not be consistent with the most humane and cost-effective provision of care. And despite much recent hand-wringing, it still remains to be seen whether physicians will be edged aside from their positions of institutional authority.

There are many equities to be maximized in the hospital, many interests to be served, but the collective interest does not always have effective advocates. The discipline of the marketplace will not necessarily speak to that interest; the most vulnerable will inevitably suffer. In any case, I see little prospect of hospitals in general becoming monolithic cost minimizers and profit maximizers. Social expectations and well-established interests are both inconsistent with such a state of things. We will support research and education, we will feel uncomfortable with a medical system that does not provide a plausible (if not exactly equal) level of care to the poor and socially isolated. Health care policy will continue to reflect the special character of our attitudes toward sickness and society.

Bibliographical Note

Despite our late twentieth-century assumption that the hospital is a necessarily central social institution, historians have told us comparatively little about the evolution of American hospitals, especially during the critical period between the mid-nineteenth century and the Second World War, which is the focus of this book. We have no synthesis of American hospital history comparable to Brian Abel-Smith's *The Hospitals, 1880–1948: A Study in Social Administration in England and Wales* (Cambridge, Mass.: Harvard University Press, 1964) or his companion study, *A History of the Nursing Profession* (London, Melbourne, Toronto: Heinemann, 1960). Only in the past decade has there been a vigorous scholarly interest in the historical development of the hospital, reflecting the ongoing debate over the role and authority of medicine. It has reflected as well the growth of social and institutional history; prisons, asylums, and public schools, for example, have all been the focus of academic inquiry. The hospital is, in fact, a latecomer to this movement. Interest in the "insane asylum," for example, was manifested earlier and has influenced a far greater number of historians. The general hospital has always seemed a necessary and unambiguously benevolent institution; it was less easily construed as an engine of social control.

Of course we have a goodly number of chronicles of individual hospitals. Yet, even the most detailed and reliable of these are by intent monuments to far-sighted philanthropists and discerning clinicians. This is hardly an accident, nor is it happenstance that such histories are written from a narrow internal perspective. This inward-looking canon is entirely consistent with the hospital's evolution. It is to be expected that we should have numerous histories of hospitals but no history of *the* hospital in America. To write about *the* hospital is to see it as a social institution, but to write about *a* hospital has normally been to chronicle its internal development. Most hospital histories, including many of recent vintage, define their scope, logically enough, in terms of the accomplishments and dedication of skilled clinicians, the adoption of an increasingly sophisticated set of therapeutic and diagnostic tools, and, of course, the building of buildings.

Many histories of individual hospitals remain enormously valuable. Of the older studies, I have found the following particularly useful: Nathaniel T. Bowditch, *A History of the Massachusetts General Hospital, 2nd. ed.* (Boston: The Hospital, 1872); Frederic A. Washburn, *The Massachusetts General Hospital. Its Development, 1900–1935* (Boston: Houghton Mifflin, 1939); Thomas G. Morton, assisted by Frank Woodbury, *The History of the Pennsylvania Hospital. 1751–1895* (Philadelphia: Times Printing House, 1895); Charles Lawrence, *History of the Philadelphia Almshouses and Hospitals . . . Showing the Mode of Distributing Public Relief through the Management of the Boards of Overseers of the Poor, Guardians of the Poor and the Directors of the Departments of Charities and Correction* (Philadelphia: The Author, 1905); David W. Cheever et al., *A History of the Boston City Hospital from its Foundation until 1904* (Boston: Municipal Printing Office, 1906). There are scores of useful hospital histories of more recent vintage, usually written by senior staff members or sometimes professional writers. Examples of those that I have found particularly useful in presenting a rounded picture of an institution's development are: Fenwick Beekman, *Hospital for the Ruptured and Crippled. A Historical Sketch . . .* (New York: Privately Printed, 1939); Joseph Hirsh and Beka Doherty, *The First Hundred Years of the Mount Sinai Hospital of New York* (New York: Random House, 1952); Frank B. Woodford and Philip P. Mason, *Harper of Detroit. The Origin and Growth of a Great Metropolitan Hospital* (Detroit: Wayne State University, 1964); William C. Posey and Samuel Horton Brown, *The Wills Hospital of Philadelphia. The Influence of European and British Ophthalmology upon It, and the Part It Played in Developing Ophthalmology in America* (Philadelphia, Montreal, and London: J.B. Lippincott, 1931); Dorothy Levenson, *Montefiore, The Hospital as Social Instrument, 1884–1984* (New York: Farrar, Straus & Giroux, 1984); Charles Snyder, *Massachusetts Eye and Ear Infirmary. Studies on its History* (Boston: The

Infirmary, 1984); Alan M. Chesney, *The Johns Hopkins Hospital and the Johns Hopkins University School of Medicine. A Chronicle . . .*, 3 vols. (Baltimore: Johns Hopkins University, 1943, 1958, 1963.)

Since at least the 1920s, however, some physicians and medical historians have been writing a history informed by an awareness of the profession's social and economic context. (For an attempt to reconstruct this thread of interest in medicine's social history, see Susan Reverby and David Rosner, "Beyond the Great Doctors," in Rosner and Reverby, eds., *Health Care in America: Essays in Social History* [Philadelphia: Temple University Press, 1979].) For a discussion of trends in the history of American medicine during the past generation, see in addition, Ronald L. Numbers, "The History of American Medicine: A Field in Ferment," *Reviews in American History* 10 (1982): 245–63. Numbers' footnotes provide a useful guide to the controversy occasioned by much of this new and often critical scholarship. The past generations' interest in the social and economic has also resulted in the publication of a number of collections and symposia. Judith W. Leavitt and Ronald L. Numbers, eds., *Sickness and Health in America: Readings in the History of Medicine and Public Health,* 2nd. ed. (Madison: University of Wisconsin, 1986) contains a useful bibliography. See also Charles E. Rosenberg, "Bibliographical Note," in George Rosen, *The Structure of American Medical Practice. 1875–1941* (Philadelphia: University of Pennsylvania, 1983), pp. 141–46. As an aspect of this expanding interest in medicine's economic and social history, the hospital has gradually become a focus of concerted scholarly investigation.

Important local studies reflecting this point of view include: Morris Vogel, *The Invention of the Modern Hospital: Boston 1870–1930* (Chicago and London: University of Chicago Press, 1980) and David Rosner, *A Once Charitable Enterprise: Hospitals and Health Care in Brooklyn and New York, 1885–1915* (Cambridge, London, New York: Cambridge University Press, 1982). Rosner emphasizes the economic impact of the panic of 1893 and the consequent desire by hospitals and municipalities to rationalize costs. Vogel is particularly concerned to underline the social and political contrasts between Massachusetts General and Boston City hospitals, and the medicalization of the hospital enterprise generally. Joan Lynaugh's "The Community Hospitals of Kansas City, Missouri, 1870–1915," Ph.D. diss., University of Kansas, 1982, and Jon M. Kingsdale's "The Growth of Hospitals: An Economic History in Baltimore," Ph.D

diss., University of Michigan, 1981, provide valuable parallel studies of other cities. Leonard K. Eaton's older study, *New England Hospitals, 1790–1833* (Ann Arbor: University of Michigan Press, 1957) is
a pioneer study of the hospital as social institution, placing particular emphasis on the motivations of their founders. It should be read
in conjunction with William Williams's *America's First Hospital: The
Pennsylvania Hospital, 1751–1841* (Wayne, Pa.: Haverford House,
1976). For English precedents and influences, see also, Guenter B.
Risse, *Hospital Life in Enlightenment Scotland. Care and Teaching at the Royal
Infirmary of Edinburgh* (Cambridge, London, and New York: Cambridge University Press, 1986) and John Woodward, *To Do the Sick No
Harm. A Study of the British Voluntary Hospital System to 1875* (London and
Boston: Routledge & Kegan Paul, 1974). M. Jeanne Peterson's *The
Medical Profession in Mid-Victorian London* (Berkeley, Los Angeles, and
London: University of California Press, 1978) provides a valuable
study of career patterns, paralleling yet contrasting with realities in
American cities and hospitals. An important study by John D.
Thompson and Grace Goldin focuses on the ward and the hospital
as physical as well as social artifact: *The Hospital: A Social and Architectural History* (New Haven and London: Yale University Press, 1975).
In many ways, municipal hospitals represent a peculiar problem in
terms of the balance between the hospital's welfare and technical
functions, as well as their sensitive political identity. Harry Dowling's recent study of *City Hospitals. The Undercare of the Underprivileged*
(Cambridge and London: Harvard University Press, 1982) provides
a useful introduction. Technology has become central to diagnosis
and therapeutics in the late twentieth-century hospital; for a useful
introduction to this area, see Stanley Reiser, *Medicine and the Reign of
Technology* (Cambridge, London, and New York: Cambridge University Press, 1978). Virginia G. Drachman's *Hospital with a Heart. Women
Doctors and the Paradox of Separatism at the New England Hospital, 1862–1969*
(Ithaca and London: Cornell University Press, 1984) evaluates the
distinctive history of care and professional identity in one of the
minority of female-oriented and administered hospitals. In this connection, Regina Markell Morantz-Sanchez's *Sympathy and Science.
Women Physicians in American Medicine* (New York and Oxford: Oxford
University Press, 1985) offers a well-balanced introduction to the
problems of women physicians in general and their relationship to
hospitals in particular. Although not directed specifically at the
development of American hospitals, a number of other recent stud-

ies provide valuable context for the understanding of that develop-ment and constitute evidence for the rapid maturing of professional scholarship in the social history of medicine. Particularly relevant are: Kenneth M. Ludmerer, *Learning to Heal. The Development of American Medical Education* (New York: Basic Books, 1985); Judith M. Leavitt, *Brought to Bed. Child-Bearing in America, 1750–1950* (New York and Oxford: Oxford University Press, 1986); Martin S. Pernick, *A Calculus of Suffering. Pain, Professionalism, and Anesthesia in Nineteenth-Century America* (New York: Columbia University Press, 1985); John Harley Warner, *The Therapeutic Perspective. Medical Practice, Knowledge, and Identity in America, 1820–1885* (Cambridge and London: Harvard University Press, 1986). Two recent comparative studies of American and En-glish policy will prove valuable to students of twentieth-century health care. They are Daniel M. Fox's *Health Policies, Health Politics: The British & American Experience, 1911–1965* (Princeton: Princeton Univer-sity Press, 1986) and J. Rogers Hollingsworth's *A Political Economy of Medicine: Great Britain and the United States* (Baltimore and London: Johns Hopkins University Press, 1986).

Rosemary Stevens, the author of an indispensable overview, *American Medicine and the Public Interest* (New Haven: Yale University Press, 1971) is completing a study of the American hospital in the twentieth century. She has already published two valuable arti-cles: " 'A Poor Sort of Memory': Voluntary Hospitals and Govern-ment before the Great Depression," *Health and Society,* 60(1982): 551–584 and "Sweet Charity: State Aid to Hospitals in Pennsyl-vania, 1870–1910," *Bulletin of the History of Medicine* 58(1984): 287–314, 474–495. For a description and interpretation of medical care in twentieth-century America, Stevens's work should be supple-mented by sociologist Paul Starr's influential and policy-oriented study, *The Social Transformation of American Medicine* (New York: Basic Books, 1982).

Sociologists have played an important role in focusing scholarly interest on the hospital. Rose Coser, Renée Fox and Erving Goff-man, among others, have emphasized the need to understand the hospital as a social environment, characterized by stylized roles, interactions, and expectations. They have also devoted a good deal of attention to evaluating and understanding the place of the professions in modern society. For influential works in this area, see Eliot Freidson, *Profession of Medicine* (New York: Dodd, Mead, 1970); Freidson, *Professional Powers. A Study of the Institutionalization of Formal*

Knowledge (Chicago and London: University of Chicago Press, 1986);
Magali Sarfatti Larson, *The Rise of Professionalism: A Sociological Analysis*
(Berkeley and Los Angeles: University of California Press, 1977);
Jeffrey L. Berlant, *Profession and Monopoly: A Study of Medicine in the*
United States and Great Britain (Berkeley and Los Angeles: University
of California Press, 1975), and Starr, *Social Transformation.*

Related to the increased interest in the hospital, as well as labor
and women's history, has been a parallel concern with the history
of nursing. For recent studies that provide an introduction to this
literature, see Celia Davies, ed., *Rewriting Nursing History* (London:
Croom, Helm, 1980); Barbara Melosh, *"The Physician's Hand": Work,*
Culture and Conflict in American Nursing (Philadelphia: Temple Univer-
sity Press, 1982); Abel-Smith, *A History of Nursing;* Ellen Condliffe
Lagemann, ed., *Nursing History: New Perspectives and Possibilities* (New
York: Teachers' College Press, 1983); Susan Reverby, *Ordered to*
Care. The Dilemma of American Nursing, 1850–1945 (Cambridge, Lon-
don, and New York: Cambridge University Press, 1987); Karen
Buhler-Wilkerson, "False Dawn: The Rise and Decline of Public
Health Nursing, 1900–1930," Ph.D. diss., University of Pennsyl-
vania, 1984.

I have been working on this book (for more years than I like to
recall), at first as part of a more general history of medicine in
America. In the course of those years I have written a number of
articles that have functioned, at least in retrospect, as "working
papers." Some deal with issues in much greater length or with a
different emphasis than in the present book. They include: "The
Practice of Medicine in New York a Century Ago," *Bulletin of the*
History of Medicine 41(1967): 223–253 (in which I first began to think
systematically about the central role of the hospital in elite medical
careers); "Social Class and Medical Care in Nineteenth-Century
America: The Rise and Fall of the Dispensary," *Journal of the History*
of Medicine 29(1974): 32–54; "And Heal the Sick: The Hospital and
Patient in 19th Century America," *Journal of Social History* 10(1977):
428–447; "The Therapeutic Revolution. Medicine, Meaning and Social Change in Nineteenth-Century America," *Perspectives in Biology*
and Medicine 20(1977): 485–506; "Inward Vision and Outward
Glance: The Shaping of the American Hospital, 1880–1914," *Bulletin*
of the History of Medicine 53(1979): 346–391; "Florence Nightingale on
Contagion: The Hospital as Moral Universe," in C. E. Rosenberg,
ed., *Healing and History: Essays for George Rosen* (New York: Science
History Publications, 1979), pp. 116–136; "From Almshouse to Hos-

pital: The Shaping of Philadelphia General Hospital," *Milbank Memorial Fund Quarterly* 60(1982): 108–154; "Disease and Social Order in America: Perceptions and Expectations," *Milbank Memorial Fund Quarterly* 64, suppl. 1(1986): 34–55. I have used ideas, data, and on occasion passages from these essays. Where they are quoted, it is with the kind permission of the original copyholders.

Notes

AR   annual report
BCH   Boston City Hospital
BM&SJ   *Boston Medical and Surgical Journal*
CGHA   Cincinnati General Hospital Archives
CPP   Historical Collections, College of Physicians of Philadelphia
EHA   Episcopal Hospital Archives, Philadelphia
HCC   Rare Book Department, Countway Library of Medicine, Harvard University
JAMA   *Journal of the American Medical Association*
JHH   Alan Mason Chesney Archives of the Johns Hopkins Medical Institutions, Baltimore
MCP   Archives and Special Collections on Women in Medicine, Medical College of Pennsylvania
MCV   Medical College of Virginia Archives, Richmond
MGH   Massachusetts General Hospital
MGHA   Massachusetts General Hospital Archives
NHR   *National Hospital Record*
NYHA   The Medical Archives, New York Hospital–Cornell Medical Center
NYHS   New-York Historical Society
PCA   Philadelphia City Archives
PGH   Philadelphia General Hospital
PHA   Pennsylvania Hospital Archives, Philadelphia
PNY   Presbyterian Hospital, New York City
SCC   South Caroliniana Library, University of South Carolina, Columbia
SCHS   South Carolina Historical Society, Charleston
SHSW   State Historical Society of Wisconsin, Madison
SLA   Lane Medical Library, Stanford University
TAHA   *Transactions of the American Hospital Association*
TAMA   *Transactions of the American Medical Association*

Introduction

1. Valentine Mott Francis, *A Thesis on Hospital Hygiene* (New York: J.F. Trow, 1859), pp. 145–46. "When they cross the threshold," Francis continued, "they are found not only suffering from disease, but in a half-starved condition, poor, broken-down wrecks of humanity, stranded on the cold bleak shores of that most forbidding of all coasts, charity."

2. J.M. Toner, "Statistics of Regular Medical Associations and Hospitals of the United States," *Transactions of the American Medical Association* (hereafter *TAMA*) 24 (1873): 285–333. The data are not complete, but provide a fair picture of the limited scale of the American hospital enterprise.

3. I have presented this argument in greater detail in: "The Therapeutic Revolution: Medicine, Meaning, and Social Change in Nineteenth-Century America," *Perspectives in Biology and Medicine* 20 (1977): 485–506.

4. E.H.L. Corwin, *The American Hospital* (New York: The Commonwealth Fund, 1946), p. 8.

5. C.E. Rosenberg, "Inward Vision and Outward Glance: The Shaping of the American Hospital, 1880–1914," *Bulletin of the History of Medicine* (hereafter *BHM*) 53 (1979): 346–91.

6. Although I have spoken of the American hospital, many aspects of the institution are international But not all, of course. Ecological differences—in values, political systems, economies, and cultures—alter the forms in which technological possibilities are employed (or ignored). English hospitals are in some ways very much like their American counterparts; in other ways, they differ. Such differences are clues to the historian and policy-maker—and warn of the temptation to place the development of hospitals in a rigid stepwise pattern from something called the traditional to something called modern.

1. To Heal the Sick: The Antebellum Hospital and Society

1. E.S. Ely, *The Journal of the Stated Preacher to the Hospital and Almshouse, in the City of New-York, for the Year of Our Lord 1811* (New York: Whiting and Watson, 1812), p. 7.

2. Ely, I:26; E.S. Ely, *The Second Journal of the Stated Preacher to the Hospital and Almshouse, in the City of New-York, for a Part of the Year of Our Lord 1813 . . .* (Philadelphia: M. Carey, 1815), p. 43.

3. Ely, I:204, 156; II:100, 67–68. On another occasion, Ely distributed cookies to prostitutes: "Gain the good-will of a dog," he explained, "and you may teach him: kick him and he will bite you." II:102.

4. Ely, II:65.

5. Ely, II:x; on blacks, II:89, 168; on sailors, II:78; on Catholics, II:18, 75–76.

6. Ely, I:75. Ely called for the establishment of so-called Lock hospitals on the London model, where female venereal disease cases could be segregated.

7. Ely, I:51 for quote; II:137 on insanity; I:76–77 on idiocy.

8. Ely, I:94. Referring to one such patient, Ely noted that she no longer showed symptoms of venereal disease. "The effects of mercury alone remain in her system; but her cure is but a protracted death." II:139.

9. U.S. Bureau of the Census, *Historical Statistics of the United States, Colonial Times to 1970* (Washington: GPO, 1975), Series A 57–72.

10. Ely, I:18–19, 74.

11. William H. Williams, *America's First Hospital: The Pennsylvania Hospital, 1751–*

1841 (Wayne, Pa.: Haverford House, c. 1976), pp. 8–14. This followed traditional English precedent. In some early hospitals subscribers were responsible for ensuring that patients arrived free from vermin—at once a real and symbolic acting out of accepted class relationships. Cf. John Woodward, *To Do the Sick No Harm. A Study of the British Voluntary Hospital System to 1875* (London and Boston: Routledge & Kegan Paul, 1974), p. 40.

12. *Constitution of the Philadelphia Lying-In Charity* (n.p., n.d., [1834]), p. 3.

13. N.I. Bowditch, *A History of the Massachusetts General Hospital. [To August 5, 1851.] Second Edition . . .* (Boston: The Hospital, 1872), p. 3n., citing a circular letter of 1810 soliciting support for a proposed general hospital in Boston. For recent discussions of motivations in the founding of Massachusetts General Hospital (hereafter MGH), see: Leonard K. Eaton, *New England Hospitals. 1790–1833* (Ann Arbor: University of Michigan Press, c. 1957); Margaret Gerteis, "The Massachusetts General Hospital, 1810–1865: An Essay on the Political Construction of Social Responsibility During New England's Early Industrialization," Ph.D. diss., Tufts University, 1985.

14. Entry for July 7, 1809, Board of Governors' Minutes, New York Hospital Archives (hereafter NYHA). The phrase is extracted from the board's annual report to the state legislature. Samuel Bard, *A Discourse upon the Duties of a Physician, with some Sentiments, on the Usefulness and Necessity of a Public Hospital . . .* (New-York: A. & J. Robertson, 1769), pp. 15–18.

15. *Address of the Trustees of the Massachusetts General Hospital to the Subscribers and to the Public* (n.p., n.d. [Boston, 1822]), p. 22. All of the early appeals and addresses made in behalf of MGH underlined the importance of the hospital to clinical training. Cf. Richard Sullivan, *Address Delivered before the Governour and Council, Members of the Legislature, and other Patrons of the Massachusetts General Hospital* (Boston: Wells and Lilly, 1819). I will return to the question of clinical education in chapter 8.

16. J. Jackson and J.C. Warren to Richard Sullivan and Theodore Lyman, October 30, 1822, Venereal Disease File, Massachusetts General Hospital Archives (hereafter MGHA).

17. W.G. Malin, *Some Account of the Pennsylvania Hospital, Its Origin, Objects and Present State* (Philadelphia: Thomas Kite, 1831), p. 7; "The Massachusetts Hospital," *Boston Medical & Surgical Journal* (hereafter *BM&SJ*) 3 (May 4, 1830): 194–95. The second quote is from Jackson's letter to the editor, dated April 27, 1830, and printed with the editor's introductory remarks.

18. Entries for June 28, December 27, 1841, September 29, 1845, May 29, 1848, Minutes, Board of Managers, Pennsylvania Hospital Archives (hereafter PHA).

19. New York Dispensary, *Annual Report* (hereafter *AR*), 1829, 6.

20. [Mrs. T. Mason], "Account of Organization of the Society of the New York Asylum for Lying-in Women," Ms. Div., New-York Historical Society (hereafter NYHS).

21. MGH, *Address to Subscribers, . . . 1822*, pp. 6–7; Benjamin Rush to Ashbel Green, April 26, 1803, *Letters of Benjamin Rush*, ed. L.H. Butterfield, two vols. (Princeton: Princeton University for the American Philosophical Society, 1951), 2:863.

22. James Jackson, Walter Channing, John Ware, et al. to Trustees, MGH, December [8], 1833, "Wards, Isolation & Pavilion File," MGHA.

23. Samuel Jackson to the Managers, August 18, 1853, Box 155, Medical Staff Papers, PHA.

24. *Charter and By-Laws of the New-York Dispensary* (New York: Van Winkle and Wiley, 1814), p. 11; Nathan Gurney (Supt.) to Trustees, January 22, 1826, "Administration—Care of Patients, Charges Made to, File," MGHA.

25. Lowell Hospital Assoc., *AR, 1900,* p. 11.

26. Female Medical Casebooks, 1837–40, Cincinnati General Hospital Archives (hereafter CGHA).

27. The Almshouse census is included among the papers of the Philadelphia Board of Guardians of the Poor, Philadelphia City Archives (hereafter PCA); Samuel C. Hopkins, House Pupil to Board of Managers, January 25, 1808, Medical Staff Papers, PHA; Entry for July 25, 1853, Minutes, Board of Managers, PHA; "Report of the Committee appointed to meet with the trustees of the Jefferson College," October 27, 1834, Minutes, Board of Guardians, PCA; Testimony of Drs. Courcillon and Hooker before Committee on Internal Affairs, January 22, 1858, House Officers-Administration File, MGHA. I should like to thank Priscilla Clement for her analysis of the 1807 almshouse census. Cf. Priscilla Clement, *Welfare and the Poor in the Nineteenth-Century City. Philadelphia, 1800–1854* (Rutherford, N.J.: Fairleigh Dickinson University Press, c. 1985), esp. pp. 83–86.

28. Entry for October 27, 1826, Minutes, Inspecting Committee, MGHA; John Roberts, "Notes of Life in a Hospital by a Resident Physician, January, 1877," Historical Collections, College of Physicians of Philadelphia (hereafter CPP).

29. Thomas Markoe to Board of Governors, December 3, 1858, Papers, Board of Governors, The New York Hospital Archives (hereafter NYHA).

30. Entry for May 8, 1809, Minutes, Board of Physicians, Board of Guardians, PCA; "Report on Women's Wards," July 20, 1835, Minutes, Board of Guardians PCA. Chronic neurological and epileptic cases presented a similar dilemma: were they sick or dependent? paupers or patients? When Charleston, South Carolina opened a new hospital and moved the sick from the almshouse to its wards, a number did not fit easily into the category of sick (suitable for transfer to the hospital) or dependent (and thus appropriately left in the almshouse). Entry for August 17, 1842, Almshouse Minutes, South Carolina Historical Society (hereafter SCHS).

31. Entry for December 3, 1832, Minutes, Board of Managers, PHA; March 23, 1827, Visiting Committee Minutes, MGHA. For the unwillingness of the New York Hospital to receive female venereal patients, see: New York Hospital, *Report of a Committee of the Governors . . . on the Occasional Prevalence of Erysipelas . . .* (New York: William H. Colyer, 1836).

32. Entry for January 29, 1821, Minutes, Board of Managers, PHA.

33. Entry for September 19, 1828, Visiting Comm. Minutes, MGHA. MGH bylaws (1821, p. 20) had explicitly empowered the superintendent to provide relief in the form of money or clothing to patients about to be discharged. Traditional views of paternalistic responsibility could not end abruptly at the hospital's gate. The task of caring for the sick implied at least some responsibility for the body in health (while contemporary medical theory emphasized the ways in which health could shade into sickness as a result of deprived circumstances).

34. Entry for April 7, May 5, 1818, Minutes, Board of Governors, NYHA; entry for May 21, 1857, Medical Board, Episcopal Hospital, Episcopal Hospital Archives, Philadelphia (hereafter EHA); Communication from Dr. R. Levis, September 9, 1859, Hospital Committee, Board of Guardians, PCA.

35. Thomas [Lyell] to Board of Governors, February 12, 1842, Papers, Board of Governors, NYHA.

36. For references to scurvy, see Thomas Akin, chairman, Commissioners of the Poorhouse to the Mayor, October 21, 1840, Almshouse Corresp., 1822–52, SCHS and September 28, 1853, Minutes, Charleston Almshouse, SCHS; Charles Law-

rence, *History of the Philadelphia Almshouses and Hospitals* . . . ([Philadelphia]: Privately
Printed, 1905), p. 20; October 23, 1844, Minutes, Hospital Committee, PCA.

37. Only the Royal Infirmary of Edinburgh, which treated a few pay patients and
a good number of His Majesty's troops, constituted a conspicuous exception in the
late eighteenth century. The poorest among the British populated workhouses
when sick, not voluntary hospitals. Brian Abel-Smith, *The Hospitals. 1800–1948. A
Study in Social Administration in England and Wales* (Cambridge: Harvard University
Press, 1964); Guenter B. Risse, *Hospital Life in Enlightenment Scotland. Care and Teaching
at the Royal Infirmary of Edinburgh* (Cambridge, London, and New York: Cambridge
University Press, 1986); Gwendoline M. Ayers, *England's First State Hospitals and
Metropolitan Asylums Board 1867–1930* (London: Wellcome Institute, 1971), chap. I.

38. Entry for March 27, 1854, Minutes, Board of Managers, PHA. Throughout
the antebellum years, the Philadelphia Almshouse always treated a far greater
number of patients than did its prestigious voluntary counterpart. Many had in fact
been referred or transferred from the Pennsylvania Hospital. As its endowment
grew, however, the Pennsylvania Hospital's managers approved a larger proportion
of free admissions. By midcentury, the balance had shifted decisively; for the three
years ending in December of 1852, the average number of patients in the hospital
was 154, only 39 of whom paid for all or part of their care. Entry for April 25, 1852,
Minutes, Board of Managers, PHA. Like most voluntary hospitals, the Pennsylvania Hospital routinely sought to recover its costs from local governments in the
case of indigent patients who were not Philadelphia residents.

39. Harry J. Campbell, "The Congressional Debate over the Seaman's Sickness
and Disability Act of 1798," *Bulletin of the History of Medicine* (hereafter *BHM*)
48(1974): 423–26; Robert Strauss, *Medical Care for Seamen. The Origin of Public Medical
Service in the United States* (New Haven, Conn.: Yale University Press, 1950).

40. *Report of the President and Directors of the General Hospital Society to the General Assembly,
May, 1850. Doc. No. 17* (New Haven, Conn.: Osborn & Baldwin, 1850), pp. 2, 6;
Governors of the New York Hospital, *State of New York Hospital . . . for the Year 1844*
(New-York: Egbert, Harvey & King, 1845), pp. 6–7.

41. Nancy Tomes, *A Generous Confidence. Thomas Story Kirkbride and the Art of Asylum-
Keeping, 1840–1883* (Cambridge, London, New York: Cambridge University Press,
1984), provides an excellent account of these developments.

42. The trustees promised to keep funds for the general and insane hospitals
separate and to open that branch "which the discrimination of private munificence
shall thus designate as the most worthy or interesting object of general benevolence. It being the purpose of the Trustees, should the amount of their funds
authorize it, to keep these two branches of a General Hospital distinct, in separate
buildings and under separate management, and in locations sufficiently distant, to
preclude all inconvenience from each other." *The Trustees of the Massachusetts General
Hospital, to the Public* ([Boston] Tileson and Weld, [1816]), pp. 4–5.

43. Municipal and county almshouses had, of course, no such options, and they
continued into the twentieth century to face problems posed by the chronic insane.

44. Entry for January 2, 1816, Minutes, Visiting Committee, NYHA; Governors
of New York Hospital, *By-Laws and Regulations, 1826*, p. 26.

45. Entry for March 27, 1828, March 13, 1829, Minutes, Commissioners of the
Poor House, Almshouse Records, SCHS; March 30, 1868, Minutes, Board of
Managers, PHA; June 5, 1827, Minutes, Board of Managers, New-York Asylum for
Lying-In Women, NYHA.

46. Case of Margaret Henry, November 6, 1851, Casebook kept at Bellevue
Hospital, R.L. Brodie, Waring Historical Library, Medical University of South
Carolina; Charles E. Rosenberg, "The Practice of Medicine in New York a Century
Ago," *BHM* 41 (1967): 239; Entry for December 11, 1846, Hospital Committee

Minutes, Board of Guardians, PCA; Entries for November 9, 20, 1813, Minutes, Inspecting Committee, NYHA. The "black book" in which the names and infractions of those punished at the Philadelphia Hospital were entered was maintained as late as the 1890s. Surviving volumes are preserved in PCA. Minutes of the antebellum Charleston almshouse indicate that it followed similar policies, employing "showers" and punishment cells.

47. Entry for January 6, 1852, Minutes, NYHA; Entries for January 23, June 26, 1863, April 15, 1864, Minutes, Hospital Committee, Board of Guardians, PCA.

48. Nicholas Shields, for example, 24, laborer, said he had taken *"four hats full of medicine,"* suffered through a blister to the epigastrum and: " . . . feeling somewhat uneasy under & apprehending a repitition . . . Swore by J————s he would stand it no more he would so he took French leave." Male Medical Casebook, June 7, 1837, CGHA.

49. Mary Falconer's executrix asked payment of her salary for the years between 1802 and 1805. Entry for August 26, 1805, Minutes, Board of Managers, PHA; N.I. Bowditch to Marcus Morton, February 29, 1844, N.I. Bowditch Biographical File, MGHA; for information on MGH ward see Bowditch, *History,* pp. 184–85; for 1871 letter of MGH Superintendent see Benjamin S. Shaw to Board of Trustees, August 31, 1871, Personnel File, MGHA. The New York Hospital provided in 1821 for an increase in salary of 50 percent for nurses after five years' service, an increase of another third after ten years' service, and after twenty years an annuity of $25.00 and, in case of need, "support in the hospital during life." In 1845, the New York Hospital employed three female nurses with over ten years' service, and three female and two male nurses with more than five years' service. T.R. Smith and W.A. Stewart, "Report of Committee of Revision on 13th Chapter: also resolution respecting nurses passed Feb. 6, 1821," Papers, Board of Governors, NYHA.

50. Charles Lawrence, *History of Philadelphia Almshouse,* pp. 52, 123.

51. The description of the hospital's network of relatives is drawn from the testimony of house physician Hasket Derby, fragment dated 1857–58, "Statements of House Physicians &c," House Officers-Administration of File, MGHA.

52. Elizabeth Blackwell to Sara Elder, October 16, 1857, Archives of Women in Medicine, Medical College of Pennsylvania (hereafter MCP). A recent study has documented the way in which class, ethnicity, and gender all played a role in mid-nineteenth-century decisions to use anesthesia after its discovery in 1846. Martin S. Pernick, *A Calculus of Suffering. Pain, Professionalism, and Anaesthesia in Nineteenth-Century America* (New York: Columbia University Press, 1985).

53. Entry for January 28, 1846, Minutes, Hospital Committee, Board of Guardians, PCA. At a meeting to comment on proposed building plans, Philadelphia's Episcopal Hospital medical staff urged that rooms for "colored persons" should be in rooms smaller than those suggested and separated from the main building. Entry for May 21, 1857, Minutes, Medical Board, Episcopal Hospital Archives (hereafter EHA).

54. Entry for May 11, 1842, Minutes, Almshouse Commissioners, SCHS; D. Hayes Agnew, *Lecture on the Medical History of the Philadelphia Almshouse. . . . October 15th, 1862* (Philadelphia: Holland & Edgar, 1862), p. 9.

55. Entry for May 29, 1848, Minutes, Board of Managers, PHA.

56. Howard Payson Arnold, *Memoir of Jonathan Mason Warren, M.D.* (Boston: Privately Printed, 1886), p. 85. Antebellum American hospital records do provide occasional instances of brutality toward patients as well as formal prescriptions against disciplining patients without the concurrence of steward or managers; however, it is difficult to judge the actual frequency of such physical abuse.

57. Philadelphia, Almshouse Census for 1807, PCA; Robert J. Carlisle, ed., *An Account of Bellevue Hospital with a Catalogue of the Medical and Surgical Staff from 1736 to 1894*

(New York: Society of the Alumni of Bellevue Hospital, 1893), p. 10; Charles Jackson to N.I. Bowditch, October 1, 1851, Administration, Care of Patients, General Statements File, MGHA.

58. Bowditch, *History*, pp. 366, 454–55; Surgeons of the New-York Ophthalmic Hospital, *AR*, 1855, 11; J. Roosevelt Bayley, Secretary, Roman Catholic Diocese of New York, to Board of Governors, January 6, 1851, Papers, NYHA; Entry for May 24, 1841, Hospital Committee Minutes, PCA; *Auditor's Reports of the Accounts of the Blockley Alms-House*, 1850–1; Society of the Alumni of City (Charity) Hospital, *Report for 1904 together with a History of the City Hospital and a Register of its Medical Officers* . . . (New York: Published by the Society, 1904), p. 60.

59. John Duffe, Diary, Ms. Div., NYHS.

60. Ibid., April 1, 1844.

61. Ibid., March 30, 1844.

62. Ibid., April 19, 1844.

63. Ibid., June 12, March 24, 1844.

64. Entry for June 6, 1837, J.M. Howe, Diary, Ms. Div., NYHS.

65. Ibid., June 13, July 2, September 5, 1837.

66. Ibid., July 24, 1837.

67. Ibid., June 10, 1837.

68. Ibid., November 25, 1837.

69. Ibid., July 31, April 18, 1837.

2. *Vocation and Stewardship: Inconsistent Visions*

1. February 22, 1846, cited in N. I. Bowditch, *A History of the Massachusetts General Hospital [to August 5, 1851.] Second Edition, with a Continuation to 1872* (Boston: The Trustees, 1872), p. 197.

2. Entry for February 1, 1820, Minutes, Board of Governors, The New York Hospital Archives (hereafter NYHA).

3. MGH, *Rules and Regulations for the Government of the Hospital, Adopted November 17, 1822* . . . (Boston: Russell and Gardner, 1822), p. 13; Entry for December 18, 1828, Minutes, Charleston Almshouse Commissioners, South Carolina Historical Society (hereafter SCHS); *An Account of the New-York Hospital* (New York: Mahlon Day, 1820), p. 7; Society of the New York Hospital, *By-Laws and Regulations . . . April 5th, 1825* (New York: Mahlon Day, 1826), p. 6. At the Pennsylvania Hospital, a committee of "attending managers" met every Wednesday and Saturday at ten to approve admissions and discharges. entry for May 29, 1848, Minutes, Pennsylvania Hospital (hereafter PHA). The New York Hospital Inspecting Committee also kept a record of attendance by their visiting staff physicians. Cf. entry for February 15, 1811, Minutes, Board of Governors, NYHA.

4. Bowditch, *History*, p. 383; Entry for May 13, 1822, Minutes, PHA, repassed May 29, 1848; Entry for November 17, 1826, Visiting Committee Minutes, MGHA.

5. Visiting Committee's Record and Asst. Physician's Report, April, 1839–November, 1842, Box 9, MGH Papers, Countway Library of Medicine, Harvard (hereafter HCC). Prominent local citizens might serve as "security" for patients not admitted to a free bed.

6. This sentence is based on a reading of the minute books kept by the Hospital's Inspecting Committee for the period between 1809 and 1818. NYHA.

7. Entry for January 6, 1824, Minutes of Monthly Meetings, New-York Asylum for Lying-In Women, NYHA; Bowditch, *History*, pp. 394–95.

8. George Newbold to the Governors of the New York Hospital, October 5, 1857; Swan to Governors, January 5, 1857, Filed Papers, Board of Governors, NYHA.

9. Samuel Spring to Trustees, May 21, 1825, Nathan Gurney Biographical File, MGHA. It was assumed that the superintendent's wife would serve as the hospital's "matron," overseeing the "woman's work" of cleaning, sewing, cooking, and nursing. It was natural, for example, that a superintendent of New York Hospital declined consideration for reelection when his wife became too sick to serve as matron. Charles Starr to George Newbold, April 14, 1845, Papers, Board of Governors, NYHA.

10. MGH, circular signed by James Jackson and Johns Collins Warren, *The Subscribers . . . Rules for the Admission and Conduct of Pupils, May, 1824* (Boston: MGH, 1824); Charles Lawrence, *History of the Philadelphia Almshouses and Hospitals . . .* ([Philadelphia:] Privately Printed, 1905), pp. 156–57. The Board of Guardians kept making such statements of principle which indicates that their restrictions might not have been observed in practice.

11. D.B. St. John Roosa, *The Old Hospital and Other Papers,* 2nd ed. (New York: William Wood, 1889), p. 13; *Address of the Trustees of the Massachusetts General Hospital, to the Subscribers and to the Public* (n.p.; n.d. [Boston: MGH, 1822]), p. 21. On experimentation, see James Jackson's candid depiction of it as an unavoidable aspect of medical care. "The patient's assurance," he explained, is "grounded on this, . . . that in each case, the physician will try that experiment, which, in the present state of his knowledge, appears most likely to be successful." *A Report Founded on the Cases of Typhoid Fever, . . . Which Occurred in the Massachusetts General Hospital . . .* (Boston: Whipple & Damrell, 1838), p. 23. Jackson was no average practitioner, but Boston's most prominent consultant and clinical teacher.

12. For an example, see Stephen Smith, "Hospital Appointments," *Doctor in Medicine: And Other Papers on Professional Subjects* (New York: William Wood, 1872), pp. 247–50.

13. Entry for February 24, 1806, Minutes, Board of Managers, PHA; Resident Students to Faculty, May 10, 1860, Faculty Minutes, Medical College of Virginia, Archives (hereafter MCV). At mid-century, the Massachusetts General Hospital trustees resolved to engage medical students rather than graduates as house staff; the graduates had been less amenable to discipline and, in addition, the object of patient charges of brutality. S. Parkman and H.I. Bowditch, [1849], undated memorandum, bound in "Surgical Staff Correspondence, 1847–77," Countway Library (hereafter HCC).

14. Boston Dispensary, Circular to Visiting Physicians, n.d. 1812 File, Boston Dispensary Papers, HCC.

15. "The Committee to whom was referred the subject of the increasing expenditure of the Hospital", Visiting Committee, January 6, 1845, Papers, Board of Governors, NYHA.

16. Dr. Prioleau, house physician, in entry for September 28, 1853, Minutes, Charleston Almshouse, SCHS; Cf. entries for August 21, October 12, 1853.

17. House pupils to Board of Attending Managers, February 27, 1852, copy in "Surgical Staff Correspondence, 1847–77," March 7, 1852, Minutes, Board of Trustees, MGHA.

18. Samuel Eliot and S.G. Howe, "Report of Committee on Autopsies, December 27, 1872," Autopsy File, MGHA. This file contains much illuminating detail. A key element in the autopsy problem was the practical matter of returning the body to the family promptly and in a condition suitable for viewing and burial.

19. Statement of J.C. Warren to Henry B. Rogers, Frances C. Lowell, and Charles

Amory, committee, "Report on a Lying-In Department, October, 1845," Obstetrics Department File, MGHA.

20. Cf. *Charter and By-Laws of the Marshall Infirmary* (Troy, N.Y.: Wm. H. Young, 1859), p. 21.

21. "Report of the Committee to consider the expediency of altering the By-Laws . . . ," December 6, 1842, Papers, Board of Governors, NYHA.

22. S.L. Mitchill to Lyman Spalding, October 31, 1799, James A. Spalding, ed., *Dr. Lyman Spalding* (Boston: W.M. Leonard, 1916), p. 20. Cf. R.H. Shryock, *Medical Licensing in America, 1650–1965* (Baltimore: The Johns Hopkins University Press, 1967).

23. William H. Williams, *America's First Hospital: The Pennsylvania Hospital, 1751–1841* (Wayne, Pa.: Haverford House, 1976), pp. 104–105, 136–37.

24. G.C. Shattuck to J. Bigelow, January 26, 1810, Bigelow Papers, Massachusetts Historical Society; Charles Bonner to J.Y. Bassett, October 21, 1842, J.Y. Bassett Papers, Southern Historical Collection, University of North Carolina.

25. Entry for September 24, 1804, Minutes, Board of Managers; Stephen R. Hooker, Edenton, North Carolina to Samuel Coates, June 7, 1806, Medical Staff Papers, PHA. House pupils were expected to attend medical school lectures in their free hours during the brief winter school year. J.W. Moore to Board of Managers, October 29, 1809, Medical Staff Papers, PHA.

26. The position of apothecary was also ordinarily filled by a medical student or recent graduate in search of clinical experience.

27. Russell M. Jones, ed., *The Parisian Education of an American Surgeon, Letters of Jonathan Mason Warren (1832–1835)* (Philadelphia: American Philosophical Society, 1978), p. 88.

28. Entry for October 19, 1835, Minutes, Board of Guardians, Philadelphia City Archives (hereafter PCA); Nathan Hatfield to the Managers of the Alms House of Philadelphia, draft, [1824], Hatfield Papers, College of Physicians of Philadelphia, (hereafter CPP); New York Hospital, *By-Laws and Regulations, . . .* (New York: Mahlon Day, 1826), pp. 19–20; Entry for November 3, 1812, Minutes, Board of Governors, NYHA, noting that only students of visiting staff members could serve as dressers on the wards.

29. Thomas Wharton to Board of Managers, April 28, 1827, Medical Staff Papers, PHA.

30. Alfred Stillé to James R. Greaves, March 3, 1856, Medical Staff Papers, PHA.

31. J.H. Griscom to Visiting Committee, May 1, 1858, Griscom to R.L. Kennedy, April 6, 1859, Papers, Board of Governors, NYHA.

32. On the symbiosis between professional careers and the outpatient dispensary, see Charles E. Rosenberg, "Social Class and Medical Care: The Rise and Fall of the Dispensary in Nineteenth-Century America," *Journal of the History of Medicine* 29 (1974): 32–54.

33. Simon Wickes, Journal entries for April 22, June 4, and October 14, 1833, Maryland Historical Society.

34. Robert J. Carlisle, ed., *An Account of Bellevue Hospital with a Catalogue of the Medical and Surgical Staff from 1736 to 1894* (New York: Society of the Alumni of Bellevue Hospital, 1893); p. 47; Entry for November 2, 1835, Minutes, Board of Guardians, PCA.

35. Benjamin Rush et al., to Board of Managers, September 2, 1807, December 19, 1808, Medical Staff Papers, PHA; S. Abbott to Trustees, Massachusetts General Hospital, 14 January 1853, Admitting Physician File, MGHA.

36. "Duties of Resident Physician," adopted July 17, 1856, Faculty Minutes, MCV. Cf. also April 11, 1849, Faculty Minutes, Hampden-Sydney Medical College, MCV.

37. Philadelphia, Board of Guardians of the Poor, *Rules for the Government of the Board of Guardians of the Poor . . .* (Philadelphia: McLaughlin Bros., 1859), pp. 53, 55–56. It might be noted, as an informal index of increasing bureaucracy, that these *Rules* occupied 144 pages.

3. The Medical Mind: Tradition and Change in Antebellum America

1. Alden March, *Semi-Centennial Address Delivered Before the Medical Society of the State of New-York . . .* (Albany: C. Van Benthuysen, 1857), p. 17.

2. For a fuller discussion, see Charles E. Rosenberg, "The Therapeutic Revolution: Medicine, Meaning, and Social Change in Nineteenth-Century America," *Perspectives in Biology and Medicine* 20 (1977): 485–506.

3. The phrase is taken from the title page of A. Bitner, "Notes taken from the Philadelphia Almshouse, 1824," College of Physicians of Philadelphia (hereafter CPP).

4. Although we tend to associate quacks with the sale of panaceas, contemporary physicians tended at least as frequently to see them as vendors of "specifics"—a term used in fact as a pejorative by regular medical men at the beginning of the nineteenth century.

5. D.B. St. John Roosa describes the mid-nineteenth-century hospital physician's ward rounds and his dependence on the pulse and "putting his hands on [the patient's] face to note the temperature . . ." *The Old Hospital and Other Papers.* 2nd. rev. and enl. ed. (New York: William Wood, 1889), p. 15. Reading the pulse was considered particularly important; skill in managing it could "alone ensure a successful practice." J.P. McKelpech, "Notebook on the Practice of Physick, from Lectures of Nathaniel Potter," November 12, 1816, Ms. Dept., Perkins Library, Duke University.

6. Flinn was admitted on November 20, 1809, Register, Medical Cases, 1809–1834, The New York Hospital Archives (hereafter NYHA); Hospital Casebook, 1824–27, Philadelphia City Archives (hereafter PCA).

7. "It has long been believed," as a contemporary medical man explained, "that the cinchona [bark, the source of quinine] produced its effects in intermittents [that is, malaria] through the combined agency of a bitter, an astringent, and an aromatic principle." Editorial, "Quinine and the New Medicines," *Boston Medical & Surgical Journal:* (hereafter *BM&SJ*) 3 (March 23, 1830): 111.

8. E.B. Haskins, *Therapeutic Cultivation: Its Errors and its Reformation. An Address delivered to the Tennessee Medical Society, April 7, 1857* (Nashville: Cameron and Fall, 1857), p. 22. Cf. Rosenberg, "Therapeutic Revolution," p. 491; Rosenberg, "Medical Text and Social Context: Explaining William Buchan's *Domestic Medicine,*" *Bulletin of the History of Medicine* (hereafter *BHM*) 57 (1983): 22–42; Max Neuburger, *Die Lehre von der Heilkraft der Natur im Wandel der Zeiten* (Stuttgart: Ferdinand Enke, 1926). The most detailed treatment of midnineteenth-century therapeutics is to be found in John Harley Warner, *The Therapeutic Perspective. Medical Practice, Knowledge, and Identity in America, 1820–1885* (Cambridge and London: Harvard University Press, 1986).

9. Rosenberg, "Therapeutic Revolution," p. 492.

10. Entry for March 20, 1838, Female Medical Casebooks, 1837–40, Cincinnati General Hospital Archives (hereafter CGHA).

11. Case of W. Griffith, Aet. 37, Carpenter, August 11, 1837, Male Medical Casebook, 1837–38, CGHA.

12. Case of George Devert, November 15, 1826, Hospital Casebook, 1824–27, PCA.

13. Soon after the turn of the nineteenth century, for example, a twenty-five-year-old sailor was admitted to the Pennsylvania Hospital with a "Fractured Scull." After the attending physician had removed a piece of bone, the young man was treated by being kept on a "low diet," bled twenty ounces, and had his "bowels . . . opened." With recurring infection and lengthy healing, the postoperative aspects of this, and most aspects of other than superficial surgery, were at least as important as the surgery itself. Hospital Cases, vol. I, pp. 74–75, Pennsylvania Hospital Archives (hereafter PHA).

14. The very lack of formal institutional structures underlined the significance of less formal signs of status. Learning legitimated the pretensions of ambitious young medical men; it was important that a physician dress, talk, hold himself— and be educated—as a gentleman if he were to move and practice in respectable circles.

15. "No arguments, surely," a prominent Scottish medical teacher argued in 1780, "are necessary at this day to recommend experimental pursuit. No one is now ignorant, that it is the only road to genuine science; and that nothing is intitled to the denomination of philosophy, which rests not on this foundation." Had it not been for the Baconian spirit of experimentation, he argued, we would still be bound by the toils of Aristotelian scholasticism. Andrew Duncan, *Account of the Life and Writings of the Late Alexr. Monro Senr. M.D. . . . Delivered as the Harveian Oration at Edinburgh, for the Year 1780* (Edinburgh: C. Elliot and C. Dilly, 1780), p. 37. For early American interest in physiological experimentation, see Edward C. Atwater, " 'Squeezing Mother Nature'; Experimental Physiology in the United States before 1870," *BHM*, 52(1978): 313–35; Donald G. Bates, "The Background to John Young's Thesis on Digestion," *BHM* 36(1962): 341–61.

16. On digitalis, see: J. Worth Estes, *Hall Jackson and the Purple Foxglove. Medical Practice and Research in Revolutionary America 1760–1820* (Hanover, N.H.: University Press of New England, 1979); on vaccination, John B. Blake, *Benjamin Waterhouse and the Introduction of Vaccination. A Reappraisal* (Philadelphia: University of Pennsylvania, c. 1957); James A. Spalding, *Dr. Lyman Spalding . . .* (Boston: W.M. Leonard, 1916).

17. Entry for August 3, 1819, Minutes, Board of Governors, NYHA.

18. The phrase is drawn from a petition by the institution's resident physicians, to the Hospital Committee, Board of Guardians of the Poor, August 13, 1852, PCA.

19. Entry for February 10, 1827, Minutes of the Physicians (Medical Staff), Board of Guardians, PCA. The same medical staff had been requesting postmortem facilities for some time. Entry for September 18, 1815, Minutes of Physicians. Cf. also James Jackson et al. to Trustees, MGH, December [8], 1833, asking for a room "out of the reach of patients and properly supplied with water" for postmortems. "Wards, Isolation and Pavillion File," Massachusetts General Hospital (hereafter MGHA).

20. G.C. Shattuck to Roswell Shurtleff, July 20, 1804, Shattuck Papers, Massachusetts Historical Society; S.W. Butler Diary, Entry for April 24, 1850, CPP.

21. A small minority of medical school professors at the largest schools did realize a substantial income from student fees.

22. On the nature and influence of the Paris Clinical School, see: Knud Faber, *Nosography: The Evolution of Clinical Medicine in Modern Times,* 2nd ed. rev. (New York: Paul B. Hoeber, 1930); Erwin H. Ackerknecht, *Medicine at the Paris Hospital 1794–1848* (Baltimore: The Johns Hopkins University Press, 1967); Michel Foucault, *The Birth of the Clinic. An Archaeology of Medical Perception,* trans, A.M. Sheridan Smith (New York: Pantheon, 1973); Russell M. Jones, "American Doctors and the Parisian Medical World, 1830–1840," *BHM* 47 (1973): 40–65, 177–204.

23. Ackerknecht *(Medicine at the Paris Hospital)* emphasizes this distinction, as well as the positive skepticism toward the laboratory felt by many of the leaders in French clinical medicine.

24. For a striking instance of Louis's work and his influence on an American acolyte, see: James Jackson, *A Memoir of James Jackson, Jr., M.D. With Extracts from his Letters to his Father* . . . (Boston: I.R. Butts, 1835). Cf. also the often-quoted essay by William Osler: "The Influence of Louis on American Medicine," *Johns Hopkins Hospital Bulletin* 8 (1897): 161–67.

25. For a useful account, see Stanley J. Reiser, *Medicine and the Reign of Technology* (Cambridge, London, New York: Cambridge University Press, 1978), pp. 23–44. R.T.H. Laennec pioneered in the use of the stethoscope; his classic study *On Mediate Auscultation in Diseases of the Chest* appeared in 1819 (Paris: Brosson, 1819), the first American printing in 1823.

26. Russell Jones, "American Doctors," pp. 43, 199.

27. W.W. Gerhard to James Jackson, January 1, 1835, Jackson Papers. Countway Library (hereafter HCC). Gerhard felt that reports based on American clinical experience would "attract the attention of American physicians more than the thousands collected in Paris, against which there is an absurd feeling of distrust." His opinion reflected contemporary belief in the power of environmental circumstances to shape the clinical manifestations of disease.

28. Casebook of R.L. Brodie, Bellevue Hospital, 1851, p. 26, Waring Historical Library, Medical University of South Carolina.

29. O.W. Holmes, *Valedictory Address, delivered to the Medical Graduates of Harvard University, . . . March 10, 1858* (Boston: David Clapp, 1858), p. 5. Cf. John Harley Warner, " 'The Nature-Trusting Heresy': American Physicians and the Concept of the Healing Power of Nature in the 1850s and 1860s," *Perspectives in American History* 11 (1977–78): 291–324.

30. T.G. Thomas, *Introductory Address Delivered at the College of Physicians and Surgeons, New York, October 17th, 1864* (New York: Trafton, 1864), p. 31; Jacob Bigelow, *Brief Expositions of Rational Medicine, to Which is Prefixed the Paradise of Doctors* . . . (Boston: Phillips, Sampson & Co., 1858), p. iv.

31. C.W. Parsons, *An Essay on the Question, Vis Medicatrix Naturae, How Far Is It to Be Relied On in the Treatment of Disease?* . . . (Boston: Printed for the Rhode Island Medical Society, 1849), p. 7.

32. Alexander H. Stevens to James Jackson, April 14, 1836, Jackson Papers, HCC.

33. See Martin S. Staum, *Cabanis. Enlightenment and Medical Philosophy in the French Revolution* (Princeton: Princeton University Press, 1980).

34. Elisha Bartlett to Gentlemen, September 3, 1844, Box 26, Case 7, Gratz Coll., Historical Society of Pennsylvania; E.H. Ackerknecht, "Elisha Bartlett and the Philosophy of the Paris Clinical School," *BHM* 24 (1950): 43–60; Bartlett, *An Essay on the Philosophy of Medical Science.* . . . (Philadelphia: Lea and Blanchard, 1844).

35. J.H. Miller, ed., A.P.W. Philip, *A Treatise on the Nature and Cure of those Diseases, either Acute or Chronic, Which Precede Change of Structure* . . . (Baltimore: E.J. Coale and Coale & Co., 1831), p. 251n. By the late 1840s, physicians were more willing to incorporate auscultation and percussion into their practice. Cf. Henry I. Bowditch, *Young Stethoscopist* (New York: J. & H.G. Langley, 1846), p. vii.

36. Nathan Hatfield, "Notes on the Practice of Physic by N. Chapman, November 1823," Hatfield Papers, CPP. "In the first place," he explained, "never examine the pulse on first entering the room of the patient, for the appearance of a Physician seldom fail [sic] to excite some alarm, but first allow the patient to become composed . . ."

37. Editorial, "Moral Treatment in Disease," *BM&SJ.* 3 (August 31, 1830): 469.

38. *Philadelphia Dispensary, Rules of the Dispensary with the Annual Report for 1862*

(Philadelphia: J. Crummill, 1863), pp. 12–13; O.W. Holmes, *Medical Essays* (Boston and New York: Houghton Mifflin, 1911 [orig. pub. 1861]), p. 258.

39. For a detailed study of the introduction of anesthesia in the United States, see Martin Pernick, *A Calculus of Suffering. Pain, Professionalism, and Anaesthesia in Nineteenth-Century America* (New York: Columbia University Press, 1985).

4. Expanding a Traditional Institution: Social Sources of Hospital Growth, 1850–1875

1. The standard accounts are: George W. Adams, *Doctors in Blue, The Medical History of the Union Army in the Civil War* (New York: Schuman, 1952); H.H. Cunningham, *Doctors in Gray. The Confederate Medical Service* (Baton Rouge: Louisiana State University Press, 1958); Richard H. Shryock, "A Medical Perspective on the Civil War," *American Q.* 14 (1962): 161–73; William Q. Maxwell, *Lincoln's Fifth Wheel. The Political History of the United States Sanitary Commission* (New York, London, Toronto: Longmans, Green, 1956).

2. Adams, *Doctors in Blue*, p. 134, cf. 131.

3. Cf. the influential study by George Fredrickson, *The Inner Civil War. Northern Intellectuals and the Crisis of the Union* (New York: Harper, 1965).

4. U.S. Bureau of the Census, *Historical Statistics of the United States. Colonial Times to 1970. Bicentennial Edition. Part 2* (Washington, D.C.: Government Printing Office, 1975), Series A 6–8.

5. Ibid., Series A 57–72.

6. Ibid., Series A 105–18.

7. Cf. James H. Cassedy, *American Medicine and Statistical Thinking, 1800–1860* (Cambridge and London: Harvard University Press, 1984), esp. chaps. 8 and 9; John M. Eyler, *Victorian Social Medicine. The Ideas and Methods of William Farr* (Baltimore and London: Johns Hopkins University Press, 1979); M.J. Cullen, *The Statistical Movement in Early Victorian Britain. The Foundations of Empirical Social Research* (New York: Harvester Press and Barnes & Noble, 1975).

8. Cf. Charles E. Rosenberg, *The Cholera Years. The United States in 1832, 1849 and 1866* (Chicago: University of Chicago Press, 1962).

9. [Episcopal Hospital of Philadelphia], *Appeal on Behalf of the Sick* (Philadelphia: Lindsay & Blakiston, 1851), pp. 20–21, 23.

10. Ibid., p. 7; Entries for May 29, 1848, December 31, 1855, Minutes, Board of Managers, Pennsylvania Hospital Archives (hereafter PHA). Cf. Roosevelt Hospital, Annual Report (hereafter *AR*) 1878–79, 7.

11. General Hospital Society of Connecticut, *AR*, 1871, 18.

12. N.I. Bowditch, *A History of the Massachusetts General Hospital*, ... 2nd ed. (Boston: The Trustees, 1872), p. 360.

13. New York, Commissioners of Public Charities and Correction, *AR*, 1866, 15; Jersey City Charity Hospital, *AR*, 1877, 5 (reporting data from the period 1869–1875); General Hospital Society of Connecticut, *AR*, 1871, 10; Pennsylvania Hospital, *Proceedings of a Meeting Held First Month (January) 15th, 1867* (Philadelphia: Collins, 1867), p. 25. Native-born figures would in each instance include the children of recent immigrants.

14. General Hospital Society of Connecticut, *AR*, 1877, 24.

15. Henry G. Clark, *Outlines of a Plan for a Free City Hospital* (Boston: Rand & Avery, 1860), p. 7.

16. Presbyterian Hospital (New York), *AR*, 1869, 22.

17. Woman's Hospital of Philadelphia, *AR*, 1866, 13.

18. The quotes are, in order, from: Children's Hospital, Boston, *AR,* 1874, 10; Children's Hospital, *AR,* 1870, 9.

19. Homeopathic Medical & Surgical Hospital (Pittsburgh), *AR,* 1872–3, 7.

20. "Its location," the hospital's medical board had contended a few years earlier, "is all that could be desired for a city hospital; in the very centre of a manufacturing district, where accidents of a serious nature are of almost daily occurrence, it offers speedy shelter and succor to the unfortunate sufferers. Our mill and factory owners and managers have not heretofore been slow to appreciate these advantages, and it is to be hoped that they will make still greater use of them in the future." Homeopathic Medical & Surgical Hospital, *AR,* 1869, 27.

21. J. Foster Jenkins, *Tent Hospitals. Read before the American Social Science Association, May 21, 1874* (Cambridge, Mass.: Riverside Press, 1874), p. 7.

22. Illinois Charitable Eye and Ear Infirmary (Chicago), *AR,* 1860, 6.

23. [Howard Hospital] (Philadelphia), *A Few Suggestions to the Benevolent Public Kindly Thrown Out by the Managers of the Western Clinical Infirmary* (Philadelphia: Inquirer Printing Office, 1858), p. 7.

24. With the exception of a few sanitoria for alcohol and drugs and a handful of private surgical "hospitals," the latter usually a few rooms in a residential building.

25. R. Sullivan, *Address Delivered Before the . . . Patrons of the Massachusetts General Hospital . . . June 3, 1819* (Boston: Wells and Lilly, 1819), p. 19.

26. *An Account of the New-York Hospital* (New York: Mahlon Day, 1820), p. 6.

27. A Massachusetts law disallowed such state grants in the latter year. Charles Snyder, *Massachusetts Eye and Ear Infirmary. Studies on its History* (Boston: The Infirmary, 1984), p. 237; Charity Hospital (New Orleans), *AR,* 1876, 35–37; Illinois Charitable Eye and Ear Infirmary (Chicago), *AR,* 1858–9, 5; *AR,* 1867, 7; New-York Ophthalmic Hospital, *AR,* 1854, 7.

28. Hartford Hospital, *AR,* 1854, 7–10. The Hospital's twenty-fifth annual report (Hartford: Case, Lockwood & Brainard, 1881) contains a brief historical account.

29. Hartford Hospital, *AR,* 1854, 8.

30. Hartford Hospital, *Addresses delivered on the Occasion of the Dedication . . . On the 18th of April, 1859* (Hartford: Case, Lockwood & Co., 1859), p. 25; *AR,* 1863, 12.

31. Hartford Hospital, *AR,* 1856–7, 5.

32. Ibid.; Hartford Hospital, *AR,* 1868, 9, 8.

33. Hartford Hospital, *AR,* 1866, 6–7.

34. Ibid., *AR,* 1856–7, 7.

35. Ibid., *AR,* 1870, 10–11, 19.

36. For a contemporary discussion of this expansion, see: *History of the Hospital Saturday and Sunday Movement in New York City, 1880* (New York: The Hospital Saturday and Sunday Association, 1880).

37. Charles E. Rosenberg, "The Practice of Medicine in New York a Century Ago," *Bulletin of the History of Medicine* (hereafter *BHM*), 41 (1967): 238–39. A *Medical Register of the City of New York* was published annually during these years and provides thumbnail descriptions of the various hospitals and dispensaries. Brief historical sketches are to be found in James J. Walsh, *History of Medicine in New York,* 5 vols. (New York: National Americana Society, Inc., 1910), vol. 3. Cf. John Duffy, *A History of Public Health in New York City 1625–1866* (New York: Russell Sage, 1968), ch. 22, "The Rise of the Hospital," pp. 481–514.

38. Thomas N. Bonner, *Medicine in Chicago, 1850–1950. A Chapter in the Social and Scientific Development of a City* (Madison, Wis.: American History Research Center, 1958); Chicago Medical Society, *History of Medicine and Surgery and Physicians and Surgeons of Chicago* (Chicago: The Biographical Publishing Corp., 1922), pp. 233–338;

Timothy Walch, "Catholic Social Institutions and Urban Development: The View from Nineteenth-Century Chicago and Milwaukee," *Catholic Historical Review* 64(1978): 16–32.

39. [Episcopal Hospital], *Appeal on Behalf of the Sick*, p. 26. As might have been expected, however, the low-church supporters of Episcopal hospitals soon found that comparatively few fellow churchmen filled the denomination's hospital beds.

40. Aaron I. Abell, *American Catholicism and Social Action: A Search for Social Justice, 1865–1950* (Garden City, N.Y.: Hanover House, 1960), p. 36.

41. New York Hospital, *Report of the Committee of the Board of Governors, Appointed to Enquire into the Practicability of Extending the Usefulness of the Hospital* (New York: Baker & Godwin, 1858), p. 7.

42. German Hospital of Philadelphia, *A Short History and Description . . .* (Philadelphia: Girard Printing House, 1895), p. 49.

43. Jewish Hospital (Philadelphia), *AR,* 1867, 10.

44. Circular dated August 18, 1864. In bd. vol. of Jewish Hospital publications, Edwin Wolfe Collection, Library Company of Philadelphia.

45. Cited in Morris Vogel, *The Invention of the Modern Hospital. Boston 1870–1930* (Chicago and London: University of Chicago Press, 1980), p. 73.

46. St. Luke's Hospital (Chicago), *AR,* 1866, 9.

47. Episcopal Hospital, Philadelphia, *AR,* 1880, 12.

48. *Articles of Agreement of the Lowell Hospital Association. November, 1839* (Boston: Cassady and March, 1839), p. 3.

49. Walter Licht, "Nineteenth-Century American Railwaymen: A Study in the Nature and Organization of Work," Ph.D. diss., Princeton University, 1977, p. 302.

50. Cf. Rosemary Stevens, "Sweet Charity: State Aid to Hospitals in Pennsylvania, 1870–1910," *BHM* 58(1984): 287–314.

51. Regular physicians did not provide the only impetus toward hospital growth; zealous advocates of homeopathy demanded access to existing hospital facilities for practitioners of their system and when denied often sought to create their own institutions.

52. W.W. Goodell to Visiting Committee, Preston Retreat, 14 August, 1866, Mary Ann Forsyth File, Preston Retreat Documents, PHA.

53. Harriot Hunt, *Glances and Glimpses: Or Fifty Years Social, Including Twenty Years Professional Life* (Boston: John P. Jewett, 1856), p. 172.

54. John Green, *City Hospitals* (Boston: Little, Brown, 1861), p. 11.

55. St. Luke's Hospital (New York), *AR,* 1866, 30–31.

56. "No patient shall leave the house without permission of the Superintendent," New York's Roosevelt Hospital warned. "When desiring to go beyond the Hospital bounds, patients must obtain a card from the House Physician or Surgeon at his morning round, stating that he has no objections, which card, when countersigned by the Superintendent, will serve as a pass, and will be valid for the day upon which it is given, but must be surrendered to the doorkeeper when the patient goes out." *AR,* 1871-2, 30–31.

57. Boston Dispensary, *AR,* 1871, 8.

58. "The familiarity which hospital practice begets," a prominent London practitioner warned, ". . . among women whose sensibilities are not always as keen as those of persons in a higher class of life, or the circumstance that they do not venture to express the pain which want of consideration in these respects on the part of men who would yet shrink from the idea of inflicting a moment's unnecessary suffering upon any one." Charles West, *Diseases of Women* (London: Churchill, 1858), pp. 24–25.

59. Jewish Hospital, *AR,* 1867, 5; Entry for January 2, 1862, Minutes, Board of

Managers, Woman's Hospital, Archives of Women in Medicine, Medical College
of Pennsylvania (hereafter MCP). Women's committees often had as one of their
goals the provision of clothing for destitute patients.

60. Cf. Charles E. Rosenberg, "From Almshouse to Hospital: The Shaping of
Philadelphia General Hospital," *Milbank Memorial Fund Q.* 60 (1982): 118.

61. Entry for October 11, 1861, Minutes, Hospital Committee, Board of Guardians, Philadelphia City Archives (hereafter PCA).

62. Entry for October 5, 1852, Minutes, Medical Board, Episcopal Hospital Archives (hereafter EHA).

63. Valentine Mott Francis, *A Thesis on Hospital Hygiene* (New York: J.F. Trow,
1859), p. 194.

64. Roosevelt Hospital, *AR,* 1877, 7–9.

65. Entries for May 29, 1848, October 31, 1859, Minutes, Board of Managers,
PHA.

66. William D. Purple, "On the Morbid Condition of the Generative Organs,"
New York J. Medicine 3 (1849): 207–208.

67. Joseph A. Eve, *A Report on Diseases of the Cervix Uteri; Read Before the Medical Society
of the State of Georgia* . . . (Augusta: McCafferty's, 1857), p. 38.

5. Ventilation, Contagion, and Germs

1. James Y. Simpson, *Anaesthesia, Hospitalism, Hermaphroditism, and a Proposal to Stamp
Out Smallpox and other Contagious Diseases,* ed. W.G. Simpson (New York: D. Appleton,
1872), p. 291.

2. Ibid., p. 340. Simpson's study was based on published hospital statistics and
a survey of physicians in private practice.

3. George W. Norris, "Statistical Account of the Cases of Amputation Performed
at the Pennsylvania Hospital from January 1, 1850, to January 1, 1860, . . ."
Pennsylvania Hospital Reports 1 (1868): 149–64; Thomas G. Morton, "Statistical Ac-
count of the Cases of Amputation Performed at the Pennsylvania Hospital from
Jan. 1 1860 to Jan. 1 1870 . . . ," *American Journal of Medical Science* 60 (1870): 313;
Thomas G. Morton and William Hunt, *Surgery at the Pennsylvania Hospital. Being an
Epitome of the Practice of the Hospital since 1756* . . . (Philadelphia: J.B. Lippincott, 1880),
pp. 9, 17. For similar figures on amputation results at the Massachusetts General
Hospital, see George Hayward, *Surgical Reports, and Miscellaneous Papers on Medical
Subjects* (Boston: Phillips, Sampson, 1855), pp. 142–60.

4. See, for example, Florence Nightingale, *Introductory Notes on Lying-In Institutions.
Together with a Proposal for Organizing an Institution for Training Midwives and Midwifery
Nurses* (London: Longmans, Green & Co., 1871); A.B. Steele, *Maternity Hospitals; Their
Mortality, and What Should Be Done with Them* (London: J. & A. Churchill; Liverpool:
A. Holden, 1874).

5. Simpson, *Anaesthesia* (1872), pp. 289–90.

6. See, for example, Donald Monro, *An Account of the Diseases Which Were Most
Frequent in the British Military Hospitals in Germany. . . . to Which Is Added, an Essay on the
Means of Preserving the Health of Soldiers, and Conducting Military Hospitals* (London: A.
Millar, D. Wilson and T. Durham . . . , 1764), pp. 355–408. Contemporaries were
also well aware of the seemingly greater mortality in large hospitals as opposed to
private practice. Thomas Percival, *Philosophical, Medical, and Experimental Essays* (Lon-
don: Joseph Jefferson, 1776), p. 174n; John Jones, *Plain Concise Practical Remarks, on the
Treatment of Wounds and Fractures* (Philadelphia: Robert Bell, 1776), pp. 102–14.

7. Or even hospitals built of unfinished logs with dirt floors. Benjamin Rush,
"The Result of Observations made upon the Diseases which Occurred in the
Military Hospitals of the United States, during the Revolutionary War between

Great Britain and the United States," *Medical Inquiries and Observations* (Philadelphia: M. Carey, 1815), I:150.

8. Margaret Pelling, *Cholera, Fever and English Medicine 1825–1865* (Oxford: Oxford University Press, 1978). The doctrine that diseases generally not contagious would become so through the aggregated contamination of confined spaces was termed "contingent contagionism" by contemporaries. See also Charles E. Rosenberg, "The Cause of Cholera: Aspects of Etiological Thought in Nineteenth-Century America," *Bulletin of the History of Medicine* (hereafter *BHM*) 34 (1960): 331–54.

9. William Robert Smith, *Lectures on Nursing* (Philadelphia: Lindsay & Blakiston, 1876), p. 27.

10. It is ironic that most twentieth-century medical readers would regard the often-commented upon connection between erysipelas and childbed fever as a reasonable conclusion (the reflection of an underlying empirical reality—that both are dependent upon the presence of the same organism) while ignoring the theoretical framework that made the connection plausible to mid-nineteenth-century physicians.

11. God could hardly have designed it that women should inevitably die of infections in childbed; in a properly ordered environment, some reformers charged, maternal mortality rates should approach zero—as they would in a state of nature.

12. Venereal disease was also seen as allied to smallpox, both being characterized by skin lesions and contagiosity. Its sexual aspect, moreover, added an additional element of moral ambiguity; there seemed little reason to help those who had brought disease upon themselves.

13. For an example of a physician making the connection explicit, see John Watson, *Thermal Ventilation, and Other Sanitary Improvements, Applicable to Public Buildings, and Recently Adopted at the New York Hospital* (New York: Wm. W. Rose, 1851), p. 6.

14. John Green, *City Hospitals* (Boston: Little, Brown, 1861), p. 13.

15. Hartford Hospital, Annual Report (hereafter *AR*), 1857, 10.

16. Hartford Hospital, *Addresses Delivered on the Occasion of the Dedication . . . 18th of April, 1859* (Hartford: Case, Lockwood and Co., 1859), p. 20.

17. John C. Cheeseman to Board of Governors, December 4, 1849, Papers, Board of Governors, NYHA.

18. John D. Thompson and Grace Goldin, *The Hospital: A Social and Architectural History* (New Haven and London: Yale University Press, 1975), p. 118. Chapter five ("The Pavilion Hospital: A Designed Plan," pp. 118–69) provides an excellent introduction to the subject. The history of the pavilion form can be traced directly to late eighteenth-century French debates on hospital reform. The debate was also influenced by the seeming efficacy of barrack hospitals in certain military situations. Cf. Robert Bruegmann, "Architecture of the Hospital: 1770–1870. Design and Technology," Ph.D. diss., University of Pennsylvania, 1976.

19. The very conventionality of these ideas and procedures emphasizes that the primary historical issue is not explaining the currency of these ideas at mid-century, but rather the energy and emotionality with which they were used by a zealous and self-conscious group of reformers. It is tempting to see their commitment in terms of a reaction to unsettling urban change; the hospital was a microcosm within which rationality and volition could bring order to a sample of the larger disorder outside its walls.

20. London: John W. Parker and Son., 1859. An enlarged edition was published in 1863. This book has a complex bibliographical history; for details, see W.J. Bishop, ed., *A Bio-Bibliography of Florence Nightingale,* completed by Sue Goldie (London: Dawsons for the International Council of Nurses, 1962), pp. 92–96.

21. This section is adapted from Charles E. Rosenberg, "Florence Nightingale on Contagion: The Hospital as Moral Universe." In: *Healing and History, Essays for George*

Rosen, ed. Charles E. Rosenberg (New York and London: Science History Publications and Dawson, 1979), pp. 116–36. The most recent biography of Nightingale is unrelentingly revisionist in tone: F.B. Smith, *Florence Nightingale. Reputation and Power* (London & Canberra: Croom Helm, c. 1982).

22. Although the relevant publications of Pasteur and Lister date from the 1860s, the germ theory of infectious disease did not become a central question in the medical world until the 1870s and, as we shall see, was not generally understood and accepted until the 1880s and 1890s.

23. For the best study of Farr, see John M. Eyler, *Victorian Social Medicine. The Ideas and Methods of William Farr* (Baltimore and London: The Johns Hopkins University Press, c. 1979), esp. chap. 5, "The Zymotic Theory and Farr's Studies of Epidemic Disease," pp. 97–122. Contemporaries associated the fermentation idea with the prestige and publications of the German chemist Justus von Liebig, but the notion was far older.

24. *Notes on Nursing: What it is, and What it is Not* (New York: D. Appleton, 1861), p. 25n., for citation; see also 17n., 26–27.

25. Florence Nightingale, *Notes on Hospitals,* third ed, enlarged (London: Longman, Green, Longman, Roberts and Green, 1863), p. 22.

26. At this time, it was still assumed that the ward nurse would sleep in proximity to his or her patients. Nightingale's concern both with the hospital's ventilation specifically and with the allocation of space more generally is entirely consistent with this interpretation of her moral and medical views.

27. *Notes on Hospitals,* pp. 49, 52, 114.

28. Medicine, as she put it, ". . . is the surgery of functions, as surgery proper is that of limbs and organs." Nightingale, *Notes on Nursing,* p. 133, and for parallel arguments, pp. 74, 131.

29. It need hardly be noted that this point of view magnified the nurse's role, while necessarily deemphasizing that played by the physician.

30. Henry G. Clark, *Outlines of a Plan for a Free City Hospital* (Boston: George C. Rand & Avery, 1860), p. 11.

31. Harold N. Cooledge, "Samuel Sloan and the Philadelphia School of Hospital Design, 1850–1880," *The Charette,* June, 1964, pp. 6–7, 18. The most important model for self-conscious hospital designers in the late 1850s was the Lariboisiere in Paris. Both Henry G. Clark (cf. n. 30 above), for example, and the designers of Philadelphia's Episcopal Hospital referred to it specifically. *AR,* 1860, 28ff.

32. The Confederacy's Chimborazo Hospital in Richmond accommodated some seven thousand patients in an accumulation of detached barrack-wards. Thompson and Goldin, *The Hospital,* p. 170. Some of the larger Northern hospitals built in a true corridor-connected pavilion plan held as many as three thousand patients. George W. Adams, *Doctors in Blue. The Medical History of the Union Army in the Civil War* (New York: Henry Schuman, c. 1952), pp. 149–73; H.H. Cunningham, *Doctors in Gray. The Confederate Medical Service* (Baton Rouge: Louisiana State University Press, c. 1958), pp. 45–98. Most contemporary authorities were, of course, convinced believers in the atmospheric origins of hospital infection, and the military hospitals were designed in conscious accordance with these teachings. For examples of such consensus, see: John Ordronaux, *Hints on Health in Armies, for the Use of Volunteer Officers,* 2nd ed. (New York: D. Van Nostrand, 1863), pp. 106–11; William A. Hammond, ed., *Military Medical and Surgical Essays prepared for the United States Sanitary Commission* (Philadelphia: J.B. Lippincott, 1864); Charles A. Lee, *Hospital Construction, with Notices of Foreign Military Hospitals* (Albany: C. Van Benthuysen, 1863). Lee, for example, concluded that ". . . PAVILION HOSPITALS are the only ones suited for military purposes; . . ." p. 27.

33. [W.S. Edgar], "Editorial. Hospitals," *St. Louis Medical & Surgical Journal* 11 (1874): 567.

34. From remarks of Gulian C. Verplanck, In: New York State, Commissioners of Emigration, *An Account of the Proceedings of the Laying of the Corner-Stone of the State Emigrant Hospital, on Ward's Island* . . . (New York: John F. Trow, 1865), pp. 8–9.

35. The best documentation of such planning processes is that surrounding the new Johns Hopkins Hospital: Cf. Gert Brieger, "The Original Plans for the Johns Hopkins Hospital and Their Historical Significance," *BHM*, 39 (1965): 518–28; Johns Hopkins Hospital, *Hospital Plans. Five Essays relating to the Construction, Organization & Management of Hospitals, Contributed by their Authors for the Use of the Johns Hopkins Hospital of Baltimore* (New York: William Wood, 1875); *Review of "Hospital Plans" by John R. Niernsee, Architect, of the Johns Hopkins Hospital* (n.p., n.d. [Baltimore: Trustees of the Johns Hopkins Hospital, 1876]).

36. J. Foster Jenkins, *Tent Hospitals* (Cambridge, Mass.: The American Social Science Association, 1874), pp. 5–6.

37. See, for example, J. Matthews Duncan, *On the Mortality of Childbed and Maternity Hospitals* (New York: William Wood, 1871), pp. 108–9, 115. Following in the steps of Thomas McKeown and his emphasis on diet in the decrease of late nineteenth-century mortality rates, a revisionist scholar has recently contended that much of the improvement in surgical outcomes conventionally understood to be a consequence of antiseptic surgery was, in fact, a result of improved living conditions. David Hamilton, "The Nineteenth-Century Surgical Revolution—Antisepsis or Better Nutrition?," *BHM* 56(1982): 30–40.

38. J.S. Billings, *A Report on Barracks and Hospitals, with Descriptions of Military Posts.* Circular No. 4, War Department, Surgeon General's Office (Washington: Government Printing Office, 1870).

39. Ibid., p. vi. Because of the tendency of such organic contaminants to accumulate, Billings went so far as to urge that no civil hospital be a permanent stone structure. If half the money appropriated for such pretentious buildings were invested at 6 percent, he suggested, and a frame building of the same capacity built with the remainder, it could be pulled down after a dozen years and replaced with an entirely new and healthier structure paid for with the accumulated interest. P. xxii–xxiii.

40. J.S. Billings, *A Report on the Hygiene of the United States Army, with Descriptions of Military Posts.* Circular No. 8. War Department, Surgeon-General's Office (Washington: Government Printing Office, 1875).

41. Ibid., p. lvi. See the similar remarks by the prominent English physician Jonathan Hutchinson. In: Douglas Galton, *An Address on the General Principles Which Should Be Observed in the Construction of Hospitals. . . .With the Discussion Which Took Place Thereon* (London: MacMillan, 1869), pp. 62–63.

42. Billings, "Hospital Construction and Organization.", In: Johns Hopkins Hospital, *Hospital Plans*, p. 12.

43. Ibid., p. 13. Billings was not alone in employing this particular battlefield metaphor. See, for example, Thomas J. Maclaglan, *The Germ Theory Applied to the Explanation of the Phenomena of Disease. The Specific Fevers* (London: Macmillan & Co., 1876), pp. 9–10.

44. There were two distinct causes of hospital infection, as one Englishman casually expressed a widely held and serviceably eclectic position: "First, ill ventilation; second, multiplication of organizable germs, and consequent contagion." Charles Langstaff, *Hospital Hygiene. Being the Annual Address to the Southampton Medical Society* (London: J. and A. Churchill, 1872), pp. 12–13.

6. The Promise of Healing: Science in the Hospital

1. Green, *City Hospitals* (Boston: Little, Brown, 1861), p. 9.
2. W. Gill Wylie, *Hospitals: Their History, Organization, and Construction* (New York: D. Appleton, 1877), p. 35. An earlier report on the hospital had summarized contemporary teachings by concluding that all modern experience indicated that a hospital building should never consist of more than three stories and that two were preferable to three. New York Hospital, *The Financial Condition and Restricted Charitable Operations* . . . (New York: Wm. C. Bryant, 1866), p. 7.
3. Van Buren, "An Address Delivered on the Occasion of the Inauguration of the New Building of the New York Hospital, On the 16th of March, 1877," pp. 8–23. In: New York Hospital, *Report of the Building Committee* (New York: L.W. Lawrence, 1877), p. 20. Unlike many of his contemporaries, Van Buren emphasized the logical dependence of Lister's antiseptic method on Pasteur's more fundamental work. "Pasteur's demonstration that putrefaction is a fermentative process, that certain organic particles floating in the air as dust constitute the ferment or yeast, and that the destruction or exclusion of these germs will infallibly prevent septic change in substances prone to take on putrefaction, promises to alter many of the present methods of practical surgery." (Lister had just visited the United States to attend the International Medical Congress in Philadelphia the previous year.)
4. Before fastening on antisepsis, the hospital's attending staff had already urged that ". . . the preventable causes of mortality in Hospitals, . . . depend more upon a defective internal police, than upon the salubrity of location." Physicians and Surgeons to Governors, January 1870, Board of Governors Papers, New York Hospital Archives (hereafter NYHA). Van Buren was by no means the first to find in Lister's work a defense of the hospital. Cf. J. Matthews Duncan, *On the Mortality of Childbed and Maternity Hospitals* (New York: William Wood, 1871), p. 97.
5. The grasshopper image was described as an Italian turn-of-phrase. The editor did not intend to dismiss Lister's method out-of-hand, but saw it as only one among many tactics that could shape a hospital's incidence of infection. Although skeptical about the New York Hospital's new building, he conceded that it provided ". . . the opportunity to show what comparatively perfect ventilation can accomplish for patients, combined with cleanliness, excellent sanitary regulations, and the Lister method . . ." "New York Hospital," *Medical Record* 13 (February 9, 1878): 113.
6. This is not to say that some advocates had not always claimed special therapeutic advantages for the hospital. Benjamin Franklin promised that his planned Pennsylvania Hospital would have ". . . hot and cold baths, sweating rooms, chirurgic machines, bandages, etc., which can rarely be procured in the best private lodgings, . . ." Cited in William H. Williams, "The Pennsylvania Hospital, 1751–1801," (Ph.D. diss., Univ of Delaware, 1971), p. 72.
7. For general accounts, see Gert H. Brieger, "American Surgery and the Germ Theory of Disease," *Bulletin of the History of Medicine* (hereafter BHM) 40 (1966): 135–45; Owen H. and Sarah D. Wangensteen, *The Rise of Surgery. From Empiric Craft to Scientific Discipline* (Minneapolis: University of Minnesota Press, c. 1978).
8. For the most detailed treatment of anesthesia's introduction, see: Martin S. Pernick, *A Calculus of Suffering. Pain, Professionalism and Anaesthesia in Nineteenth-Century America* (New York: Columbia University Press, 1985).
9. Cf. *Rules and Regulations for the Government of the Jersey City Hospital* (Jersey City: Pangborn, Dunning & Dear, 1871), p. 20. The rules also called for the notification of all staff surgeons so that they might observe.

10. Abraham Jacobi, "Phases in the Development of Therapy," *Medical News* 87 (October 28, 1905): 824.

11. Society of the Alumni of City (Charity) Hospital, *Report for 1904 together with a History of the City Hospital . . .* (New York: Published by the Society, 1904), p. 85.

12. America did not have a group of practitioners formally trained and identified as "surgeons" as England did. By the time of the Civil War, however, a number of urban practitioners had become de facto surgical specialists, monopolizing teaching posts, hospital attending positions, and referrals in major surgery. Although general practitioners were anxious to treat their own patients in almost every kind of situation, the comparatively uncommon operable surgical problem promised more danger than profit. As ordinarily nonrecurring ailments, they provided a perfect occasion for calling upon the specialist's skills.

13. Cf. James Carmichael Smyth, *The Effect of the Nitrous Vapour, in Preventing and Destroying Contagion; Ascertained, from a Variety of Trials, Made Chiefly by Surgeons of His Majesty's Navy, in Prisons, Hospitals, and on Board of Ships; . . .* (Philadelphia: Thomas Dobson, 1799); S. Selwyn, "Sir John Pringle: Hospital Reformer, Moral Philosopher and Pioneer of Antisepsis," *Medical History* 10 (1966): 266–74.

14. An early advocate could, for example, list "ten articles to put us in readiness for work . . .": a spray producer, solution of carbolic acid, 1 to 20, another of 1 to 40, antiseptic gauze, rubberized cloth, oiled silk, rubber drainage tubes, antiseptic gauze, catgut ligatures, and carbolized waxed ligatures. And all this in a generation still accustomed to washing and reusing the natural sponges and gauze used in operations and dressings. Edwin M. Fuller, *Lister's Antiseptic Method, with Cases . . .* (Bath, Me.: E. Upton & Son, 1881), p. 8.

15. Letter of Rufus King Browne to the Editor, *American Medical Times* 6 (May 2, 1863): 215.

16. Thomas G. Morton and William Hunt, *Surgery in the Pennsylvania Hospital* (Philadelphia: J.B. Lippincott, 1880). Cf. Edward D. Churchill, ed., *To Work in the Vineyard of Surgery. The Reminiscences of J. Collins Warren (1842–1927)* (Cambridge: Harvard University Press, c. 1958), pp. 167–68. Some hospitals improved their statistics by refusing to allow their surgeons to operate in cases where there was a strong likelihood of subsequent infection. In 1874, for example, MGH trustees approved the renting of a private room outside the hospital for a prospective ovariotomy patient. "The Surgical Staff agree," the hospital's superintendent explained, "that the chances of saving the patient would be much greater if a room were obtained outside of the Hospital for her." P. 168n.

17. Charles R. Walker, *Surgical Cleanliness. Read Before the N.H. Medical Society, June, 1884* (Manchester, N.H.: John B. Clarke, 1884), p. 4. Lister was knighted the same year.

18. William Stewart Halsted, the Johns Hopkins surgeon, described an operation he performed during the winter of 1884–1885 ". . . in a large tent which I built on the grounds of Bellevue Hospital, having found it impossible to carry out antiseptic precautions in the general amphitheatre of Bellevue where the numerous anti-Lister surgeons dominated and predominated." *Surgical Papers* (Baltimore: Johns Hopkins University Press, 1924), I: 174.

19. See, for example: Arthur A. Bliss, *Blockley Days. Memories and Impressions of a Resident Physician 1883–1884* (Philadelphia: Privately Printed, 1916), pp. 21–22; Joseph C. Aub and Ruth K. Hapgood, *Pioneer in Modern Medicine. David Linn Edsall of Harvard* ([Boston]): Harvard Medical Alumni Association, 1970), p. 15; Guy Hinsdale, "Episcopal Hospital, 1881–83," Episcopal Hospital of Philadelphia Archives (hereafter EHA).

20. Carl Beck, *A Manual of the Modern Theory and Technique of Surgical Asepsis* (Philadelphia: W.B. Saunders, 1895), p. 16.

21. Committee of Conference, Surgical Staff to Trustees, undated memorandum, [May, 1886]; Thornton Lathrop (for Trustees) to J. Collins Warren, July 10, 1886, Visiting Staff Correspondence, Box 1, MGH. Papers, Countway Library (hereafter HCC).

22. M.H. Richardson to Dr. Eliot, March 29, 1888. MGHA.

23. See, for example, Henry B. Palmer, *Surgical Asepsis Especially Adapted to Operations in the Home of the Patient* (Philadelphia: F.A. Davis, 1903).

24. Frederick Shattuck, "Specialism in Medicine," *Journal of the American Medical Association* (hereafter *JAMA*) 35 (September 22, 1900): 724. Like many of his cautious contemporaries, Shattuck warned of the growing tendency to use the knife as a diagnostic tool.

25. In 1895–1896, for example, Chicago's Mercy Hospital treated 59 appendicitis cases (42 acute, 15 recurrent, and 2 of general peritonitis), 113 fractures, 28 hernias, and 45 carcinoma. And this was less than a decade after the first publication of appendectomy. Mercy Hospital, Annual Report (hereafter *AR*), 1895–6, 20–32.

26. Twenty percent were abdominal, with the exception of occasional ovariotomies, procedures essentially nonexistent before the last two decades of the century. Leo O'Hara, "An Emerging Profession: Philadelphia Medicine 1860–1900," Ph.D. diss., University of Pennsylvania, 1976, p. 198.

27. This story is well told in Fenwick Beekman, *Hospital for the Ruptured and Crippled. A Historical Sketch Written on the Occasion of the Seventy-Fifth Anniversary of the Hospital* (New York: Privately Printed, 1939), esp. pp. 13–65.

28. Like a number of other activist physicians of his generation, Knight as a young man had been a volunteer visitor for the New York Association for Improving the Condition of the Poor. Beekman, *Hospital,* p. 13; Knight, *Rules and Regulations of the New-York Surgeon's Bandage Institute* (New York: The Institute, 1842).

29. In his first year, Gibney performed 237 operations; previous to this there had been no more than 60 or 70 a year, all superficial. Twelve years later, in 1899, the figure had increased to 522 operations, only 12 percent relatively minor. Beekman, *Hospital,* pp. 46, 64–65.

30. A late-1920s survey found that 55 percent of hospital admissions were surgical, 15 percent obstetrical, and only 30 percent medical. W.C. Rappelye, "Survey of Medical Education," *JAMA* 88 (1927): 843. Michael M. Davis and C. Rufus Rorem, probably America's leading authorities on hospital economics, estimated in 1932 that surgical cases constituted 60 to 75 percent of admissions in "most of the smaller general hospitals, while in the more fully developed hospitals in the larger cities the proportion is about 50 per cent." *The Crisis in Hospital Finance and Other Studies in Hospital Economics* (Chicago: University of Chicago, 1932), p. 84.

31. S.S. Goldwater, "Planning for Private Patients," *Modern Hospital* 1 (1914): 11.

32. The connection between the rationale for Listerian antisepsis and the germ theory of infectious disease that seems so plausible in retrospect was by no means clear to contemporaries. The world of surgery with its unavoidable debates over the necessities of wound treatment was insulated from other areas of medicine; to presume a connection between wound infection and cholera, anthrax, or typhoid was to be an ardent, sophisticated, and convinced advocate of a theory that remained controversial for a generation.

33. For an extremely influential discussion, see: Owsei Temkin, "The Scientific Approach to Disease: Specific Entity and Individual Sickness." In: A.C. Crombie, ed., *Scientific Change* (New York: Basic Books, 1963), pp. 629–47, reprinted in Temkin, *The Double Face of Janus and Other Essays in the History of Medicine* (Baltimore: Johns Hopkins University Press, c. 1977), pp. 441–55.

34. The best balanced account of the Paris Clinical School is still to be found in

Erwin H. Ackerknecht, *Medicine at the Paris Hospital, 1794–1848* (Baltimore: Johns Hopkins University Press, 1967).

35. In using the phrase "experience of medical care," I imply the aggregate sum of doctor-patient interactions; morbidity patterns are obviously one major factor in determining that aggregate.

36. The "home" might have been the physician's, for most offices were still in the physician's residence.

37. We need a careful study of the hospital record as genre. But it is clear even from an impressionistic reading of late nineteenth- and early twentieth-century records, that an increase in uniformity (often connected with the use of printed forms for cases and laboratory reports) is associated with a decrease in personal impressionistic content. In 1884, for example, a Pennsylvania Hospital house officer described a patient as "worn to a shadow." A month later, he noted that "a light breeze would blow him out of the window. Looks as if he had been passed through a patent clothes-wringer." Some days later, the record concluded: "All that was left of John went to Heaven this day." Case of John Ayres, Case #1014, vol. 29, PHA. Two decades later such personal comments had become far less common. For a recent discussion of the case record, see: Stanley J. Reiser, "Creating Form Out of Mass: The Development of the Medical Record." In: Everett Mendelsohn, ed., *Transformation and Tradition in the Sciences. Essays in Honor of I. Bernard Cohen* (Cambridge, London, New York: Cambridge University Press, 1984), pp. 303–16.

38. Roosevelt Hospital, *AR,* 1878, 18; *AR,* 1882, 22. In the latter year, however, three patients were admitted with "senility." p. 26.

39. S. Weir Mitchell, *The Early History of Instrumental Precision in Medicine. An Address before the Second Congress of American Physicians and Surgeons* (New Haven: Tuttle, Morehouse & Taylor, 1892).

40. This change had taken place gradually during the middle third of the century. At the Cincinnati General Hospital, for example, auscultation and percussion seem not to have been used at all in the late 1830s, while they had become routine in 1865–1866. This observation is based on a comparison of the "Female Medical" ledgers for 1837–1840 and 1865–1866, CGHA. Other hospitals showed different patterns; at MGH, for example, house staff employed auscultation and percussion earlier.

41. For a useful inventory of midcentury observations linking pathology and "animal chemistry," see: J. Franz Simon, *Animal Chemistry with Reference to the Physiology and Pathology of Man*, trans. and ed. by George E. Day (Philadelphia: Lea and Blanchard, 1846).

42. Benjamin Silliman, Jr., *A Century of Medicine and Chemistry. A Lecture Introductory . . . to the Medical Class in Yale College* (New Haven: Charles C. Chatfield, 1871), p. 65.

43. "Account of Observations made under the Superintendence of Dr. Bright, on Patients whose Urine was Albuminous: By George H. Barrow, . . . with a Chemical Examination of the Blood and Secretions by G.O. Rees," *Guy's Hospital Reports.* Second Series. No. 1., April 1843, pp. 189–316. For a study emphasizing the therapeutic context of such work, see: Steven J. Peitzman, "Bright's Disease and Bright's Generation—Toward Exact Medicine at Guy's Hospital," *BHM* 55 (1981): 307–21.

44. I have used the term "scholarship" rather than "research," advisedly. "Research" conjures up patterns of systematic clinical or laboratory investigation that are misleading and anachronistic.

45. Stacy Collins and Gurdon Buck to Board of Governors, February 6, 1855, NYHA. Four years later, another promising young man resigned his curatorship, explaining that it ". . . requires more time than my general professional engage-

ments will permit." C.R. Agnew to Gentlemen of the Cabinet Committee, March 26, 1859, Board of Governors Papers, NYHA.

46. As early as 1859, the editor of Philadelphia's *Medical and Surgical Reporter* called for the appointment of a pathologist in every hospital. By 1880, six of the city's hospitals had pathologist members on their medical boards. O'Hara, "Emerging Profession," p. 192.

47. Entry for November 11, 1870, Board of Managers Minutes, PHA. Like the microscopist and pathologist already on the hospital's table of organization, the pathological chemist was to examine materials from both wards and autopsies, thus gradually adding clinical pathology to a more traditional postmortem pathology.

48. "Recent discoveries in Medical Science," as Pennsylvania Hospital staff members contended in 1849, "have clearly indicated the great utility of microscopic and chemical examinations of the different structures and fluids of the human body—both in a healthy and diseased condition . . ." William Pepper et al. to Board of Managers, May 23 1849, Box 155, Medical Staff Papers, PHA. A half century later, the University of Pennsylvania's first clinical laboratory was to be named after Pepper.

49. "Medical Progress," *Medical Record* 6 (September 1, 1871): 303.

50. James Tyson, Report of the Microscopist, Philadelphia, Guardians of the Poor, *AR,* 1868, 96.

51. Cf. Edward T. Morman, "Clinical Pathology in America, 1865–1915: Philadelphia as a Test Case," *BHM* 58(1984): 198–214.

52. Executive Committee Minutes, January 26, 1903, Board of Governors, NYHA. Despite efforts to categorically distinguish clinical from "dead-house" pathology, the two tended in practice to be so "intermingled," in the words of one hospital superintendent, "that it is difficult to assign any definite space to the different branches." Daniel Test to Renwick Ross, November 20, 1908, Superintendent's Letterbooks, PHA. The "province" of Boston City Hospital's clinical pathologist included "urine, faeces, stomach, blood and sputum . . ." Meeting of Surgical Section, January 22, 1908, Records of Surgical Staff, 1906–17, Boston City Hospital (hereafter BCH).

53. The Pennsylvania Hospital, for example, had been fortunate to receive an endowment to establish a clinical laboratory; it paid for the salaries of a director and his assistant, but did not cover the $2,500–3,000 it cost to operate the laboratory each year. This was, as the superintendent put it in 1908, ". . . a tax on the already insufficient funds of the Hospital." Daniel Test to Stacy B. Collins, June 3, 1908, Superintendent's Letterbooks, PHA.

54. "Report of Microscopical Department," Cincinnati General Hospital, *AR,* 1888, 89–90.

55. It is safe to generalize that laymen were increasingly impressed with scientific credentials in this period. The *content* of that science was, of course, problematic and certainly varied in terms of class and region. This was precisely the period during which osteopathy grew with enormous rapidity, frequently boasting the support of influential state legislators. It is equally significant, however, that the fledgling medical sect soon adopted the institutional forms and educational requirements of regular medicine. Cf. Norman Gevitz, *The D.O.'s. Osteopathic Medicine in America* (Baltimore and London: The Johns Hopkins University Press, 1982).

56. And quinine and digitalis were more likely to be used in appropriate clinical situations. Aspirin was probably the most important and widely-used drug introduced during the second half of the nineteenth century.

57. Cf. Joel D. Howell, "Early Use of X-ray Machines and Electrocardiographs at the Pennsylvania Hospital. 1897 through 1927," *JAMA* 255 (May 2, 1986): 2320–23.

58. Lionel Smith Beale, *The Medical Student as a Student in Science. The Introductory Lecture Delivered at the Opening of the Twenty-Fourth Session of the Medical Department of King's College* (London: John Churchill, 1855), pp. 29, 12.

59. Stephen Smith, *Doctor in Medicine: And other Papers on Professional Subjects* (New York: William Wood, 1872), pp. 130–32.

60. Paraphrased from Jeffreys Wyman to S.W. Mitchell, February 22, 1863, Mitchell Papers, Trent Collection, Duke University. Cf. also C.E. Brown-Séquard to S.W. Mitchell, February 7, 1862. An internationally known physiologist, Brown-Séquard complained that his London practice was so extensive he had hardly time to breathe. "I hope, however, to be soon able to give up a part of this practice and devote one-half of my time to science." Mitchell himself had done work in experimental physiology and pharmacology, but failing to find an appropriate teaching position turned to clinical specialism—becoming a founder of neurology in America. "I have missed you in the field of letters recently," Oliver Wendell Holmes wrote to Mitchell in 1872, "I suppose because you are working in the mine of practice for I have heard that you have become a great doctor." Holmes to Mitchell, April 16, 1872, Mitchell Papers, Trent Collection, Duke University.

61. William Osler, "Letters to My House Physicians. Letter V," *New York Medical Journal* 52 (September 20, 1890): 334.

62. S. Weir Mitchell, *Annual Address before the Medico-Chirurgical Faculty of Maryland* (Baltimore: Innes & Co, 1877), p. 17. Although an ardent spokesman for science, Mitchell was a realist, convinced by his own experience that science was not in itself a viable career for an American physician. "I dare now to counsel any young and able man," he added, "that to spend a few years in such work is not only to give himself the best of intellectual training, but is also one of the best means of advancing himself and fortifying his position when by degrees he becomes absorbed in clinical pursuits and daily practice. . . ."

63. Roberts Bartholow, *The Present State of Therapeutics: A Lecture Introductory to the Fifty-Sixth Annual Course in Jefferson Medical College* (Philadelphia: J.B. Lippincott, 1879), p. 20.

64. "Some of the Uses of Hospitals," *Philadelphia Medical Times* 4 (February 7, 1874): 298–99.

65. "The Uses of Hospitals," *Philadelphia Medical Times* 4 (April 18, 1874): 458.

66. See, for example, John S. Billings, "Hospital Construction and Organization." In: Johns Hopkins Hospital, *Hospital Plans. Five Essays Relating to the Construction & Management of Hospitals, Contributed by their Authors for the Use of the Johns Hopkins Hospital of Baltimore* (New York: William Wood, 1875), p. 5.

67. Morris C. Ernst, *Some Fermentations in Medical Education. The Annual Address Delivered before the Massachusetts Medical Society, June 8, 1904* (Boston: The Society, [1904]), p. 24.

68. J.S. Billings. In: *Opening Exercises of the Institute of Hygiene of the University of Pennsylvania* (Philadelphia: [The University of Pennsylvania], 1892), p. 28; Henry M. Hurd, "Laboratories and Hospital Work," *Bulletin of the American Academy of Medicine* 2 (1895–6): 493.

69. New Orleans' Charity Hospital promised in 1901 that greater aid to its laboratories would "redound to the pride of our Southern country. Investigation upon abstruse medical subjects, out of which can be evolved great human blessings, . . . would be comfortingly assured." *AR*, 1901, 32.

70. "Scientific Use of Hospitals," *JAMA* (February 23, 1901): 510. For an example of the interaction between medical reform and disciplinary strategies, see Robert E. Kohler, *From Medical Chemistry to Biochemistry. The Making of a Biomedical Discipline* (Cambridge, London, New York: Cambridge University Press, 1982).

71. Presbyterian Hospital (New York), *AR*, 1907, 17.
72. Putnam to F.A. Washburn, June 6, 1911, MGH Papers, Box 12, HCC.

7. A Marriage of Convenience: Hospitals and Medical Careers

1. Blake to Dear Pater, April 2, 1866, February 8, 1866, Blake Papers, Countway Library (hereafter HCC).
2. See, for example, Blake to Dear Pater and Mater, February 8, 1866; Blake to Dear Pater, June 8, 1869. He was aware that an immediate public declaration of exclusive devotion to special practice would be foolhardy; it is clear, however, that Blake planned ultimately to practice an "exclusive specialism." Blake to Dear Pater and Mater, April 11, 1869.
3. Blake to Dear Mater, May 13, 1866; the details on the hospital are drawn from Blake to Dear Pater, October 24, 1865; Cf. also June 19, 1866. He was particularly impressed with the numbers of autopsies, nine or even more each evening. Blake to Dear Pater and Mater, October 10, 1865.
4. Blake to Dear Pater, March 9, 1866.
5. "With regard to nervous diseases," he agreed, "they indeed seem to be rapidly on the increase in the States; they are a most interesting study and from the field for discovery they present, and as a majority rule the class of patients in which they are more generally found, offer the inducements of a name and a goodly living to the practitioner who particularly studies them." Blake to Dear Pater and Mater, February 8, 1866.
6. The phrases are from Blake to Dear Pater and Mater, April 11, 1869 and Blake to Dear Pater, May 19, 1869.
7. Blake to Dear Pater, March 19, 1866; Cf. also Blake to Pater, March 9, 1866.
8. Blake to Dear Mater and Pater, May 4, 1869.
9. Blake to Dear Pater, June 8, 1869. In the same letter, Blake regretted not having published more in American journals, a failing he obviously hoped to remedy.
10. Cf. Charles Snyder, *Massachusetts Eye and Ear Infirmary. Studies on Its History* (Boston: The Hospital, c. 1984). The key actors in this group were associated, among other activities, in an eating club, the members of which were to play an extraordinarily important role in Boston medicine. Henry A. Christian, "Kappa Pi Eta Dinner Club 1871–1946." In George C. Shattuck, *Frederick Cheever Shattuck, M.D. 1847–1929. A Memoir* ([Boston]; Privately Printed, 1967).
11. Blake to Dear Pater, November 9, 1865. He is explaining to his father that he no longer plans to use available family funds for travel and sightseeing.
12. The classic formulation of the factors relevant to the development of special practice is to be found in George Rosen, *The Specialization of Medicine with Particular Reference to Ophthalmology* (New York: Froben Press, 1944); the past century is covered in far greater detail by Rosemary Stevens, *American Medicine and the Public Interest* (New Haven and London: Yale University Press, 1971).
13. For a recent synthesis of a growing literature, see Ivan Waddington, *The Medical Profession in the Industrial Revolution* (Dublin: Gill and Macmillan, c. 1984), pp. 1–49; Irvine Loudon, *Medical Care and the General Practitioner, 1750–1850* (Oxford: Oxford University Press, 1986); for the situation in France, see Matthew Ramsey, *Professional and Popular Medicine in France, 1770–1830* (Cambridge: Cambridge University Press, 1987).
14. As we have seen, attending responsibilities were rotated among two or three senior practitioners, so that each would be on duty only three, four, or six months at a time. Thus, the status and duties could be shared more widely among a community's elite practitioners.

15. William H. Williams, *America's First Hospital: The Pennsylvania Hospital, 1751–1841* (Wayne, Pa.: Haverford House, 1976), p. 131.

16. Here and elsewhere, I have used male pronouns or referred to "men." This is meant to reflect, not endorse, nineteenth-century practice. Women were, of course, excluded from the regular medical profession in this period, and all such consultants were male, although there had been some early attempts to teach midwifery to females, most notably by Valentine Seaman in New York. Cf. Valentine Seaman, *The Midwives Monitor, and Mother's Mirror: Being Three Concluding Lectures of a Course of Instruction on Midwifery* (New York: Isaac Collins, 1800).

17. Cf. Erwin H. Ackerknecht, *Medicine at the Paris Hospital. 1794–1848* (Baltimore: Johns Hopkins, 1967), esp. pp. 163–82; Hans-Heinz Eulner, *Die Entwicklung der medizinischen Spezialfacher an den Universitaten des deutschen Sprachgebietes* (Stuttgart: Ferdinand Enke, 1970). Ophthalmology and orthopedics had even earlier roots in practice.

18. The best study is still Thomas N. Bonner's *American Doctors and German Universities. A Chapter in International Intellectual Relations 1870–1914* (Lincoln: University of Nebraska Press, 1963).

19. Howard Kelly, "Letter from Bremen," *Pittsburgh Medical Review,* cited in Audrey W. Davis, *Dr. Kelly of Hopkins. Surgeon, Scientist, Christian* (Baltimore: Johns Hopkins University Press, 1959), pp. 58–59.

20. Charles Newman, "The Rise of Specialism and Postgraduate Education," in F.N.L. Poynter, ed., *The Evolution of Medical Education in Britain* (London: Pitman, 1966), p. 172.

21. Such conflict is emphasized in Brian Abel-Smith's still standard history of English hospitals: *The Hospitals. 1800–1948. A Study in Social Administration in England and Wales* (Cambridge: Harvard University Press, 1964); Cf. also Lindsay Granshaw's exemplary study: *St. Mark's Hospital, London. A Social History of a Specialist Hospital* (London: King Edward's Hospital Fund, 1985).

22. John Watson, a prominent attending at the New York Hospital, referred in 1858 to ". . . those special hospitals which almost all grow out of the enthusiasm, the caprice, or the industrial enterprise of private individuals, who, to carry out their own views, enlist the sympathy or cooperation of the public . . ." New York Hospital, *Report of the Committee of Governors . . . on Extending the Usefulness of the Hospital* (New York: Baker & Godwin, 1858), p. 9.

23. When, for example, the Worcester, Massachusetts, Memorial Hospital opened in 1888, its dispensary included hours for orthopedic, eye and ear, gynecological, skin, and nose and throat, as well as general medicine and surgery. Annual Report (hereafter *AR*), 1888–1890, 3. Those outpatient dispensaries unconnected with general hospitals, were quick to reorganize their clinics according to specialty. Cf. Charles E. Rosenberg, "Social Class and Medical Care in Nineteenth-Century America: The Rise and Fall of the Dispensary," *Journal of the History of Medicine* 29 (1974): 37, 41.

24. Surgery and medicine were in fact to remain the highest status fields at America's most prestigious hospitals and medical schools. Highest-ranking medical school graduates usually sought medical and surgical house officerships; the specialties had ordinarily to be content with those who had been somewhat less successful as undergraduates.

25. Cf. entry for May 31, 1878, Minutes, Medical Board, EHA.

26. Statement of Resident Physician, Northern Dispensary, Philadelphia, *AR,* 1880, 13–14.

27. Frederick Shattuck, "Specialism in Medicine," *JAMA* 35 (September 22, 1900): 725–26. Such sentiments did not necessarily describe contemporary reality at the level of everyday practice; many general practitioners, even attending surgeons and physicians in hospitals, undertook procedures for which they were ill

equipped even by contemporary standards. To refer a patient was to lose a fee—and possibly the patient's confidence as well.

28. It must be emphasized that opposition remained, and individual specialists and specialties had to keep advancing their case in new contexts. In 1905, for example, the Johns Hopkins Medical Board tabled the suggestion that beds in their new surgical building be alloted to their eye and ear, throat, and skin specialists (Minutes, February 6, 1905, Medical Board, Johns Hopkins Hospital [hereafter JHH]). Harvard did not establish a pediatrics service until 1910, to cite another example, despite repeated earlier requests. Cf. Frederic A. Washburn, *The Massachusetts General Hospital. Its Development, 1900–1935* (Boston: Houghton, Mifflin Co., 1939), pp. 336–38. Washburn's study includes much valuable material relating to the gradual acceptance of the specialties at MGH.

29. Entry for March 8, 1910, Minutes, Board of Trustees, JHH. As early as 1887, the United States Bureau of Pensions had required that the ophthalmoscope and "auroscope" be used in disability examinations. U.S. Department of the Interior, Bureau of Pensions, *Instructions to Examining Surgeons . . .* (Washington: Government Printing Office, 1887), p. 11.

30. Beatrice Fox Griffith, *Pennsylvania Doctor* (Harrisburg, Pa.: The Stackpole Co., 1957), pp. 66–67. "I have introduced several new things in the treatment of ophthalmia, and as soon as my 100 cases are complete will publish my results. . . . My greatest aim is to become a thorough man with the ophthalmoscope."

31. Charles E. Rosenberg, "Doctors and Credentials—The Roots of Uncertainty," *Transactions and Studies. College of Physicians of Philadelphia* ser. v. 6 (1984):295–302.

32. James Jackson Putnam to Trustees, August 8, 1912, Box 12, MGH Papers Countway Library HCC. In this period it was also assumed that young men would not and could not marry while they served as House officers. Some institutions made married men explicitly ineligible for house staff positions. Entry for April 17, 1901, Minutes, Medical Board, Presbyterian Hospital of New York Archives (hereafter PNY), H. Hurd to R.R. Ross, October 28, 1890, Hurd Letterbooks, JHH.

33. Middleton Goldsmith to Lewis Sayre, April 2, 1870. In Virginia Kneeland Frantz, "Middleton Goldsmith . . . 1818–1887," *Academy Bookman* 7 (1954): 12–13.

34. In the period 1880–1910, especially, when wealthy private patients were still unwilling to enter hospitals, a young associate's services remained extremely valuable. He could stay at a patient's home overnight and supervise nurses, or pay routine calls, thus freeing his patron to visit other clients. In a period before formal research support, hospital-centered relationships could function in the same symbiotic way. For a particularly revealing example of such patronage see the relationship between Howard A. Kelly and Thomas S. Cullen at the Johns Hopkins Hospital. Cullen served as Kelly's research assistant and clinical stand-in, while Kelly worked systematically to find a place for Cullen on the hospital staff. Kelly File, Cullen Papers, JHH.

35. ". . . universally so," he continued, "except in the case of the Philadelphia Hospital, where an examination is held, whose results, although they do not absolutely decide in all cases, influence very greatly, the decision." "The Appointment of Resident Physicians in our Hospitals," *Philadelphia Medical Times* 3 (August 2, 1873): 697.

36. [James] to Alice James, Cambridge, December 12, 1866, Ralph B. Perry, *The Thought and Character of William James* (Boston: Little, Brown, 1935), I:231.

37. Guy Hinsdale, "Episcopal Hospital. 1881–1883," EHA; Ella M. E. Flick, *Beloved Crusader Lawrence F. Flick. Physician* (Philadelphia: Dorrance, 1944), pp. 66, 69, 111.

Flick, who was a Catholic, could not well have expected appointment at any of the city's Protestant hospitals.

38. Daniel Test to G.H.R. Ross, February 25, 1910, Superintendent's Letterbooks, PHA. Applicants routinely served as "vacation substitutes" and thus became acquainted with the attending staff; this, Test explained, was one reason non-Philadelphians would have a difficult time competing. Test to P.C. Jeans, January 30, 1909, Superintendent's Letterbook, PHA. In 1905, the Hahnemann Hospital staff urged that the college dean be requested to reassure students that "merit alone and not 'pull,' is the factor in selecting residents." Medical Staff Minutes, May 13, 1905, Hahnemann Hospital Archives, Philadelphia.

39. George C. Wilkins to Edward Taylor, [June 25, 1901], Long Island Hospital Letterbook, HCC. See also for similar instances, A.N. Collins to E.A. Lock, February 11, 1907, Charles Mahoney to E.W. Taylor, December 18, 1910.

40. It might be argued that these practitioners all used specialization as a mechanism to bypass the normal professional hierarchy—a tactic apparent to those who regarded such men as interlopers.

41. Cf. Mary Roth Walsh, "Doctors Wanted: No Women Need Apply." Sexual Barriers in the Medical Profession, 1835–1975 (New Haven and London: Yale University Press, 1977); Virginia Drachman, Hospital with a Heart. Women Doctors and the Paradox of Separatism at the New England Hospital 1862–1969 (Ithaca and London: Cornell University Press, 1984); Regina Markell Morantz-Sanchez, Sympathy and Science. Women Physicians in American Medicine (New York: Oxford University Press, 1985).

42. Vanessa N. Gamble, "The Negro Hospital Renaissance: The Black Hospital Movement, 1920–1940," (Ph.D. diss., University of Pennsylvania, 1987).

43. For relevant case studies, see: Gail Farr Casterline, "St. Joseph's and St. Mary's: The Origins of Catholic Hospitals in Philadelphia," Pennsylvania Magazine History & Biography 108 (1984): 289–314; Leo O'Hara, "An Emerging Profession: Philadelphia Medicine 1860–1900," (Ph.D. diss., University of Pennsylvania, 1976); Morris Vogel, The Invention of the Modern Hospital, Boston 1870–1930 (Chicago: University of Chicago Press, 1980).

44. Cf. Thomas L. Bradford, History of the Homeopathic Medical College of Pennsylvania; the Hahnemann Medical College and Hospital of Philadelphia (Philadelphia: Boericke & Tafel, 1898); William H. King, History of Homeopathy and its Institutions in America, 4 vols. (New York and Chicago: The Lewis Co., 1905); Frederick M. Dearborn, The Metropolitan Hospital (New York: Privately Printed, 1937).

45. J.S. Lockhart, "Life Tenure on Hospital Boards," Medical Record 45 (January 27, 1894): 123. Such resentments had a basis in reality. For a study of the domination of the New York hospital attending system by a relatively small group of multiple place-holders, see, Charles E. Rosenberg, "The Practice of Medicine in New York a Century Ago," Bulletin of the History of Medicine (hereafter BHM) 41 (1967): 223–53.

46. In an era when most specialists were also family practitioners, it was natural that ordinary physicians might fear consultants as potential competitors. But even with increasing "exclusive" specialism at the beginning of the twentieth century, general practitioners might still be unwilling to refer patients and thus be deprived of even one or two fees. Similarly, general surgeons might be unwilling to refer patients to better qualified subspecialists.

47. Late nineteenth-century attitudes toward dependence supported and legitimated such fears; the need for "scientific" control of welfare expenditures generally was widely accepted among thoughtful Americans. Even those genuinely unable to pay might well be pauperized as a by-product of gratuitous hospital or dispensary care.

48. This bit of doggerel was entitled "The Song of the Absentees," italics as in original, *BM&SJ* n.s. 110 (January 10, 1884): 44.

49. Entry for April 2, 1886, Hospital Committee Minutes, Board of Guardians of the Poor, Philadelphia City Archives (hereafter PCA). The problem was an old one. As early as 1863, the same hospital had sought to deal with it by requiring that one old and one new resident physician be paired in each ward. April 10, 1863.

50. The Cincinnati General Hospital, for example, had begun this policy as early as 1883; the resident physician was responsible for admissions, and the position seems to have developed out of this functional necessity. By 1895, the number of interns had doubled, from six to twelve, and their term increased from a year to eighteen months. *AR,* 1883, 5; *AR,* 1895, 7.

51. Richard H. Shryock, *The Unique Influence of the Johns Hopkins University on American Medicine* (Copenhagen: Ejnar Munksgaard, 1953).

52. Entry for May 14, 1900, Minutes, Medical Board, PNY; Entry for January 22, 1908, Meeting of the Surgical Section, Records of the Surgical Staff, 1906–17, Boston City Hospital (hereafter BCH).

53. In an effort to attract staff radiologists, hospitals would sometimes allow them to use institutional facilities for an outside consulting practice. Fees would typically be shared between hospital and practitioner. For background see, E.R.N. Grigg, *The Trail of the Invisible Light . . .* (Springfield, Ill.: Charles C. Thomas, 1965).

54. New York Committee on the Study of Hospital Internships and Residencies, *Internships and Residencies in New York City, 1934–1937. Their Place in Medical Education* (New York: Commonwealth Fund, 1938), pp. 26–45, provides a useful if brief summary history.

55. Entry for April 1, 1890, Minutes, Executive Committee, Board of Trustees, JHH.

56. Arpad Gerster, "The System of Medical Service in Hospitals," *Medical Record* 45 (January 27, 1894): 124.

57. Meanwhile hospitals began to raise their standards, increasingly requiring examinations and outstanding class ranking for appointment to internships. By 1904, New York's Charity Hospital could boast that ninety men from every section of the country had competed for twelve positions. The examination included oral and practical as well as written sections, and extra credits were assigned to those applicants who had earned a college degree before medical school. City (Charity) Hospital, *Report for 1904,* pp. 100–101.

58. Simon Flexner to L. Barker, March 24, 1905, Barker Papers, JHH. The second phrase is from a letter written by Frank Billings, attempting to lure Barker to the University of Chicago, March 25, 1900. The word movement is used—among many other places—in Flexner to Barker, February 27, 1900, Barker Papers. Cf. *Time and the Physician. The Autobiography of Lewellys F. Barker* (New York: Putnam's, 1942).

59. L. Barker, "On the Present Status of Therapy and its Future," *Bulletin of the Johns Hopkins Hospital* 11 (1900): 152.

60. Joseph D. Craig to L. Barker, January 23, 1903, Barker Papers, JHH.

61. William Councilman to L. Barker, October 21, 1901, Barker Papers, JHH. For further detail on Boston hospital intransigence, Cf. Vogel, *Invention of the Modern Hospital.* Councilman felt that Boston was particularly closed and conservative.

62. For background on this tendency and its consequences, see Robert E. Kohler, *From Medical Chemistry to Biochemistry. The Making of a Biomedical Discipline* (Cambridge, London, New York: Cambridge University Press, 1982).

63. For a correspondence illustrating this pattern, see P.K. Brown to Richard Cabot, December 29, 1901, February 18, 1902, July 30, 1902, March 10, 1904, January 3, 1906. Box 22, Richard Cabot Papers, Harvard University Archives.

Brown, who had an interest in clinical pathology, found it difficult to get access to beds. Physicians in his position could be and were easily exploited.

64. Thus the symbolic and substantive significance of Johns Hopkins Hospital trustees ignoring the resentment of Baltimore practitioners in the 1880s and selecting their original chiefs of service on the basis of academic "visibility." This was certainly a landmark in the history of American medicine, if rather less dramatic and celebrated than innovations with an immediate impact on therapeutics.

65. Christian to Reginald Fitz, January 30, 1912; Cf. also Christian to Francis Peabody, January 17, 1912, "Letters from Medical Staff," bd. vol. in Christian Papers, HCC.

66. R.H. Fitz to Christian, July 14, 1906, "Miscellaneous Letters," bd. vol. in Christian Papers.

67. Peabody to Christian, February 9, 1912, Christian Papers.

68. The role of bacteriology and immunology in preventive medicine obviously brings up different questions. But with the exception of treatment for rabies and diphtheria and serological diagnoses of several other infectious ills, the explicitly therapeutic capacities of internal medicine were quite limited.

69. Joseph H. Pratt, "The Method of Science in Clinical Training," BM&SJ. 166 (June 12, 1912): 840.

70. Ibid., 842.

8. The Ward as Classroom

1. Benjamin Franklin, Some Account of the Pennsylvania Hospital. Printed in Facsimile, with an Introduction by I. Bernard Cohen (Baltimore: Johns Hopkins University Press, 1954), p. 19.

2. Francis Home, Clinical Experiments, Histories, and Dissections . . . 3rd.ed. (London: J. Murray, 1783), p. vi.

3. The best account of this formative period can be found in Kenneth M. Ludmerer, Learning to Heal. The Development of American Medical Education (New York: Basic Books, 1985). Cf. also Edward C. Atwater, " 'Making Fewer Mistakes': A History of Students and Patients," Bulletin of the History of Medicine (hereafter BHM) 57(1983): 165–197; Kenneth M. Ludmerer, "The Plight of Clinical Teaching in America," Ibid., 218–29.

4. When the Massachusetts General Hospital wrote its first bylaws in 1821, for example, they specified that attendings should ". . . receive no pay or emolument, other than that derived from the power of admitting Students to see the practice of the Hospital." By-Laws of the Massachusetts General Hospital . . . (Boston: Charles Crocker, 1821), p. 21. The practice of rotating ward responsibility among attending physicians had implications for education as well as for medical care. It almost certainly allowed a larger number of students to have some clinical experience, if for shorter periods of time.

5. W.S. Middleton, "Clinical Teaching in the Philadelphia Almshouse and Hospital," Medical Life 40(1933): 207–55; Charles Lawrence, History of the Philadelphia Almshouses and Hospitals (Philadelphia: Privately Printed, 1905); Charles E. Rosenberg, "From Almshouse to Hospital: The Shaping of Philadelphia General Hospital," Milbank Memorial Fund Q. 60(1982): 141–42.

6. Cf. R.A. Kondratas, "Joseph Frank (1771–1842) and the Development of Clinical Medicine. A Study of the Transformation of Medical Thought and Practice at the End of the 18th and the Beginning of the 19th Centuries," (Ph.D. diss., Harvard University, 1977); Phillipe Pinel, The Clinical Training of Doctors. An Essay of 1793, ed. and trans. Dora B. Weiner (Baltimore and London: Johns Hopkins Uni-

versity Press, 1980); Toby Gelfand, " 'Invite the Philosopher, as Well as the Chari-table': Hospital Teaching as Private Enterprise in Hunterian London," in W.F. Bynum and Roy Porter, eds., *William Hunter and the Eighteenth-Century Medical World* (Cambridge: Cambridge University Press, 1985), pp. 129–51; Guenter Risse, *Hospital Life in Enlightenment Scotland. Care and Teaching at the Royal Infirmary of Edinburgh* (Cambridge, London, New York: Cambridge University Press, 1986); Susan C. Lawrence, "Science and Medicine at the London Hospitals: The Development of Teaching and Research, 1750–1815" (Ph.D. diss., University of Toronto, 1985).

7. Thomas Y. Simons, *An Introductory Lecture Delivered in the Medical College of South Carolina* (Charleston: T.A. Hayden, 1835), pp. 10–11.

8. Samuel Bard, *Two Discourses Dealing with Medical Education in Early New York* (New York: Columbia University Press, 1921), pp. 16, 19–20.

9. A hospital constituted the difference between a good and a bad education, a spokesman for the proposed Massachusetts General Hospital argued in 1819: "The medical school at Philadelphia is connected with the Hospital. Hence it is that it is so thronged with students. For the same reason it is that students in medicine, to whom expense forms no obstacle, cross the ocean to perfect their education at the Hospitals in London, Edinburgh, and Paris." Richard Sullivan, *Address Delivered before the Governour and Council, . . . and other Patrons of the Massachusetts General Hospital . . .* (Boston: Wells and Lilly, 1819), pp. 17–18.

10. *The Journal of William Tully, Medical Student at Dartmouth. 1808–1809,* ed. O.S. Hayward and E.H. Thomson (New York: Science History Publications, 1977), p. 48.

11. For an example of the enticing emphasis on the availability of hospital facilities, see: [S.L. Mitchill], *The Present State of Medical Learning in the City of New-York* (New York: T. and J. Swords, 1797), pp. 12–13.

12. The phrase is drawn from, "[Astley] Coopers Surgical Lectures delivered at St. Thomas's Hospital. . . . 1801," p. 1, Matthias Spalding Papers, Trent Collection, Duke University.

13. J.C. Warren to Daniel Parker, 13 May, 1824, "Administration: Care of Patients General Statements Concerning," MGHA; *Some Account of the Medical School in Boston, and of the Massachusetts General Hospital* (Boston: Phelps and Farnham, 1824), p. 9. They proudly reported having performed twenty-two major operations "during the short period of twenty-eight months" between the opening of the hospital in September of 1821 and February, 1824, pp. 9–10.

14. William S. Dillard to John J. Dillard, Elk-Mills, Amherst Co. Va., J.J. Dillard Letters, Perkins Library, Duke University.

15. In 1810, for example, Benjamin Rush, perhaps America's most prominent teacher of medicine, urged his son, then studying in London, to keep alert to any developments in surgery. "It will be necessary for you to practice it," he warned, "in order to assist you in getting into business. It will enable you moreover to keep your business when acquired. I have lost many families by declining it." Benjamin to James Rush, February 7, 1810, ed. Lyman Butterfield, *Letters of Benjamin Rush* (Princeton: Princeton University Press for the American Philosophical Society, 1951), II:1036.

16. J. Post, Diary, Entries for October 1, 5, 8, 1792, New York Historical Society (hereafter NYHS).

17. Samuel Rezneck, "A Course of Medical Education in New York City in 1828–29: The Journal of Asa Fitch," *BHM* 42 (1968): 560.

18. Harry Hammond to James H. Hammond, March 18, 1855, Hammond-Bryan-Cumming Papers, South Caroliniana Library, University of South Carolina, Columbia (hereafter SCC).

19. Rush was certainly reflecting his student experience in Edinburgh. Benjamin

Rush to Board of Managers, October 29, 1791, Box 155, Pennsylvania Hospital Archives (hereafter PHA).

20. In 1817, for example, the University of Pennsylvania again approached the Pennsylvania Hospital, asking that a formal arrangement be made to facilitate their students' clinical work. The university suggested that its clinical professor have one male and one female ward at his disposal, containing at least fifteen beds each. By way of compensation, every medical student registered would be required to pay a ten dollar fee to the hospital for every course of clinical lectures he might attend and no student be permitted to graduate without proof of attendance. Trustees of the University of Pennsylvania to Board of Managers, November 22, 1817, PHA. Despite this promised quid-pro-quo, the hospital was still unwilling to meet university requests. The 1840s saw another round of such suggestions. Entry for December 29, 1845, Minutes, Board of Managers, PHA.

21. Dale Smith, "The Emergence of Organized Clinical Instruction in the Nineteenth-Century American Cities of Boston, New York and Philadelphia" (Ph.D. diss., University of Minnesota, 1979), p. 162.

22. "The Free Dispensary of the New Orleans School of Medicine," *New Orleans Medical News & Hospital Gazette* 3(1856–1857):735–38; Jon M. Kingsdale, "The Growth of Hospitals: An Economic History in Baltimore" (Ph.D. diss., University of Michigan, 1981), p. 205 and *passim*. For the Charleston situation, I have consulted the Almshouse Committee Minutes, South Carolina Historical Society (hereafter SCHS); Minutes, South Carolina Medical Society, transcript, SCC; "Societies-Petitions Files," Legislative Papers, 1831–1859, S.C. State Archives, Columbia. The Richmond situation can be documented in the archives of the Medical College of Virginia Archives (hereafter MCV).

23. The best account of these developments is to be found in Dale Smith, "Emergence of Organized Clinical Instruction." The most comprehensive account of antebellum American medical education is still that by William F. Norwood, *Medical Education in the United States before the Civil War* (Philadelphia: University of Pennsylvania Press, 1944).

24. The variety of special clinical courses and tutorials was, however, enormous by mid-century. See, for example: "Some Account of the Schools of Medicine, Hospitals, Dispensaries, Private Lectures, and other Means of Imparting Medical Instruction in the City of Philadelphia," *Medical and Surgical Reporter* n.s. 3 (October 1, 1859): 9–22.

25. Report of Physicians and Surgeons of the New York Hospital, October 2, 1851, Papers, Board of Governors, NYHA; Statement of John Watson, October 25, 1858, in New York Hospital, *Report of the Committee of the Board of Governors Appointed to Inquire into . . . Extending the Usefulness of the Hospital . . .* (New York: Baker & Godwin, 1858), p. 10.

26. Professional rivalries were sometimes as important as lay intransigence in closing wards to students. N.S. Davis, *Address on Free Medical Schools, . . .* (Chicago, n.p., 1849), p. 9.

27. "Alumnus of the University of La.," dated New York, December 15, 1877, *New Orleans Medical & Surgical Journal* 5 (1878): 559.

28. Cf. A.H. Stevens et al., "Report of the Committee on Education," *Transactions, American Medical Association* (hereafter *TAMA*) 1 (1848): 245–46. The committee emphasized "that an adequate course of clinical instruction can only be obtained in hospitals . . ."

29. Remarks of Mary Putnam Jacobi as reported in "Medical News and Items," *Medical Record* 7(May 15, 1872): 215.

30. William Edgar, [Review of Johns Hopkins' "Five Essays on Hospital Plans"], *St. Louis Medical & Surgical Journal* 13(1876): 43.

31. Albert Gihon, "The Hospital: An Element and Exponent of Medical Education," *JAMA* 18 (March 26, 1892): 380.

32. Walter L. Carr, "How to Obtain Clinical Material without Impoverishing the Young Doctor," *Medical Record* 27(1885): 178–79.

33. "The Medical Colleges and the Hospital," *Cincinnati Gazette,* July 29, 1872, clipping in Commercial Hospital Scrapbook, Cincinnati General Hospital Archives (hereafter CGHA).

34. Three other board members were chosen from among the school's alumni, so that a majority of the board were medical men. *Philadelphia Medical Times* 4(January 11, 1874): 255; *Account of the Inauguration of the Hospital of the University of Pennsylvania* . . . (Philadelphia: Collins, 1874); George W. Corner, *Two Centuries of Medicine. A History of the School of Medicine, University of Pennsylvania* (Philadelphia and Montreal: J.B. Lippincott, 1965), pp. 133–73; Rosemary Stevens, "Sweet Charity: State Aid to Hospitals in Pennsylvania, 1870–1910," *BHM* 58(1984): 287–314; 474–95.

35. Edward L. Bauer, *Doctors Made in America* (Philadelphia and London: J.B. Lippincott, 1963), pp. 165–70; Thomas L. Bradford, *History of the Homeopathic Medical College of Pennsylvania* (Philadelphia: Boericke & Tafel, 1898), esp. pp. 421–88; Naomi Rogers, "The Proper Place of Homeopathy: Hahnemann Medical College and Hospital in an Age of Scientific Medicine," *Pennsylvania Magazine of History & Biography* 108(1984): 179–201.

36. R.M. Doolen, "The Founding of the University of Michigan Hospital: An Innovation in Medical Education," *Journal of Medical Education* 39(1964): 50–57. All of the large urban medical schools had, of course, sponsored free clinics and a few inpatient beds much earlier.

37. Whites were charged at a rate of six dollars a week in the ward, slaves and free Negroes, five dollars, and private rooms at seven to fifteen dollars. *Catalogue of Medical College of Virginia, 1859–60, and Announcement of 1860–61* (Richmond: Charles H. Wynne, 1860), advertisement on rear wrap.

38. Ibid., pp. 13, 14, 16, 18. On hospital facilities in nineteenth-century Virginia, see Wyndham Blanton, *Medicine in Virginia in the Nineteenth Century* (Richmond: Garrett & Massie, 1933), pp. 204–23. The James River was still navigable as far as Richmond, and hence the need for a marine hospital. These plans were given particular urgency by a growing Southern nationalism that resented the dominance of Philadelphia medicine in the education of youths from Virginia, the Carolinas, and Georgia.

39. Sanger Collection, Historical Files, MCV. Cf. "City Almshouse," "Memorial Hospital," and "Hospital Division-Misc." Files; UCM, Minutes of the Advisory Committee, June 28, 1904, MCV.

40. Entry for January 23, 1864, Faculty Record, University of Louisville, School of Medicine.

41. Albany Hospital, *Report . . . Two Years ending January 31st, 1880* (New York: Burdick & Taylor, 1880), pp. 7, 10, 13.

42. Cf. agreements dated February 12, 1879, March 31, 1892, and January 30, 1895 between the Charleston City Council and the Medical College of South Carolina, Filed Papers, RG 29, Charleston City Archives.

43. Kenneth M. Ludmerer, "The Plight of Clinical Teaching in America," *BHM* 57 (1983): 227. The two hospitals were Cleveland's Lakeside (associated with Western Reserve) and Hanover, New Hampshire's Mary Hitchcock (associated with Dartmouth).

44. Entry for January, 1897, Minutes, Board of Corporators, p. 146, Archives of Women in Medicine, Medical College of Pennsylvania (hereafter MCP).

45. Cf. the discussion by Edward Atwater, " 'Making Fewer Mistakes': A History of Students and Patients," *BHM* 57(1983): 172.

46. These conclusions are drawn from Thomas N. Bonner's *American Doctors and German Universities. A Chapter in International Intellectual Relations 1870–1914* (Lincoln: University of Nebraska Press, 1963).

47. The editor's comments were more optimistic than accurate. "The New Hospital and the Post-Graduate Medical School," *Medical Record* 25(January 19, 1884): 70. For a concise account of these institutions, see Steven Peitzman, " 'Thoroughly Practical': America's Polyclinic Medical Schools," *BHM* 54(1980): 166–87.

48. By 1908, the Dean of Philadelphia's Polyclinic Medical College and Hospital, one of the leading postgraduate schools, could provide three reasons for the decline of interest in postgraduate courses in general medicine. These were the improvement in clinical teaching in the better undergraduate schools, "the multiplication of hospitals and the growth of those already in existence, giving opportunities for many more graduates to obtain positions as hospital interns than formerly," and, finally, the growth of interest in specialization. Report of the Dean, Philadelphia Polyclinic, *AR*, 1908, 37. The majority of their matriculants registered for intensive short courses of a month or six weeks in the specialties. Annual Report (hereafter *AR*), 1906, 36.

49. Entry for December 3, 1889, Minutes of the Medical Board, Johns Hopkins Hospital (hereafter JHH).

50. Charles E. Rosenberg, "From Almshouse to Hospital: The Shaping of Philadelphia General Hospital," *Milbank Memorial Fund Q.* 60(1982): 142.

51. C. M. Ellinwood, "President's Annual Report of 1905," Cooper Medical College Records, Lane Library, Stanford University (hereafter SLA). This policy had been followed for at least a decade. Cf. Entry for February 20 1895, Minutes, Board of Managers, Lane Hospital, SLA. Local physicians often resented such policies. Cf. Carl B. Cone, "History of the State University of Iowa. The College of Medicine," Ms. Typescript, 1941, p. 66, 136–41, Special Collections, University of Iowa.

52. Entry for November 30, 1899, Minutes, Board of Managers, EHA.

53. With the general introduction of clinical clerkships, the line between teaching and care grew almost indistinguishable—and such traditional admonitions against "demonstrating" patients meant even less.

54. R. L. Wilbur to Dr. N. N. Wood, December 14, 1923, carbon, Box 56A, Los Angeles Co. Gen. Hosp. File, Wilbur Papers, SLA.

55. Harold C. Ernst, *Some Fermentations in Medical Education. The Annual Address Delivered before the Massachusetts Medical Society, June 8, 1904* (Boston: The Society, n.d., p. 22.

56. Ibid., p. 26. "They should use their hospital wards and clinics as the laboratory man uses his laboratory—as places of study, teaching and research," Ernst added, "in which the constant presence of the directing head shall serve as an inspiration to the students attracted thither."

57. Abraham Flexner, *Medical Education in the United States and Canada. A Report to the Carnegie Foundation for the Advancement of Teaching,* Bulletin Number Four (New York: The Foundation, 1910). The Flexner Report has spawned an abundant and often-polemical historical literature. Cf. for example, Howard S. Berliner, *A System of Scientific Medicine. Philanthropic Foundations in the Flexner Era* (New York and London: Tavistock, 1985); E. Richard Brown, *Rockefeller Medicine Men: Medicine and Capitalism in America* (Berkeley: University of California Press, 1979); Carleton B. Chapman, "The Flexner Report by Abraham Flexner," *Daedalus* 103 (1974): 105–17; Robert P. Hudson, "Abraham Flexner in Perspective: American Medical Education, 1865–1910," *BHM* 46(1972): 185–207; Saul Jarcho, "Medical Education in the U.S., 1910–1956," *Journal of Mt. Sinai Hospital* 26(1959): 339–85; Ludmerer, *Learning to Heal.*

58. The new model education also assumed more demanding admission standards, better laboratory facilities, and higher standards of performance—as well

as bedside training. As many contemporaries were aware, these reforms were both expensive and aimed at the creation of a small and intensely trained profession, in contrast to its large and loosely trained nineteenth-century predecessor. They sought to limit access to the medical school and thus the profession; what had been a plausible poor boy's option in midnineteenth century would become available only to the most able and motivated of the upwardly mobile in the twentieth.

59. Rosemary Stevens, "Graduate Medical Education: A Continuing History," *Journal of Medical Education* 53(1978): 6–7.

60. Kenneth M. Ludmerer, "The Rise of the Teaching Hospital in America," *Journal of the History of Medicine* 38(1983): 410.

61. Leo O'Hara, "An Emerging Profession: Philadelphia Medicine 1860–1900," (Ph.D. diss., University of Pennsylvania, 1976), pp. 154, 311.

62. Even at an elite school like Johns Hopkins, there was enormous conflict over the establishment of full-time clinical positions. Hopkins professors had served for years as prominent and well-paid consultants. Many of those who opposed full-time academic appointments were undoubtedly sincere in their fears that the academicization of their positions would widen the gap between practice and teaching, between bedside and laboratory. Cf. Alan M. Chesney, *The Johns Hopkins Hospital and the Johns Hopkins University School of Medicine. A Chronicle. Volume III. 1905–1914* (Baltimore: Johns Hopkins University Press, 1963).

63. Reformers contended that teaching and research would inevitably be hindered until the chairmen of academic departments and hospital services were one and the same (an arrangement often referred to as the German system). Editorial, "Hospital Services," *BM&SJ* 56(June 6, 1907): 764.

9. Healing Hands: Nursing in the Hospital

1. Florence Nightingale, "Suggestions on the Subject of Providing, Training and Organising Nurses for the Sick Poor in Workhouse Infirmaries . . . ," 1867, reprinted in Lucy R. Seymer, *Selected Writings of Florence Nightingale* (New York: Macmillan, 1954), p. 274.

2. For a discussion of these developments, see Charles E. Rosenberg, "Recent Developments in the History of Nursing," *Sociology of Health and Illness* 4(1982): 86–94.

3. R. Girdler, Superintendent, MGHA, to F. Sheldon, January 19, 1849, Papers, Board of Governors, NYHA. See also Georgia L. Sturtevant to the Trustees, November 8, 1894, Matron File, MGHA. Sturtevant recalled that when she started work in the hospital in 1862, nurses were expected to begin work at 5 A.M. and end at 9:30 P.M.

4. Referring to the situation in Philadelphia's Episcopal Hospital before it inaugurated its training school in 1888, for example, a staff member recalled that nurses ". . . staid [sic] in the hospital year in and year out, and some had actually grown gray in its service." Elliston Morris, "Episcopal Hospital in 1888 and 1912," *Episcopal Hospital Reports* 2(1914): 102.

5. One physician described nursing at Bellevue immediately before the establishment of its training school in these terms: "At that time, with rare exceptions, the nurses were ignorant and in some cases worthless characters, who accepted the almost impossible task of attending to and nursing from twenty to thirty patients each. There were no night-nurses; the night-watchmen—three in number to a hospital of eight hundred beds—were expected to give assistance to patients re-

quiring attention during the night." W. Gill Wylie, *Hospitals: Their History, Organization and Construction* (New York: D. Appleton, 1877), pp. 3–4.

6. T.R. Smith and W.A. Stewart, "Report of . . . Revision on 13th Chapter: Also Resolution Respecting Nurses Passed Feb. 6, 1821," 1845 File, Board of Governors Papers, NYHA.

7. Society of the Alumni of City (Charity) Hospital, *Report for 1904 Together with a History of the City Hospital . . .* (New York: The Society, 1904), pp. 84, 72; Cf. also 33–34.

8. Entries for September 1, and December 1, 1840, Minutes, Board of Governors, NYHA. For earlier references to the hospital's nursing problems, see entries for April 5, 1808 and August 6, 1833.

9. [Episcopal Hospital of Philadelphia], *Appeal on Behalf of the Sick* (Philadelphia: Lindsay & Blakiston, 1851), p. 36, citing a letter from prominent local physician Joseph Carson. A few years earlier (in 1846) nursing had been included in the home-care program of the Philadelphia Dispensary. Philadelphia Dispensary, Annual Report (hereafter *AR*), 1888, 9.

10. Willard Parker to Gentlemen, [August, 1860], letter accompanying his report for July for the Second Surgical Division, Papers, Board of Governors, NYHA.

11. [Stephen Smith], "Female Nurses in Hospitals," *American Medical Times* 5 (September 13, 1862): 149–50.

12. Cf. Charles E. Rosenberg and Carroll Smith-Rosenberg, "Pietism and the Origins of the American Public Health Movement," *Journal of the History of Medicine* 23(1968): 16–35.

13. Florence Nightingale, *Notes on Nursing. What it is and What it is Not* (New York: D. Appleton, 1861), p. 9.

14. Florence Nightingale, *Notes on Nursing for the Labouring Classes,* new ed. (London: Harrison, 1876), p. 5.

15. Nightingale, *Notes on Nursing,* p. 134. The terms "lady" and "poor workhouse drudge" indicated another of Nightingale's assumptions: that nursing would reflect a two-tier division of authority and recruitment. Nightingale consistently mixed appeals to piety and self-abnegation with invocations of skill and efficiency. Nursing the sick poor in their homes, she wrote on one occasion, "is no amateur work. To do it as it ought to be done requires knowledge, practice, self-abnegation, and, . . . direct obedience to, and activity under, the highest of all Masters, and from the highest of all motives." [William Rathbone], *Organization of Nursing. An Account* (Liverpool: A. Holden, 1865), pp. 10–11.

16. "The nurse-room need not be large; sufficient to accommodate the head nurse, with her assistant, by night and day; situated at one end of the pavilion ward; with a door opening into the same, and also into the common hall; with a window, too, opening into the ward, by which a view can be commanded of the whole at any time. The medicine and liquors should be kept in her room, where she alone can be responsible for them, . . ." F.H. Brown, *Hospital Construction* (Cambridge, Mass.: n.p., 1861), p. 10. For a representative evangelical rationale for nurse training see, "The Appendix," in L.P. Brockett, ed. Agnes Jones, *Una and her Paupers* (New York: George Routledge, 1872), pp. 471–97.

17. Thomas Cullen, *Church Home and Infirmary* (Baltimore: [The Church Home], 1915), pp. 16–18. A contemporary newspaperman emphasized the *"communion of labor"* between men and women in most of the hospitals staffed by Protestant nursing orders. "In each men provide the money that is necessary, and carefully manage the finances, but, accepting as an axiom that nursing the sick is a *special* province of women, they wisely leave to women all that relates to the care of the patients . . ." "Nursing Sisterhoods," undated clipping, *Pittsburgh Commercial,* 1874,

in Children's Hospital Scrapbook, Countway Library of Medicine, Harvard (hereafter HCC).

18. Woman's Hospital of the State of Illinois, *Announcement. Charter of Incorporation, and By-Laws* (Chicago: Horton & Leonard, 1871), pp. 8–9.

19. U.S. Bureau of the Census, *Historical Statistics of the United States, Colonial Times to 1970* (Washington: Government Printing Office, 1975), Series B, 275–90.

20. Linda Richards, *Reminiscences* (Boston: Thomas Todd, 1911), p. 7. Richards's class assumptions are obvious. There were some instances of continuity between the older nursing staff and the new-style trained nurses. Miss Lucia E. Woodward, for example, had been hired as an attendant at MGH in 1864, promoted to supervisor in 1870, and made superintendent of nursing in 1885. Edward Cowles to Henry P. Walcott, June 26, 1903, MGH Trustees Documents Files, Box 1, HCC.

21. Grace F. Shryver, *A History of the Illinois Training School for Nurses 1880–1929* (Chicago: The Training School, 1930); Charles E. Rosenberg, "From Almshouse to Hospital: The Shaping of Philadelphia General Hospital," *Milbank Memorial Fund Q.* 60(1982): 143–46. At New Orleans' Charity Hospital, the Sisters were successful for a good many years in opposing the establishment of a training school that might have compromised their accustomed authority. Charity Hospital, *AR,* 1881, v.

22. Nurses were well aware that training was difficult and demanding. "Almost all the work that a nurse has to do in a hospital is drudgery of the most disillusioning kind, and only girls that have the real desire to do the work, and to succeed in it, whatever discomforts it may entail on them, even go through with it." "Editorial," *Trained Nurse* 1(1888): 25. This, America's first journal for trained nurses, articulated a rationale of dedication and self-abnegation. The editors' motto stated that it was "Consecrated to those who Minister to the Sick and Suffering" and a high proportion of its contributions were signed anonymously—"Nurse Norine" or "May"—a suppression of ego consistent both with views of women's work role and gender assumptions more generally.

23. George Ludlam, superintendent of New York Hospital, complained in 1905, for example, that graduate nurses were "wage earners" and demanded concessions from the hospital such as two hours a day absence from the hospital for rest or recreation. Students made no such demands. Report of the Training School Committee, July 25, 1906, Secretary-Treasurer's Papers, NYHA, cited in Susan Reverby, "The Nursing Disorder: A Critical History of the Hospital-Nursing Relationship, 1860–1945," (Ph.D. diss., Boston University, 1982), pp. 189–90.

24. Philadelphia, Dept. of Charity and Corrections, *AR,* 1889, 49; Worcester Memorial Hospital, *AR,* 1894, 7; Atlanta, Grady Hospital, *AR,* 1899, 7–8.

25. Cf. New Haven, General Hospital Soc., *AR,* 1874, 15, 17. In some hospitals, rules for ward assistants were simply republished as rules for students after a training school was established.

26. Elliot Hospital, Keene, N.H., *AR,* 1905, 18, 27. These figures are typical of this hospital's pattern of operation, beginning with its founding in 1893. The institution's annual report for 1893 provides a revealing table of private nursing fees, pp. 35–36.

27. Henry Hurd to A. Carey, January 2, 1891, Superintendent's Letterbook, JHH. On another occasion, Hurd explained to a prospective orderly that he would have to work under the direction of a female nurse, and ". . . for that reason, it may not be pleasant for you to accept a position here." Hurd to Robert Brown, June 15, 1891, Superintendent's Letterbook, JHH. On the failure of the system to provide career opportunities for men, cf. D. Test to Whom it May Concern (testimonial letter for Benjamin Lloyd), March, 1910, Superintendent's Letterbook, Pennsylvania Hospital Archives (hereafter PHA).

28. Even middle-class families would rarely have invested scarce savings in the

career potential of daughters, as they often did for sons, who might be provided with an education or a start in business.

29. See the excellent discussion in Reverby, "Nursing Disorder," pp. 156–58; Jane E. Mottus, *New York Nightingales. The Emergence of the Nursing Profession at Bellevue and New York Hospital* (Ann Arbor: University Microfilms, 1981), p. 211. Women with a background in domestic service were in practice denied entrance to the best nursing schools—along with the married and divorced.

30. New York State Charities Aid Assoc., *Hospital Housekeeping* (New York: G.P. Putnam's, 1877), p. 40.

31. George Ludlam to Rev. William Tucker, Wellington, Ontario, March 19, 1901, Superintendent's Letterbooks, NYHA; Levi C. Lane to Mrs. C.A. [Hull], August 27, 1897, Cooper Medical College, Letterbook, Lane Medical Library, Stanford University (hereafter SLA).

32. George Ludlam to Emma L. Stowe, Superintendent of Nurses, Connecticut Training School, New Haven, April 24, 1902, Superintendent's Letterbooks, NYHA.

33. In a survey of late nineteenth-century nursing students, Reverby found that roughly half were born in rural areas or small towns, although "only a third were still in such communities when they applied to train." Reverby, "Nursing Disorder," p. 145.

34. Lucy Walker, Report to the Board of Managers for April, 1899, PHA.

35. In a functional sense, this system paralleled the class-based differentiation originally envisaged by Nightingale. Nancy Tomes, "Little World of Our Own: The Pennsylvania Hospital Training School for Nurses, 1895–1907," *Journal of the History of Medicine* 33 (1978): 328–45, provides a case study of the way in which this two-track system worked. A handful of nursing schools were particularly prominent in the training of key nurse administrators: Johns Hopkins, Bellevue, Massachusetts General, and the Connecticut Training School were leaders in the first generations of professional nursing.

36. Cleveland's Lakeside Hospital, for example, complained that: "Of the eight head nurses who took charge of the several departments in January, 1898, only two," they noted at the year's end, "are, at present, with us, the remainder leaving to accept more remunerative positions, or to undertake work in other cities." *AR*, 1898, 27.

37. This is not meant to imply that private duty nursing might not have developed outside hospital confines—inasmuch as it existed before the 1870s and answered needs of both physicians and patients.

38. [A Hospital Nurse] "Glimpses of Hospital Life," *Trained Nurse* 1(1888):11.

39. Haverhill, Mass., Hale Hospital, *AR*, 1899, 50. Such hours were typical. See, for example, Pennsylvania Hospital, *Training School for Nurses. Announcement* (Philadelphia, n.p., n.d.); Lowell, Mass., Hospital Association, *AR*, 1901, 29. New hospitals hastened to follow the work patterns established by older institutions. "When possible," Durham, North Carolina's Watts Hospital's first annual report explained, "the nurses will have an hour to rest or exercise each day, and are frequently given an afternoon. While it is not always possible, they may usually expect part of each Sunday."*AR*, 1895, 45.

40. Hartford, Conn. Hospital, *AR*, 1879, 10.

41. Entry for January 31, 1887, Executive Committee Minutes, NYHA.

42. Worcester, Mass. Memorial Hospital, *AR*, 1895, 23.

43. *Charter and By-Laws of the Marshall Infirmary* (Troy, N.Y.: Wm. H. Young, 1859), p. 25.

44. As we have seen (chapter 5), the germ theory threatened at first to undermine this worship of cleanliness; over time, however, its impact was to intensify and

legitimate older attitudes toward the centrality of order and cleanliness. If even the tiniest fragment of "dirt" might cause infection, then no effort could be spared in promoting cleanliness.

45. "Hospital Housekeeping by Dr. Edw. Cowles," Katherine Guion Babcock, Medical Note-Book, 1889–90, Babcock Notebooks, SCC.

46. A resident at Philadelphia General Hospital, for example, noted his sympathy for a girl ". . . who, after almost two years' hard work here is sent away in disgrace without her diploma. It is too severe a punishment," he felt, "for a slight offense, but that is the way with . . . the training school run as it is by an unprincipled haughty, ignorant woman with a fine form & oily tongue who by her personal effect on men maintains the greater part of her power." Entry for February 20, 1899, Sherman Gilpin Diary, Temple University Urban Archives, Philadelphia. Cf. Albert Houston, Manuscript Autobiography, pp. 89–90, Bancroft Library, University of California, Berkeley; *Medical Record* (October 12, 19, 1895): 534, 572; "The Hospital Tyrants and their Victims the Nurses. What Doctors Say of the Oppression of Young Women in these Institutions," *New York Times,* August 22, 1909.

47. See, for example, the *Rules and Regulations of the Pennsylvania Hospital* (Philadelphia: Friend's Printing House, 1887), pp. 11–13, in which rules for "Nurses and Servants" were listed together. The phrase describing required footwear is from the Haverhill, Mass. Hale Hospital, *AR,* 1899, 50.

48. Entry for September 30, 1902, Minutes, Ladies Hospital Aid Association, Raleigh, N.C., Hinsdale Family Papers, Perkins Library, Duke University.

49. Henry M. Hurd, "Why a Nurse Should be Educated," pp. 8–9, undated ms., Hurd Papers, JHH. These outspoken remarks have been x'ed out of the typed ms. Hurd, "The Proper Length of the Period of Training for Nurses," *American Journal of Nursing* 8(1908): 671–83, outlines his reform program.

50. Charles Emerson, "The American Hospital Field." In: Charlotte Aiken, ed., *Hospital Management: A Handbook for Hospital Trustees, Superintendents, Training School Principals, Physicians, and All Who Are Actively Engaged in Promoting Hospital Work* (Philadelphia: W.B. Saunders, 1911), p. 62; John Dill Robertson, *The Ideal Training School for Nurses* (Philadelphia: Philadelphia School for Nurses, 1911), p. 5. Robertson recommended six hours of floor duty each day and three hours instruction in nursing: "None of her lecture work should be done in the evening, but these should be devoted to recreation and the time necessary for study." p. 11.

51. Entry for April 2, 1888, Executive Committee Minutes, Board of Governors, NYHA; Cincinnati General Hospital, *AR,* 1894, 34.

52. In this instance at least, ideological considerations worked against the desire to limit costs; paternalistic assumptions concerning the schools' responsibility as foster parent—allied with simple humanity—urged the need for adequate housing for student nurses. A separate residence provided a controlled moral environment reassuring to donors and administrators. Lack of adequate housing also began to serve as a disadvantage in attracting the most desirable nursing students.

53. William Dorland, *The Sphere of the Trained Nurse . . .* (Philadelphia: Philadelphia School for Nurses, 1908), p. 29.

54. N.P. Dandridge, *Hospitals. Their Work and Their Obligations . . .* (Cincinnati: R. Blake & Co., 1893), p. 14.

55. William L. Richardson, *Address on the Duties and Conduct of Nurses in Private Nursing* (Boston: G.H. Ellis, 1887), p. 20; "May," "Notes on Private Nursing," *Trained Nurse* 1(1888): 21; Eugene A. Smith, "The Observation of Symptoms," *Trained Nurse* 1(1888): 53; "The Nurse's Duty to the Doctor," NHR, 2(December, 1898): 11; "There are Nurses, and Nurses," *NHR* 3(September, 1899): 31; Seymour, "A Code of Ethics for Trained Nurses," *NHR* 3(October, 1899): 31.

56. Most prominent was Henry C. Burdett. See, for example, his *Hospitals and the State* (London: J. & A. Churchill, 1881), p. 8; H.M. Hurd, to J. Hull Browning, December 9, 1890, Hurd Letterbooks, JHH. Hurd was a self-proclaimed advocate of nurse training but a bitter foe of training schools organized outside the hospital's direct authority.

57. Joseph Buffington, "Address," Pittsburgh Homeopathic Hospital, *AR,* 1893, 66.

58. Mrs. Hunter Robb, "Address," Cleveland Lakeside Hospital, *AR,* 1898, 96; George Peabody, *Address at the Graduating Exercises . . . of the New York Hospital Training School for Nurses* (New York: New York Hospital, 1911), p. 7. See also William Osler, *Nurse and Patient* (Baltimore: John Murphy & Co., 1897), p. 12. Osler did concede that nursing could serve a special function for unmarried women; "there is a gradually accumulating surplus of women who will not or cannot fulfill the highest duties for which Nature has designed them." Such a female was "apt to become a dangerous element unless her energies and emotions are diverted in a proper channel"—among them nursing. P. 15.

59. *Souvenir History of the Virginia Hospital* (Richmond: n.p., 1901), p. [19].

60. "Nurses must," in the words of a well-trained graduate nurse, "be taught pathology & clinical medicine if they are to understand the measures of treatment wh. it is their business to apply. . . . The nurse should come to be in private cases what the house officer is in hospitals." Richard Cabot, "Journal of Western Trip," 1901, p. 5, Box 2, Cabot Papers, Harvard University Archives.

61. Entry for December 14, 190[3], Minutes, Medical Board, PNY.

62. Dorland, *Sphere of the Trained Nurse,* 1908, p. 17.

63. Administrators of small hospitals contended that graduate nurses were insubordinate and unreliable as well as expensive. Cf. Theodore MacClure, "Problems in Small Hospitals," *Hospital World* 2(July, 1912): 13.

64. See the discussion at the semi-annual meeting of the New England Association for the Education of Nurses, December 10, 1909, as to whether hospitals with fewer than twenty-five beds should be allowed to have training schools. *Trained Nurse* 44 (1910): 184–87. Frederic Washburn of the MGH argued that no hospital of this size could hope to provide an adequate education. Cf. also Reverby, "Nursing Disorder," p. 100, for a discussion of this problem.

65. The Hale Hospital in Haverhill, Massachusetts, for example, increased its course from two to three years in 1905; the third year was to be spent at the Boston Lying-In and New England Charitable Eye and Ear Infirmary. *AR,* 1905, 36.

66. Contemporaries warned, however, that such highly educated nurses would always be beyond the means of ordinary Americans and that less trained or partially trained women would inevitably find a niche in the private duty marketplace. Editorial, "The Nursing Problem," *Hospital World* 2 (1912): 214–16.

67. Worcester Memorial Hospital, *AR,* 1904, 38–42.

68. A handful of postgraduate training programs had already come into being by 1910, at MGH, Grace Hospital in Detroit, Pennsylvania Hospital, and, most conspicuously, the hospital economics program at Columbia's Teacher's College. The potential for such graduate programs was limited not only by the lack of niches in the nursing system, but by the limited pool of women with the financial resources to take advantage of them. A graduate nurse complained in 1900, for example, that the fees at Teacher's College would discourage any but a "millionairess." "Should I ever become sufficiently wealthy to attend, I would prefer to retire and live on the interest of my money." Letter, "A Course in Hospital Economics," *Trained Nurse* 24(1900): 52; Cf. Charlotte A. Aikens, "Preparation for Institutional Work," *Trained Nurse* 44(1910): 172–73.

69. In the long run, he continued, "qualities of the head and heart will outweigh

the most elaborate training and skill, however useful they may be." Thomas Satterthwaite, "Private Nurses and Nursing," *Trained Nurse* 44(1910): 212–13.

70. Italics in original. Henry Beates, *The Status of Nurses: A Sociologic Problem* (Philadelphia: Physician's National Board of Regents, 1909), pp. 18–19. Beates spoke at a meeting called to discuss a proposed state registration law.

71. Cf. Nancy Tomes, "The Silent Battle: Nurse Registration in New York State, 1903–1920." In: Ellen C. Lagemann, ed., *Nursing History. New Perspectives, New Possibilities* (New York and London: Teacher's College Press, 1983), pp. 107–32.

72. These relationships also implied a particularly ambiguous role for the training school superintendent, who had, of necessity, to side in practice with her institution's medical and lay boards if she were to solidify her own authority. It often made her an unbending disciplinarian; at points of conflict she had little ability to represent forcefully the interests of the student and graduate nurses she supervised. "The nursing authority structure," in the words of Susan Reverby, "rather than protecting the student, became the mechanism through which she experienced her oppression." Cf. Reverby, "Nursing Disorder," p. 135, and pp. 123, 129.

73. S.W. Mitchell, *Address . . . Commencement Exercises, Class '05 of the Presbyterian Hospital in the City of New York . . .* (n.p., n.d.), p. 10. Some opponents of registration and the limitation of hours on duty turned instinctively to then inflammatory analogies between trade union and nursing demands. See, for example, the response to passage of a California statute limiting student nurses to an eight-hour day. "Eight Hour Day under Fire," *Modern Hospital* 1(1913): 139. "Perhaps the most important question at issue is whether the nursing body is a trade union or a learned profession."

74. Amy Armour, "Hospital Housekeeping," *Hospital World* 2(1912): 149. Diet was a special source of resentment for nurses. "There is no more bitter or ever-smoldering indignation in any mass of people than in the minds of nurses, who see posted, or help in the diet kitchen to make up menus for the staff doctors, setting forth lordly fare, of fruits and birds, when they see them visiting assiduously all the painted, powdered, bleached patients, while the nurses go on duty many a time, eating only a dish of bread and milk, and yet upholding most ethical standards." P. 155.

75. U. S. Bureau of the Census, *Historical Statistics of the United States* (Washington: Government Printing Office, 1959), Series B, 192–94, 235–36.

76. For many such nurses, of course, this promise was not to be fulfilled, as the private duty market soon became crowded and unstable. One factor that helped maintain this tenuous equilibrium until the 1920s was the consistently high drop-out rate among training school graduates.

77. For the most recent analysis of public health nursing, see Karen Buhler-Wilkerson, "False Dawn: The Rise and Decline of Public Health Nursing, 1900–30," (Ph.D. diss., University of Pennsylvania, 1984).

10. The Private Patient Revolution

1. Statement of James Darrach, Superintendent, New York Hospital, *Report of the . . . Board of Governors . . . on Extending the Usefulness of the Hospital* (New York: Baker & Godwin, 1858), p. 25. In his study of Boston hospitals, Morris Vogel nicely documents this point by describing the way in which even victims of a train crash were treated in their homes, not in available hospitals. Vogel, *The Invention of the Modern Hospital. Boston, 1870–1930* (Chicago: University of Chicago Press, 1980), pp. 13–15.

2. A few small proprietary surgical hospitals were founded in America's largest cities in the second half of the nineteenth century, but they were few in number, minute in scale, and ordinarily ephemeral. It was not until the last decade of the nineteenth and first decade of the twentieth centuries that proprietary (ordinarily surgical) hospitals became widespread.

3. In port cities, as we have seen, hospitals often depended on fees earned in treating sick and injured seamen; in New York, the state Commissioners of Emigration at mid-century also paid a dollar a day for the care of recent immigrants. Negotiated rates tended to be as low as the collector of a particular port could manage.

4. Hospitals in smaller cities tended to have available a relatively wider spectrum of income sources and community support. The Albany hospital, for example, spent $13,466.13 for patient care in 1879–1880. Of this, individual patients paid $6,327.47, the city $4,000, and the county $502.54—leaving a burden of $2,636.12 for the care of free patients to be met by the institution's own resources. The city reimbursed the hospital at a rate of $4 per week when costs averaged $6. Both the mix of income sources and the gap between costs and reimbursement rates were typical. Albany Hospital, Annual Report (hereafter *AR*), 1879–80, 24.

5. Pennsylvania Hospital, *Proceedings of a Meeting Held First Month . . . 1867* (Philadelphia: Collins, 1867), pp. 8–9. As in many such cautiously-managed institutions, cost cutting was enthusiastically pursued. A medical staff member boasted, for example, that they used two thousand fewer yards of muslin for bandaging than they had two decades before, when they had a fourth the number of accidents to treat. "We used the bandages the second, third, and fourth time, after they had been thoroughly washed and disinfected." P. 15. In 1853 patient care expenses totaled $28,184 and investment income amounted to $23,144. April 25, 1853, Minutes, Board of Managers, Pennsylvania Hospital Archives (hereafter PHA).

6. Executive Committee Report, Pittsburgh Homeopathic Medical & Surgical Hospital, *AR*, 1872–73, 14–15. Members of the committee had been forced to serve as "financial agents"—that is solicitors. Prudent financial management dictated that any capital improvements be paid for with cash in hand; charitable institutions did not normally borrow in this period.

7. Roosevelt Hospital, *AR*, 1871–2, 7–8. Not surprisingly, the hospital had little success in maintaining such ratios.

8. In 1874, their third year of operation, the hospital reported having treated 1,177 free patients and 177 paying full or part of their "board" including 43 in private rooms. Roosevelt Hospital, *AR*, 1874, 10.

9. The distinction between "charitable" and "convenient" institutions was made by John Watson, in the New York Hospital's *Report . . . on Extending the Usefulness of the Hospital*, 1858, p. 7; Hartford Hospital, *AR*, 1857, 9. A decade later, the Hartford Hospital could report progress on a new wing in which there would be ten well-furnished and ventilated private rooms with water-closets and baths attached to each, "designed for persons willing to pay for extra accommodations. *AR*, 1868, 11. See also Massachusetts General Hospital Archives (hereafter MGHA) "Phillips House" and "Wards. Isolation & Pavilion" files for material on private patient policies; entry for July 5, 1851, Faculty Minutes, Hampden-Sydney College, Medical College of Virginia Archives (hereafter MCV).

10. J. Green, *City Hospitals* (Boston: Little, Brown, 1861), pp. 18–19, 50.

11. Even before antisepsis, surgery was the most frequent justification for an occasional respectable American entering a hospital.

12. Entry for October 5, 1852, Minutes, Medical Board, Episcopal Hospital of Philadelphia (hereafter EHA).

13. *Pocket Compendium to Presbyterian Hospital, . . . For Patients of Every Creed, Nationality and Color . . . 1882,* bound in Presbyterian Hospital Scrapbook, Public Relations Office, PNY. Five thousand was a widely, though not universally, agreed-upon figure in this period. In the 1860s, two or three thousand dollars was considered adequate as a perpetual endowment by some hospitals.

14. By the early years of the present century, rising costs had made such calculations obsolete. In 1906, the superintendent of Pennsylvania Hospital noted that the income from five thousand dollars would not even support six months of care. Test to Louis B. Robinson, October 3, 1906, Superintendent's Letterbooks, PHA.

15. Roosevelt Hospital, *AR,* 1871–2, 9. Some hospitals promised donors that their name would be displayed on a plate attached to the bed whose occupant they were entitled to designate (assuming admitting physicians concurred). The Jewish Hospital Association of Philadelphia, *Constitution, By-Laws, Regulations, and List of Members* (Philadelphia: The Hospital, 1874), p. 27.

16. In 1895, Philadelphia German (now Lankenau) Hospital offered mill and factory owners and lodge and beneficial associations a bed in the hospital for 365 days for a prepaid two hundred dollars. *AR,* 1895, 88. Prices varied from city to city; in high-priced San Francisco, for example, the Lane Hospital charged business firms and associations $2.50 a day for treating members or employees. C.N. Ellinwood to John Dougherty, August 19, 1897, Lane Hospital Letterpress Copybook, SLA.

17. "Hospital Sunday," *Medical Record* 15 (January 18, 1879): 64. The editorialist assumed that the funds would be distributed in proportion to the number of free patients in each hospital.

18. For a useful account of one city, see Joan B. Trauner, "From Benevolence to Negotiation: Prepaid Health Care in San Francisco, 1850–1950," (Ph.D. diss., University of California, San Francisco, 1977), ch. I. "Mutual Aid Associations, 1849–1915"; Jerome L. Schwartz, "Early History of Prepaid Medical Care Plans," *Bulletin of the History of Medicine,* (hereafter *BHM*) 39(1965): 450–75.

19. St. Joseph's Hospital, Chippewa Falls, Wisconsin, Misc. Ms. File, January 21, 1897, State Historical Society of Wisconsin (hereafter SHSW); Brockton Hospital, *AR,* 1901, inside of rear cover. Cf. also certificate of Marinette & Menominee Hospital Co., Marinette, Wisconsin, Misc. Ms. File, February 13, 1908, SHSW.

20. "Fifty Cent Hospitals," *Medical Record* 51(April 10, 1897): 527; Pittsburgh Homeopathic Hospital, *AR,* 1870, 9. Harvard's Stillman Infirmary provided an early example of a university prepaid clinic for students and employees. "The Stillman Infirmary," *BM&SJ,* 147 (October 30, 1902): 501.

21. V. Gibney, 1899, cited by Fenwick Beekman, *Hospital for Ruptured and Crippled* (New York: Privately Printed, 1939), p. 64.

22. At Cleveland's Lakeside Hospital, for example, per capita costs increased from $2.18 to $2.34 between 1899 and 1912, while the average hospital census climbed from 101 to 223 and thus expenses more than doubled—from $97,152.62 to $222,775.25.

23. David Rosner's recent study of Brooklyn hospitals places particular emphasis on the economic impact of the panic in reshaping the hospitals' financial strategies. *A Once Charitable Enterprise. Hospitals and Health Care in Brooklyn and New York, 1885–1915* (Cambridge, London, New York: Cambridge University Press, 1982), esp. ch. 2, "Embattled Benefactors: The Crisis in Hospital Financing." It is difficult to balance the impact of general secular trends against the specific effects of the depression in the 1890s.

24. H.M. Hurd to Board of Trustees, Annual Report dated February 17, 1894, Minutes for February 20, 1894, JHH; Worcester Memorial Hospital, *AR,* 1899, 4; Chicago, St. Luke's Hospital, *AR,* 1897–98, 9.

25. The New Haven Hospital announced proudly in 1895 that it had cut such costs almost in half the previous year. General Hospital Association of Connecticut, New Haven, *AR,* 1894, 13. For a typical thirteen-point cost containment program see, Report of Committee on Income and Expenditures, November 30, 1900, Minutes, Board of Managers, EHA. They hoped, among other things, to cut patient food costs, limit length of stays, reduce student nurse allowances, trim clerical and drug expenditures "as shall not be damaging to the welfare of the patients" and begin charging dispensary patients for their prescriptions.

26. Presbyterian Hospital, *AR,* 1904, 13. Cf. Editorial, "Against Municipal Hospitals," *NHR* 3(1900): 35. At precisely this time, New York hospitals were forced to adjust to the city's newly instituted mode of per capita reimbursement; some hospitals refused to make their records available to city auditors and would not apply for such reimbursement. Cf. Rosner, *A Once Charitable Enterprise;* Robert W. de Forest to John S. Kennedy, President, Presbyterian Hospital, January 29, 1903. In: Minutes, Executive Committee, Board of Managers, tipped in following minutes for March 24, 1903, PNY. The city reimbursed private hospitals at a rate of sixty cents a day for medical and eighty cents for surgical cases.

27. See, for example, the recent studies by Vogel, *Invention* and Rosner, *A Once Charitable.*

28. Charles Emerson, "The American Hospital Field." In: Charlotte Aikens, ed., *Hospital Management* (Philadelphia: W.B. Saunders, 1911), pp. 18–19.

29. Even the "normal" process of childbirth in respectable families was beginning to move into the hospital. New York's Sloane Maternity Hospital, for example, reported in 1897 that ". . . married women belonging to reputable families . . ." had not entered the hospital "to any great extent." It had not been customary at any of the city's hospitals. By 1900, however, the number of private patients at Sloane had "so increased as to make it almost a department in itself, . . ." J.W. McLane to T.M. Prudden, October 13, 1897; Anne D. Van Kirk to J. McLane, [December, 1900], Letters and Reports, Sloane Maternity Hospital, PNY. Cf. Judith Walzer Leavitt, *Brought to Bed. Child-Bearing in America, 1750–1950* (New York: Oxford University Press, 1986).

30. "Rex Hospital," undated [1897] clipping, in rear cover, Minutes, Ladies' Hospital Aid Association, Raleigh, Hinsdale Family Papers, Perkins Library, Duke University; Richmond, Virginia, *Memorial Hospital . . .* (1903), pp. 22, 25. Cf. also Jon M. Kingsdale, "The Growth of Hospitals: An Economic History in Baltimore," (Ph.D. diss., University of Michigan, 1981), p. 14; Charles E. Rosenberg, "Inward Vision and Outward Glance: The Shaping of the American Hospital, 1880–1914," *BHM* 53 (1979): 384–85. In the 1870s and 1880s, such descriptions tended to emphasize furniture, ventilation, meals, and attendance, rather than technical matters.

31. Entry for November 13, 1905, Minutes, Medical Board, PNY.

32. Worcester, Mass., Memorial Hospital, *AR,* 1899, 9.

33. "This arrangement," he added, "is a great help to the hospitals as it brings them wealthy and influential patients who later show a deep interest in their prosperity." Nicholas Senn to J. Collins Warren, February 28, 1894. In a letter transmitting Senn's letter to the MGH trustees' Secretary Edmund Dwight, Warren noted that: "Dr. Senn is one of the most prominent men in the country. He told me recently he 'paid no visits.' He is said to have an income of $75,000.00 a year." Phillips House File, MGH, cited in Rosenberg, "Inward Vision," p. 367.

34. S.S. Goldwater, "The Hospital and the Surgeon," *Modern Hospital* 7(1916): 373.

35. Elizabeth Greener, "Admission of Patients . . . ," *Modern Hospital* 2(1914): 19.

36. Katherine H. Billings, New York to Dearest Mother, January 29, 1909, Hammond-Bryan-Cumming Papers, South Caroliniana Library (hereafter SCC).

37. The big city demand for clinical teaching material provided another difference between small town and urban orientations toward the hospital, although many staff members at small private city hospitals had no teaching ambitions.

38. Morton Hospital, Taunton, Mass., *AR,* 1889, 7.

39. Fred C. Hubbard, *Physicians, Medical Practice, and Development of Hospitals in Wilkes County, 1830 to 1975* (n.p., 1978), p. 66.

40. Although not all physicians were surgeons—or even willing to claim they were—patient loyalties were maintained in community hospitals by having the referring physician present at or assisting in the surgical procedure, a practice normally discouraged at big city hospitals. Entry for November 25, 1904, Minutes, Board of Managers, EHA. Local physicians often made themselves useful—and earned a fee—by administering anesthesia.

41. "County Hospitals are Advocated," C.S. Miller Scrapbook, undated [1909] clipping, p. 44, Iowa State Historical Society.

42. "Wants a Hospital Tax," Waverly, Iowa *Democrat,* [1909], C.S. Miller Scrapbook, pp. 26–27.

43. Editorial, "The Small Hospital," *Modern Hospital* 1(October, 1913): 113.

44. Watts Hospital, *AR,* 1895, 11, 13, 25, 31.

45. Watts Hospital, *AR,* 1921, 3–4, 15–18, 20, 55. Physicians had to agree to abide by the hospital's rules and regulations. The fact that 258 of the appendectomies were categorized as clean, with 28 requiring drainage, raises some doubt as to the indications justifying this procedure, as does the improbably high proportion.

46. Mission Hospital of Asheville, North Carolina, *AR,* 1887, 2; *AR,* 1889, 5, 8; *AR,* 1928, 23.

47. Haverhill, Mass. Hospital, *AR,* 1888, 7–11, 15.

48. Haverhill, Mass. Hospital, *AR,* 1905, 60–61; several years later, hospital supporters arranged a "Tombola"—at which men arranged the tea tables and served as pourers; a blue ribbon was awarded to the man with the most artistic table. *AR,* 1907, 46.

49. Private patient fees accounted for $11,089.65 of a total current expenditure of $17,868.85; donations provided $2,202.84 and investments yielded $3,358.33. *AR,* 1905, 11–12, 13, 31. Like many other hospitals, appendectomies were an important surgical procedure. In 1907, for example, of 477 admissions, 395 were surgical and 102 medical, with appendectomy being by far the most frequent procedure performed at 78 and cholecystotomy second at 23. No other procedure was performed more than ten times during the year. *AR,* 1907, 11, 21f.

50. Rosner, *A Once Charitable Enterprise.* This change was most apparent in a minority of older hospitals in large Eastern cities; many smaller hospitals, denominational institutions, and those founded in the Midwest and West had never known a time when they had not had to maximize patient income.

51. Philadelphia's Episcopal Hospital provides another example of this conflict of values and authority; the medical board began seeking the right to charge private room patients in the mid-nineties, but it was not until 1901 that they were granted it. Entries for May 25, 1895, Medical Board Minutes; May 30, 1901, Board of Managers Minutes, EHA. "No chief resident," the steward of the Pennsylvania Hospital explained in 1894, "is allowed to make any charge to any patient under any pretext or circumstances. Such practice did grow up in the house to some extent but within two months the Board of Managers have adopted a new and stringent rule forbidding any charge to be made under any circumstances." J.G. Williams to J.W. Pratt, Resident Physician, MGH March 6, 1894, MGHA.

52. H.J. Bigelow, "Fees in Hospitals," *BM&SJ* 120 (April 11, 1889): 377. For a lucid analysis of the MGH conflict, see, Vogel, *Invention,* pp. 107–11.

53. Editorial, "Hospital Physicians and Pay-Patients," *Philadelphia Medical Times 14* (May 31, 1884): 643. The editorialist warned pointedly that the situation "doubt-less has had the effect of keeping patients out of the hospital who would have been better cared for in the wards." And if Pennsylvania and Episcopal refused to allow its patients to be charged, Philadelphia's St. Joseph's, German, and Jefferson hospi-tals did allow it. Editorial, "Pay-Hospitals, and a Point in Hospital Management," *Medical Record* 17 (April 10, 1880): 402 and "Philadelphia," *BM&SJ* 100(January 23, 1879): 134 present similar arguments—the former emphasizing the contention that the system was adequate for the very rich (who would never enter a hospital in any case) and the poor (who did and received excellent gratuitous care) but unfair to the middle classes who often needed hospital care but would not and should not accept charity.

54. The circular explained that a staff member performed "his duty as a charity to the sick and disabled patients under his care, and for the advancement of medical and surgical science." Circular Letter dated March 18, 1881, signed by T.H. Hall, Secretary, MGH, Admission-Care of Patients File, MGHA.

55. Frederick C. Shattuck, "Some Remarks on Hospital Abuse," *Medical Record* 53 (May 7, 1898): 649–51. It will be recalled that private patients were never used for teaching or, ordinarily, in systematic clinical investigation. For another striking illustration of the conflict between what might be called the patrician and entre-preneurial views, see the response of J. West Roosevelt to a bitter editorial attack on hospital trustees in *Medical Record* 45 (January 13, 1894): 62–63; (January 20, 1894): 96; (February 3, 1894): 134–35.

56. Egbert H. Grandin, "Address of the Retiring President," *Medical Record* 47 (December 14, 1895): 851.

57. George Gay, "Abuse of Medical Charity . . ." *BM&SJ* 152 (March 16, 1905): 295, 297, 300.

58. In a period when there were still few exclusive specialists, general practition-ers feared that turning a patient over to a hospital physician for treatment of a particular ailment might well result in the permanent loss of a whole family's patronage.

59. F.B. Kirkbride, to Solis-Cohen, March 5, 1904; W.B. Hackenburg, to Solis-Cohen, January 25, 1904. College of Physicians of Philadelphia (hereafter CPP). The Jewish Hospital, for example, had just opened a new pay hospital and, "in an effort to extend its benefits" the board had decided to offer admitting privileges to "certain physicians of repute (though not connected with the regular Hospital Staff) . . ."

60. Like most of its peers, the Pennsylvania Hospital had adopted a compromise position allowing surgeons to charge private room patients but not those treated in wards. Occasional conflict could arise over patients barely able to pay for private accommodations but, in the hospital's view, unable to pay a surgeon's fee in addition. Cf. Daniel Test to Richard H. Harte, May 6, 1905, Superintendent's Letterbook, PHA.

61. In 1897, for example, the Johns Hopkins Hospital Medical Board urged that ". . . with the hope of retaining the valuable services of Dr. Finney he be given the privilege of sending private patients to the hospital" and that his salary be in-creased from $500 to $750. Entry for May 28, 1897, Medical Board Minutes, JHH. Similar tactics were employed several years later to keep Thomas Cullen, Kelly's protégé, from accepting a Yale offer. Entry for March 7, 1900, Medical Board, Minutes. The minute's discreet referral to a "free discussion" and the inclusion of two other bright young staffers indicates that the issue was controversial.

62. Entry for December 13, 1909, Minutes, Medical Board, PNY.

63. In 1899, the Johns Hopkins Medical Board asked that the surgeon and gynecologist be asked to provide the superintendent with a sliding fee table specifying
maximum and minimum figures between which operations were to be billed. It was
also understood that the superintendent would exercise a "wise discretion" in
regard to specialist fees and be able to remit them when indicated. H.M. Hurd to
Board of Trustees, February 20, 1899, Minutes, Board, Medical Board Minutes, of
same date, JHH.

64. In wheedling patients into private room beds, for example, such physicians
might provoke conflict by making promises inconsistent with hospital rules. Cf.
Hahnemann Hospital, Medical Staff Minutes, September 4, October 2, November
6, 1896; January 4, 1897, Hahnemann Hospital, Philadelphia. In Catholic Hospitals,
of course, where nurses did not necessarily assume a physician-oriented authority
structure, admitting privileges did not necessarily imply such threats to institutional discipline. H.M. Hurd to Reuben Peterson, October 10, 1890, Hurd Letterbook, JHH.

65. Hospitals often specified nursing ratios for private patients—usually one
nurse to four patients—with the understanding that families who wished more
intensive nursing care be responsible for payment of private duty fees.

66. See also the discussion of clinical pathology in chapter 6.

67. Most urban hospitals sought to compromise with their original social mission
by insisting that ward patients never be charged a fee for medical care; difficulties
arose with the widespread adoption of modestly scaled pay wards.

68. From the very beginning, hospitals were conscious of the potential long-term
return from private patients in the form of donations and bequests. Medical care
was a way to familiarize the local elite with an institution and the work it performed. There was no better time, as one administrator summed up the accepted
wisdom, "to appeal to a person's charitable tendencies than when they are ill or
just convalescing. And here is the opportunity to bring the needs of the hospital
before the people and educate them to the giving, not only to the hospital, but also
to other philanthropic institutions." Edgar A. Vander Veer, "The Importance of a
General Hospital in the Education of the Profession and the Public," *Bulletin of the
American Academy of Medicine* 12 (1911): 162.

69. Not only market considerations, but deeply ingrained social assumptions
guaranteed that paying patients would be spared such "unpleasantness."

70. Cleveland's Lakeside and New York Hospital were pioneers in creating such
private house staffs. Cf. entry for March 3, 1903, Minutes, Executive Comm., Board
of Governors, NYHA. S.S. Goldwater warned of the danger of disrupting the ward
services in attempts to increase occupancy rates in newly built private pavilions.
"They then proceed to reorganize the whole hospital, cutting ward service to pieces
for the sake of creating a staff capable of maintaining the private pavilion." Remarks, *TAMA* 8 (1906): 129.

71. In an effort to combat this seasonality, Johns Hopkins, like some other
hospitals, offered favored junior staff members admissions privileges limited to the
summer months. Entry for January 8, 1912, Medical Board, Minutes, JHH. New
York Hospital, typically, reduced its nursing and attendant staff during the summer
months. George Ludlam to Miss Martha Palser, April 19, 1902, Superintendent's
Letterbooks, NYHA.

72. Ward patient costs rose from $2.81.33 to $3.09.6, while pay patient costs rose
from $3.64.83 to $7.10.4. The figures are derived from the relevant annual reports.
The hospital's board was well aware that income from paying patients had increased but emphasized that improved standards demanded by such patients inevitably increased costs for every patient in the hospital. *AR*, 1910, 14.

73. Polyclinic Hospital & College for Graduates in Medicine, *AR*, 1904, 41. The hospital charged $10.50 a week, well under the full cost, which they calculated to be $12.80.

74. Hurd, "Laboratories and Hospital Work," *Bulletin of the American Academy of Medicine* 2 (1896): 485.

75. Surgery was disproportionately important, even at large acute-care hospitals. The Massachusetts General Hospital, for example, admitted 1,633 patients in the quarter ending September 30, 1910—the year of the Flexner Report. Over one thousand (1056) admissions were surgical and only 577 medical; 770 were pay and 863 free. Almost 1,100 operations had been performed. F.A. Washburn to John A. Blanchard, Secretary, Board of Trustees, MGH Trustees' Papers, Box 12, HCC.

11. A Careful Oversight: Reshaping Authority

1. Entry for July 1, 1825, Minutes, Visiting Committee; Samuel Spring to Trustees of the MGH, May 14, 1825, Nathan Gurney Biographical File, Massachusetts General Hospital Archives (hereafter MGHA). For comments on the first superintendent, Nathaniel Fletcher, and his nautical career, see Fletcher Biographical File, Joseph Balch to Gamelial Bradford, March 2, 1821.

2. Entries for November 8, 1872, December 3, 1872, January 6, 1873, May 12, 1873, March 13, 1875, Inspecting Committee Minutes, Presbyterian Hospital of New York Archives (hereafter PNY).

3. Report of the Visiting Committee for the Month of August, Minutes for October 11, 1892, Board of Trustees, Johns Hopkins Hospital Archives (hereafter JHH); Report of the Visiting Committee for the Month, Minutes for December 11, 1900, Board of Trustees, JHH.

4. Cleveland, Lakeside Hospital, Annual Report (hereafter *AR*) 1898, 85; Executive Committee Minutes, June 2, 1886, Board of Governors, New York Hospital Archives (hereafter NYHA).

5. Comments of Rev. E.P. Cowan, Pittsburgh, Homeopathic Medical & Surg. Hospital, AR 1888, 13.

6. Comments of Rev. Austin M. Courtenay, Pittsburgh, Homeopathic Medical & Surg. Hospital, *AR*, 1893–94, 66.

7. Henry D. Harlan and W.T. Dixon, Visiting Committee Report, February 11, 1902, With Minutes for February 11, 1902, Board of Trustees, JHH.

8. Regulations of the Board of Lady Visitors of the Protestant Episcopal Hospital, March 1883, Minute Book, 1883–1917, Episcopal Hospital of Philadelphia Archives (hereafter EHA). This particular board consisted of twelve ladies appointed by the Bishop. Although "bound not to hide or dissemble the truth of God," the ladies were urged to avoid any sectarian interpretations, especially those that might "unnecessarily drive off Roman Catholics, or others, whose views differ from theirs."

9. At the Albany Hospital, for example, ladies committees from twelve local churches furnished twelve different rooms. "The rooms were not only made comfortable, but were hung with pictures and curtains, and furnished so tastefully that they are a constant surprise to visitors." Albany Hospital, *AR*, 1878–79, 13.

10. Editorial, "Wanted-Aid by a Distressed Community," *Philadelphia Medical Times* 4 (April 11, 1874): 442.

11. Entry for April 29, 1823, Minutes of Monthly Meetings of Board of Managers, New-York Asylum for Lying-in Women, NYHA. For a later period, see Virginia A.M. Quiroga, "Female Lay Managers and Scientific Pediatrics at Nursery

and Child's Hospital, 1854–1910," *Bulletin of the History of Medicine* (hereafter *BHM*) 60(1986): 194–208.

12. Entries for February 17, 1873, February 5, 1877, Matron's Journal, Boston Lying-In Hospital, Countway Library (hereafter HCC).

13. The object of the hospital is quoted from the Minutes, vol. 2, pp. 1–2 [1888], Minnesota Maternity Hospital, P432, Minnesota Historical Society. Other citations are from the same source, entries for June 3, 1887; November 11, 1887; June 10, 1890. Cf. Virginia G. Drachman, *Hospital with a Heart. Women Doctors and the Paradox of Separatism at the New England Hospital, 1862–1969* (Ithaca and London: Cornell University Press, c. 1984).

14. Report of Physician-in-Charge, Minnesota Maternity Hospital, *AR*, 1899, 11; Entry for August 12, 1890, Minutes, Minnesota Maternity Hospital. Such policies continued into the twentieth century. In 1910, for example, the board was still placing babies (though only "into Christian homes, and 3 mo. on trial"), and Dr. Ripley was still urging the need to separate "the married women from the girls." Entries for May 10, August 9, 1910.

15. Del Sutton, "The Modern Hospital," *Transactions American Hospital Association* (hereafter *TAHA*) (1906): 135–36; Thomas Addis Emmett, *Incidents in My Life* (New York and London: Putnam's, 1911), pp. 200, 335.

16. J.C. Biddle, "The Physician as a Hospital Superintendent," *TAHA* 6 (1904): 48; A Lay Superintendent, "Medical vs. Lay Superintendents," *National Hospital Record* 3 (1900): 37–38.

17. Editorial, "Hospital Management," *Medical Record* 18 (October 30, 1880): 492.

18. "There is very little sentiment in such a game. The bluff is higher education, the hollow echo a broader humanity," the acid medical man concluded. Editorial, "A Lack of Professional Business," *Medical Record* 49 (May 23, 1896): 730.

19. Editorial, "Filling Forced Vacancies," *Medical Record* 46 (December 22, 1894): 785–86; J.C. DaCosta, "The Old Blockley Hospital," *Journal American Medical Association* (hereafter *JAMA*) 50 (1908): 1183; Editorial, "Politics and the Medical Profession," *National Hospital Record* 3 (1899): 37–38.

20. N.P. Dandridge, *Hospitals. Their Work and their Obligations. The Valedictory Address delivered at the Commencement of the Miami Medical College, Cincinnati* (Cincinnati: Robert Clarke & Co., 1893), pp. 10–11.

21. Roosevelt Hospital, *AR*, 1873, 17.

22. Richard Cadbury, Steward to E.H. Kistler, Carbon Co., Pa., June 11, 1885, Superintendent's Letterbooks, PHA. At the same time, the hospital maintained its policy of refusing admission to "chronic, or offensive cases." Cadbury to A.S. [Raudenbush], Reading, Pa., July 14, 1885. Cases of epilepsy were also excluded categorically. Daniel D. Test to John W. Thomas, Ashland, Pa., November 12, 1898. Superintendent's Letterbooks, PHA.

23. Lakeside Hospital, *AR*, 1898, 5; H.B. Howard, Resident Physician to Charles H.W. Foster, Secretary, Board of Trustees, MGH, October 28, 1904, HCC, justifying the retention of a particular cancer patient who was receiving an experimental x-ray treatment.

24. "Minority Report to Special Committee Report on Training School & Outpatient Department," December 5, 1887, Executive Committee Minutes, Board of Governors, NYHA.

25. Remarks of Isaac Leeser, *Dedication of the Jewish Hospital of Philadelphia* (Philadelphia: Jones & Thacher, 1867), p. 17.

26. Thomas Hall to Visiting Staff, June 29, 1894; J. Collins Warren to Hall, July 5, 1894, Urology Dept. File, MGHA. For an instance of conflict between eager specialists and lay authorities, see the unwillingness of board members to allow staff physicians to treat acute venereal patients at a newly founded Hospital and

Dispensary for the Relief of the Diseases of the Rectum and Genito-Urinary Organs in Philadelphia. December 7, 1877, Minutes, 1875–1887, CPP.

27. The phrase "pure and simple inebriety" is drawn from a letter transmitting a resolution of the MGH trustees to its resident admitting physician; the phrase "immediate alcoholic poisoning" and reference to the dangers of police cells from his reply. Thomas B. Hall to Norton Folsom and Folsom to Hall, January 25, 1876, Admitting Office File, MGHA.

28. Responding to such an awkward instance, the New York Hospital Executive Committee explained in 1906 that in no case should evidence of alcoholism be considered a reason for refusing ambulance service to their emergency room when the patient was semi- or unconscious or showed evidence of a head wound. June 1, 1906, Executive Committee Minutes, vol. 3, p. 478, NYHA.

29. For instances of tardiness in outpatient clinics, for example, see: H.M. Hurd to Dr. Lafleur, December 27, 1890, Superintendent's Letterbooks, JHH; Entry for February 29, 1908, Minutes, Records of Surgical Staff, 1906–17, Boston City Hospital (hereafter BCH); George Ludlam to J.M. Mabbott, May 23, 1902, Superintendent's Letterbooks, NYHA; for examples of disciplining staff members for erratic attendance or unwillingness to respond to emergency calls, see: Entries for May 25, 1882 and June 30, 1892, Minutes, Board of Managers, EHA; Board of Trustees to George C. Stout, February 21, 1908, Polyclinic Hospital Papers, University of Pennsylvania Archives; October 28, 1907, Minutes, Executive Committee, Board of Governors, NYHA. A particularly wild party by the MGH house staff not only called for internal discipline (the related correspondence is to be found in MGH Trustees, Documents, Box 1, HCC, in June of 1903) but even reached the newspapers: *Boston Daily Globe,* June 27, 1903 and *Evening Transcript,* June 27, 1903. At St Agnes' Hospital in Philadelphia the entire house staff was dismissed for "inefficiency and insubordination" when they capped a year of truculence by refusing to appear for breakfast at the appointed time. *New York Times,* November 9, 1908.

30. Conflict often arose over the paid tutorial classes offered by junior staff members on the wards; as we have seen, this was a traditional perquisite of hospital staffers, but terms were always subject to negotiation. See, for example, entry for February 12, 1895, Medical Board Minutes, Willard Parker Hospital, New York Academy of Medicine.

31. Hartford Hospital, *AR,* 1877, 11.

32. Contemporary documents always use masculine pronouns. Chief administrators of large non-Catholic hospitals were always male in the nineteenth century.

33. At the Pennsylvania Hospital, for example, responsibility for physical plant was carefully divided between steward (their time-honored term for superintendent) and matron. The matron was to have charge of the domestics and housekeeping and the cooking and distribution of food. The steward was to have general charge of the buildings, purchasing and accounts. The head nurse's responsibility was in the wards, to see that food and medication was provided, and hired and supervised nurses (with the approval of the "attending managers," a subcommittee of the full board). *Rules and Regulations of the Pennsylvania Hospital* (Philadelphia: Friend's Printing House, 1887), pp. 10–11.

34. This was a useful arrangement for local practitioners who sought to transfer a portion of their practice to the hospital; it meant that a trained salaried physician, as well as twenty-four-hour nursing, would always be available. Taunton, Mass., *Rules and Regulations of the Morton Hospital* (Taunton: C.A. Hack, 1889), pp. 4–8. In this particular case, the physician-superintendent was not only expected to reside in the hospital and perform the duties mentioned, but administer the nurse training school, keep a record of state charges, and oversee the behavior of patients.

35. Edw. Cowles, "The Relations of the Medical Staff to the Governing Bodies in Hospitals." In: J.S. Billings and H. Hurd, eds., *Hospitals Dispensaries and Nursing.* . . . (Baltimore: Johns Hopkins Press; London: The Scientific Press, 1894), p. 70.

36. Book Review, *Hospital World* 1 (January, 1912): 78.

37. Editorial, "The Superintendent," *Hospital World* 1 (April, 1912): 228.

38. By 1914, three handbooks for American hospital administrators had been published: Charlotte A. Aikens, ed., *Hospital Management* (Philadelphia: W.B. Saunders, 1911); Albert J. Ochsner and Meyer J. Strum, *The Organization, Construction and Management of Hospitals* (Chicago: Cleveland Press, 1909); John Hornsby and Richard Schmidt, *The Modern Hospital* (Philadelphia: W.B. Saunders, 1913). A related specialty of hospital architecture was developing at the same time and deserves separate and more detailed attention.

39. "The authority should be highly centralized, for then only can unity of plan and action be obtained; but this presupposes that the superintendent shall have the power and ability to gather about him assistants each of whom is capable of handling his or her own department successfully." Russell, "The Duties and Responsibilities of a Hospital Superintendent," *National Hospital Record* 4 (November, 1900): 3.

40. Daniel Test to Charles Noble, November 2, 1908, Superintendent's Letterbook, PHA.

41. Test to Heber S. Thompson, January 11, 1908, Superintendent's Letterbooks, PHA.

42. Russell, "The Duties and Responsibilities of a Hospital Superintendent," *National Hospital Record* 4 (November, 1900): 5. Russell compared the hospital executive's situation with the far more satisfactory relationship he imagined subsisting between a college president and his trustees.

43. TAHA 8 (1906): 48–53. Those opposed wanted full membership limited to superintendents and their assistants.

44. Editorial, "Another Political Investigation," *Modern Hospital* 1 (1913): 187; "Hints for Hospital Superintendents," *Modern Hospital* 1 (1913): 268.

45. Hospitals were a convenient target of sensationalist journalism. "Burned and Kept in Awful Agony," a *New York Evening Telegram* headline reported on February 25, 1897; "Ambulance Surgeon from Presbyterian Hospital Insisted that Freda Ziebold should go to Bellevue." Clipping in Presbyterian Hospital Scrapbooks, PNY. For examples of the executive's need to handle such difficulties, see entries for June 24–26, 1896, October 4, 1898, Executive Committee Minutes, Papers, Board of Governors, NYHA.

46. C. Irving Fisher, "The Superintendent Himself," *National Hospital Record* 5 (October, 1901): 13.

47. May 22, 1907, Minutes, Records of the Surgical Staff, BCH.

48. H.B. Howard, "The Medical Superintendent: His Advantages, His Duties and His Limitations," *Hospital World* 2 (July, 1912): 34. Howard was willing to concede that in earlier years the medical superintendent "of general hospitals was in disrepute because he was usually someone who had failed in the practice of medicine and in every other avenue of life, and held his position as superintendent as a somewhat active pensioner."

49. Daniel Test, the lay superintendent of Pennsylvania Hospital, argued for example that a medical superintendent would inevitably become involved in medical politics. "There are so many cliques and clans in the medical profession, which, if allowed to be carried into the hospital organization, must, necessarily do it injury." Test to A.B. Tipping, December 28, 1909, Superintendent's Letterbooks, PHA; see also Maud Banfield to Francis R. Bond, November 15, 1909, Polyclinic Hospital Papers, University of Pennsylvania Archives.

50. Contemporaries were well aware of the problem. When the new Peter Bent Brigham Hospital was being planned, its chief of medicine, Henry Christian, wanted resident clinicians and physician administrators to have rooms close together. "I myself believe it is important to have the administrative officers in no wise separated in their feelings and attitude from the medical and surgical men . . ." Christian to H. B. Howard, March 2, 1912, copy in "Letters to Superintendents of Brigham Hospital," Christian Papers, HCC. Christian and Howard, ironically, were soon at loggerheads about Howard's attempts to impose bureaucratic controls over the Brigham's medical wards.

51. [New York] State Charities Aid Association, *Hospital Housekeeping* (New York: Putnam's, 1877), pp. 5, 7.

52. Entry for November 24, 1806, Minutes, Board of Managers, PHA. The Charleston Almshouse did not discontinue its whiskey ration to workers until 1828. Entry for June 19, 1828, Minutes, Almshouse Commissioners, SCHS. In mid-nineteenth century, even the Quaker Pennsylvania Hospital served "stout ale, ale and beer" to its workers. Daniel D. Test to Florence M. Greim, November 29, 1933, typescript, PHA.

53. John W. Pratt to S. Eliot, Chairman, Board of Trustees, January 13, 1893; November 2, 1894, Minutes, Board of Trustees; Ellen Richards to Edmund Dwight, November 14, 1895; Edmund Dwight and H.P. Walcott to Board of Trustees, December 13, 1895, all in Dietary Department File, MGHA. Richards promised that she could reduce food costs per patient day to twenty-eight cents without lessening palatability or nutritional value.

54. The assumption that workingmen and women should live in the institution coupled with the generally wretched accommodations provided were a particular problem. In 1908, for example, the Pennsylvania Hospital's well-meaning superintendent asked the managers to allow the hospital's male employees to use a large empty room as a lounge. "The sleeping rooms of the male employees are not heated," he explained, "and smoking is not allowed, and in cold weather we offer them no encouragement to spend a quiet evening at home." Test to Board of Managers, September 28, 1908, Monthly Reports, PHA. A high rate of employee turnover remained a hospital problem throughout this period. New York's Metropolitan Hospital, for example, had to make 7,400 changes in order to keep 1,200 places filled in one year. "Hospital Intelligence," *Hospital World* 1 (1912): 416. See also, Editorial, "The Orderly," *Ibid.*, 84–85.

55. The following material is cited from the one-man committee report in the September 10, 1907 minutes of the hospital's executive committee, pp. 180–82, NYHA.

56. The average pay of orderlies was twenty-five dollars a month; in addition they received a salary supplement of four dollars a month for lodging. Unlike most of its peers, the New York Hospital did not provide rooms for its orderlies, and the lodging supplement was a vestigial recognition of the traditional assumption that hospitals should provide room as well as board for its lay employees.

57. On workers subsidizing the hospital "in the form of wages earned and not fully paid," see the remarks of S.S. Goldwater, *TAHA* 8 (1906): 94.

12. Life on the Ward

1. The phrase quoted is from the entry for June 8, 1874, Officer of Hygiene, Daily Report Ledger, PHA. Other observations are drawn from entries made between early June and November of 1874.

2. New Haven, Gen. Hosp. Soc. Conn, Annual Report (hereafter *AR*) 1874, 18–19; Philadelphia, Jewish Hospital, *Constitution, By-Laws, Regulations and List of Members* (Philadelphia: [The Hospital], 1874), pp. 29, 31. Cf. also Hartford, Conn, Hospital, *AR*, 1865, 25.

3. Entry for September 7, 1883, Hospital Committee Minutes, Board of Guardians of the Poor, 1882–7, Philadelphia City Archives (hereafter PCA). A contemporary manual listed appropriate light work for convalescents, ranging from washing dishes and dusting to serving meals and watering plants. [N.Y.] State Charities Aid Assoc., *Hospital Housekeeping* (New York: G.P. Putnams, 1877), p. 29. Other institutions boasted that even carpentry, plumbing, and painting were undertaken by convalescent patients.

4. Dr. Clark Bell to Mr. Macy, October 19, 1876, Papers, Board of Governors, New York Hospital Archives (hereafter NYHA). This was the prestigious New York Hospital; expectations were even more brutal in considering the amenities appropriate to paupers and blacks. "It is undeniably true," a report summarizing an investigation of Washington's Freedmen's Hospital explained in 1878, "that vermin of a certain class do exist in the beds and wainscoting of the walls, but it was not found that they existed in excessive numbers when the character of the inmates and their associations are considered." U.S. Senate, Committee on Appropriations, *Report on the Affairs of the Freedmen's Hospital in the District of Columbia, 45th Cong., 2nd Session, Report No. 209, 1878*, p. iii.

5. John B. Roberts, "Notes of Life in a Hospital by a Resident Physician, January, 1877," p. 17, College of Physicians of Philadelphia (hereafter CPP).

6. At Philadelphia's Episcopal Hospital, for example, average lengths of stay were reduced from thirty-four days in 1890 to nineteen in 1910. Hospital authorities were much concerned about such trends. See, for example, data collected by John Shaw Billings: "Hospital and Vital Statistics, 1875–1888," folder, Box 49, Billings Papers, New York Public Library. Cf. also, Morris Vogel, *Invention of the Modern Hospital. Boston, 1870–1930* (Chicago: University of Chicago Press, 1980), pp. 73–75.

7. The trend, as one hospital authority viewed it, was for hospitals to aim at wards of roughly twenty beds, far less than the thirty-six or so assumed in the Nightingale ward. A.C. Abbott, "Some of the Objects, Aims, and Needs of Modern Hospitals," *Pennsylvania Medical Journal* 5 (1902): 229.

8. Stanley J. Reiser, *Medicine and the Reign of Technology* (Cambridge, London, and New York: Cambridge University Press, 1978) emphasizes this shift.

9. Entry for January 19, 1874, Inspecting Committee Minutes, Presbyterian Hospital of New York Archives (hereafter PNY). They also recommended that whistles be placed on the speaking tubes where necessary.

10. Clinical case records had a much older history, and even in the United States, hospitals such as New York and MGH kept such case records almost from their establishment. In the last quarter of the century, however, such records were kept more systematically, tied increasingly to the use of thermometers, laboratory tests, and other "objective" data, as well as being entered on printed forms rather than as discursive and personal narratives on a blank ledger page. See also the discussion in ch. 6.

11. A patient at Cincinnati General Hospital complained later of being roused at four each morning so that his ward could be cleaned. Letter, S. Hechinger to Editor, *Commercial Tribune,* January 16, 1899, Cincinnati Commercial Hospital Scrapbook, Cincinnati General Hospital Archives (hereafter CGHA). By the end of the century, some hospitals had begun to maintain a temperature chart "conspicuously

at the head of each patient's bed . . ." May 9 1899, Medical Board Minutes, Willard Parker and Riverside Hospital, New York Academy of Medicine.

12. Orderlies and other workers were usually the last to be uniformed. See, for example: April 30, 1896, Minutes, Board of Managers, Episcopal Hospital of Philadelphia (hereafter EHA); December 19, 1908, Meeting of Surgical Section, Records of Surgical Staff, Boston City Hospital (hereafter BCH); May 31, 1898, Minutes, Executive Committee, Board of Governors, NYHA. On municipal hospital policies on patients wearing "uniforms," see: September 8, 1882, Minutes, Hospital Committee, Board of Guardians of the Poor, PCA; October 4, 1881, Minutes, Board of Commissioners, City Hospital, RG 29, Charleston City Archives.

13. "Formerly, invalids brought in the Ambulance," one hospital boasted at the end of the century, "were received at the door in front of the building, thus exposing them to the public, which was often very trying—now the Ambulance drives to the rear, where the patient is carried quickly and easily into the new and fully equipped Receiving Ward . . . ," Germantown Dispensary and Hospital, AR, 1897, 7–8.

14. J.B. Roberts, "Notes of Life in a Hospital," p. 5.

15. Entry for November 5, 1897, Medical Staff Minutes, Hahnemann Hospital, Philadelphia.

16. New York, Presbyterian Hospital, AR, 1891, 19; Entry for May 31, 1906, Minutes, Board of Managers, EHA. See also entry for September 4, 1896, Medical Staff Minutes, Hahnemann Hospital, Philadelphia.

17. By the 1870s, that is before the acceptance of antiseptic surgery, it was assumed that any painful or protracted procedure should if possible be removed from the ward. Entry for October 31, 1872, Minutes, Board of Managers, EHA.

18. Report of Inspection by Heber R. Bishop for November, 1896, Minutes of the Inspecting Committee, 1872–99, pp. 221–22, PNY. At Philadelphia's Lying-In Charity, when nurses received boiled codfish, private patients received beef steak, when private patients received lamb chops, nurses ate corned beef. Entry for December 16, 28, 1905, Minutes, House Committee, Philadelphia Lying-In Charity, PHA.

19. At Philadelphia's Stetson Hospital, for example, private room patients could entertain visitors any day between eleven in the morning and eight in the evening; ward patients were permitted visitors on Tuesdays and Thursdays from two to three P.M. and 7 to 8 P.M. and on Sundays from two to four P.M. only. AR, 1910, 56.

20. Editorial, "Floors," Hospital World 2 (August, 1912): 82. On heat see entries for October 9, 1905 and June 11, 1906, Minutes, Medical Board, PNY.

21. Daniel Test to Dr. John Gibbon, March 24, 1910, Superintendent's Letterbook, PHA. On students not being able to observe operations on private patients, see C.J. Huguenin, to Board of Commissioners, City Hospital, February 27, 1886, tipped in Minute Book, 1883–6, RG29, Charleston City Archives; Clara P. Bateman to H.M. Hurd, February 20, 1892, Superintendent's Correspondence, Johns Hopkins Hospital Archives (hereafter JHH). The Charleston case refers to a surgeon's bill protested because students had observed the operation and the second referred to the practice at the University of Michigan of not charging for operations that students were allowed to observe.

22. Anna Baird to H. Hurd, July 2, 1892, Superintendent's Correspondence, JHH. In an earlier letter Miss Baird had noted that her father's entire income was $100. per annum from the church's invalid fund. February 23, 1892.

23. Cincinnati General Hospital, AR, 1904, 11.

24. Thus, a Philadelphia physician endorsing such a proposal could point to the

experience of a fellow medical man's brother-in-law suffering from smallpox who ". . . was obliged to lie in the general ward of the Municipal Hospital with only the privacy afforded by a screen about his bed. The emanations arising from 40 to 50 other smallpox cases could not have been but obnoxious to him." J. Madison Taylor, "Report of a Committee on a Private Pay Hospital for Contagious Diseases . . . ," *Proceedings of the Philadelphia County Medical Society* 21 (1900): 93. The most important need, as another advocate charged, was for the endowment of private contagious disease hospitals with modest charges "in which a family of moderate means may place their sick without prohibitive charges." Wayne Smith, "Model Contagious Hospital," *Hospital World* 1 (February, 1912): 89.

25. Maude Banfield to Francis Bond, President, Board of Trustees, November 15, 1909, "On the Proposed Reorganization of Hospital," Polyclinic Hospital Correspondence, University of Pennsylvania Archives.

26. Entry for February 19, 1889, Committee on Clinics, Cooper Medical College, San Francisco, Lane Medical Library, Stanford University (hereafter SLA).

27. J. McLane to T.M. Prudden, on verso of p. 6 of copy of F.A. Dorman to McLane, February 18, 1901, Letters and Reports, Sloane Maternity Hospital, PNY. Dorman had noted that: "The women dread nothing so much as the knowledge that students are to be present, . . ."

28. Cf. A. McGehee Harvey, *Science at the Bedside. Clinical Research in American Medicine, 1905–1945* (Baltimore and London: Johns Hopkins University Press, 1981).

29. "The waifs of humanity," he continued, "who seek in their weakness and distress the wards of a hospital, should find in the medical attendants men whose hearts respond to their helplessness, and whose most skilled efforts will be rendered with tenderest consideration." Hunter H. Powell, "The Ideal Medical Staff of a Modern Hospital," Lakeside Hospital, *AR,* 1898, 92.

30. Samuel D. Gross, "Nature's Voice in Disease," *American Practitioner* 1(1870): 269; J. McVean, "Hints for Nurses," *Trained Nurse* 1 (1888): 8; Louise Coleman, "The Relative Authority of the Superintendent and the Staff in the Control and Discipline of Patients," *TAHA* 9 (1907): 97; "Hospitals for Bluejackets," *National Hospital Record* 1 (September, 1897): 20.

31. Jane Addams, "The Layman's View of Hospital Work among the Poor," *TAHA* 9 (1907): 58.

32. David Cheever, *Boston Medical & Surgical Journal* (hereafter *BM&SJ*) 135 (1896): 614, cited in Vogel, *Invention,* p. 127; L.E. Gretter, "Glimpses of Hospital Life," *Trained Nurse* 1 (1888): 45; George Henry Fox, *Reminiscences* (New York: Medical Life Press, 1926), pp. 157–58.

33. In a notebook preserved in the Rare Book Department at the New York Academy of Medicine. The Librarian's Office at the Pennsylvania Hospital has preserved a scrapbook of "Resident Physician Memorabilia" beginning in 1901; it contains many examples of similar patient whimsies.

34. Amy Armour, "Hospital Housekeeping," *Hospital World* 2 (September, 1912): 153.

35. Sara E. Greenfield, "The Dangers of Menopause," *Woman's Medical Journal* 12 (1902): 183.

36. Thus a contemporary could emphasize the need for more labor in a children's hospital because the patients could not be expected to help as they would "in a charity hospital for adults." J.W.H. Lovejoy, Children's Hospital, Washington, D.C. to James McMillan, December 7, 1897, copy in H.M. Hurd Papers, JHH. See also Jon M. Kingsdale, "The Growth of Hospitals: An Economic History in Baltimore," (Ph.D. diss., University of Michigan, 1981), pp. 12–13; Entry for March 4, 1898, Medical Staff Minutes, Hahnemann Hospital, Philadelphia.

37. Nurses on private duty faced a rather different sort of dilemma, defining a

social space tolerable to the employing family, above that of the family's domestic servants yet acceptable to them.

38. Eugene B. Elder, "The Management of the Race Question in Hospitals," *TAHA* 9 (1907): 128. For examples of separate but unequal treatment in hospital facilities, see: Cincinnati General Hospital, *AR*, 1893, 28; Entry for May 19, 1880, Minutes, Board of Commissioners of City Hospital, RG 29, Charleston City Archives; A.F. Jones to the Visiting Committee, January 6, 1885, tipped in Minutes, Board of Commissioners, City Hospital, RG 29, Charleston City Archives; Entry for September 25, 1901, Minutes, Business Committee, UCM, Medical College of Virginia Archives (hereafter MCV).

39. George Ludlam to Howard Townsend, April 22, 1902, Superintendent's Letterbooks, NYHA.

40. Grady Hospital, *AR*, 1899, 6–7; *AR*, 1901, 6, 15.

41. Remarks of Dr. Wayne Smith, after paper by J.W. Fowler, "Scientific Economic and Humane Conduct of Municipal General Hospitals in the Southern States," *TAHA* 16 (1914): 280. For the earlier history, Cf. Todd L. Savitt, "The Use of Blacks for Medical Experimentation and Demonstration in the Old South," *Journal of Southern History* 48 (1982): 331–48.

42. J.S. Billings to Katherine Hammond, August 9, 1894, Hammond-Bryan-Cumming Papers, South Caroliniana Library (hereafter SCC).

43. N.P. Dandridge, *Hospitals. Their Work and Their Obligations* (Cincinnati: Robert Clarke & Co., 1893), pp. 21–22.

44. New York *World*, June 25, 1886, clipping in Babies' Hospital Scrapbook, Public Relations Department, PNY; Edward P. Davis, "The Practical Value of Modern Methods of Antisepsis in the Care of Infants, Including the Preparation of Infant Foods," *Philadelphia Hospital Reports* 1 (1890): 219.

45. Report of Physician to Branch and Annex Hospitals, Cincinnati General Hospital, *AR*, 1906, 14.

46. Report of Visiting Committee for December, 1898, filed with Minutes for December 13, 1898, Trustee's Minutes, JHH. Some hospitals were limited by bylaws or terms of bequest to the admission of married lying-in patients only.

47. Daniel W. Cathell, *The Physician Himself* (Baltimore: Cushings & Bailey, 1882), p. 186.

48. Daniel Test to J.R. Coddington, December 8, 1910, Superintendent's Papers, PHA, explains their typical policy of excluding potentially infectious cases while admitting cases with tertiary symptoms.

49. Quoted from a letter written by Lawrence Flick, cited in Ella Flick, *Beloved Crusader* (Philadelphia: Dorrance & Co., c. 1944), p. 108.

50. Entries for October 11, 1906, Minutes, Board of Trustees, Hahnemann Hospital; December 9, 1901, Minutes, Medical Board, PNY; January 7, 1902, Executive Committee Minutes, Board of Governors, v. 2, p. 265, NYHA.

51. See Morris Vogel's discussion of Carney Hospital as an example of this trend. *Invention*, pp. 73–74.

52. Thomas Addis Emmett, *Incidents in my Life* (New York: G.P. Putnam's, 1911), p. 196n. Cancer was so feared that even the private "memorial hospital" was forced to employ the euphemistic term "because the term 'Cancer Hospital' was objected to by the 'class of patients' received." P. 196.

53. Or even in the handful of well-run voluntary hospitals specializing in chronic disease. Cf. Dorothy Levenson, *Montefiore. The Hospital as Social Instrument, 1884–1984* (New York: Farrar, Straus & Giroux, c. 1984).

54. Wyndham Blanton to W.T. Sanger, February 8, 1939, W.T. Sanger Files, MCV.

55. H.B. Howard to Charles Foster, January 21, 1904, Box 4, MGH Trustees Doc.

File, HCC; Daniel Test to Messrs Wm. Sullivan, September 13, 1907, Superintendent's Letterbooks, PHA.

56. Hammond's mother lived in South Carolina; the correspondence is preserved
in the Hammond-Bryan-Cumming Papers, SCC. A selection of Hammond family
letters have been recently annotated and reprinted by Carol Bleser, ed., *The Ham-
monds of Redcliffe* (New York: Oxford University Press, 1981). This volume includes
only a few of the letters describing Hammond's Johns Hopkins experience.

57. Ibid., March 31, 1894. Hammond-Bryan-Cumming Papers, SCC.

58. Ibid., May 14, 1893.

59. Ibid., October 13, 1893. Some days later she referred to the same surgeon as
a "cruel brute—besides being a very nervous irritable fool. . . . His cruelty is
outrageous—and I feel sometimes as if I could not stay in the ward with him."
October 22, 1893.

60. Ibid., May 1, 1893.

61. Ibid., May 14, 1893.

62. E. Flick, *Beloved Crusader,* pp. 76–77. "I have noticed," Flick recorded in his
diary, "several times that when these children who have been in for some time are
punished or reprimanded they do not burst out into open or loud cry but suppress
it just as if they knew that they have no sympathy. Even children from 18 months
to 2 years old do so." Cf: "A Night in a Ward," *Cincinnati Enquirer,* December 13,
1885, clipping in Cincinnati Commercial Hospital Scrapbook, CGHA.

63. [March 29], 1893. Hammond-Bryan-Cumming Papers, SCC.

64. Ibid., August 16, 1893.

65. Ibid., June 11, 1894. In the same letter she referred to her ward as an
". . . awful place for such cases indeed there is hardly one of the pts. . . . whose
morals you can inquire into."

66. Ibid., August 11, 1893.

67. Ibid., April 24, 1894.

13. The New-Model Hospital and Its Critics

1. Mrs. [Joan Smith] to Henry P. Walcott, M.D., August 16, 1911, Box 12,
Trustees Filed Papers, Massachusetts General Hospital (hereafter MGH) Papers,
Countway Library (hereafter HCC). The letter writers' name has been changed to
maintain privacy. The writer reflected the attitudes of that large group of "respectable" Americans uncomfortable with the ward's demeaning associations, yet unable to afford private accommodations. Her letter indicates how important it was
to distance herself from the hospital's "normal" clientele.

2. "The hospital must," as this critic put it, "realize itself to be a great social force
and not content itself to be, as unfortunately it frequently is, the mere adjunct,
laboratory or experiment station of some medical school or coterie of men." Leo
Franklin, "Some Social Aspects of the Hospital," *TAHA* 14 (1912): 105. This
passage and some others in this chapter are adapted or reprinted from the author's
"Inward Vision and Outward Glance: The Shaping of the American Hospital,
1880–1914," *BHM* 53 (1979): 346–91.

3. Ida Cannon, *Social Work in Hospitals,* rev. ed. (New York: Russell Sage, 1923),
p. 27.

4. Richard Cabot, *The Achievement, Standards and Prospects of the Massachusetts General
Hospital. Ether Day Address* (Boston: The Hospital, 1919), p. 19.

5. Richard Cabot, "Why Should Hospitals Neglect the Care of Chronic Curable
Disease in Out-Patients?," *St. Paul Medical Journal* 10 (1908): 6. For a more extended
exposition of Cabot's position, see *Social Service and the Art of Healing* (New York:

Moffat, Yard, 1909) and *Social Work: Essays on the Meeting-Ground of Doctor and Social Worker* (Boston and New York: Houghton Mifflin, 1919). His social service activities are described in Ida M. Cannon, *On the Social Frontier of Medicine: Pioneering in Medical Social Service* (Cambridge: Harvard University Press, 1952).

6. For a valuable insight into the ideas and relationships of this tightly-knit group of reformers, see: Barbara Sicherman, *Alice Hamilton. A Life in Letters* (Cambridge and London: Harvard University Press, 1984).

7. Editorial, "An Ounce of Prevention," *Hospital World* 1 (1912): 204–205, reporting the gift of $100,000 to New York's Mt. Sinai Hospital for the support of social service.

8. Cf. [William Rathbone], *Organization of Nursing. An Account of the Liverpool Nurses' Training School, its Foundation, Progress, and Operation in Hospital, District, and Private Nursing. . . . With an Introduction and Notes by Florence Nightingale* (Liverpool: A Holden; London: Longman, Green, Reader and Dyer, 1865).

9. Boston's Instructive District Nursing Association began its work late in 1886. As indicated by its name, the organization hoped to "instruct" and prevent, as a consequence in part of the visitor's "refinement and higher social standing." Annual Report (hereafter *AR*), 1893, 10–11. For the most recent history of public health nursing, see Karen Buhler-Wilkerson, "False Dawn: The Rise and Decline of Public Health Nursing, 1900–30," (Ph.D. diss., University of Pennsylvania, 1984).

10. Aiding in diagnosis and treatment remained a key rationale for such programs; they were not aimed at relieving poverty in general. "It is concerned only with those whose poverty," as Richard Cabot carefully put it, "is the cause, or an important cause of their illness." Richard C. Cabot, "Some Functions of Social Work in Hospitals," *Modern Hospital* 4 (1915): 188; Mary E. Wadley, "Hospital Social Service," *TAHA* 13 (1911): 321–22.

11. Jane Addams, "The Layman's View of Hospital Work among the Poor," *TAHA* 9 (1907): 59–60. Such criticisms were commonplace and often turned on the mindlessly uniform treatment of patients no matter what their complaint.

12. Editorial, "The Patient—A Personality, Not a Case," *Hospital World* 1 (1912): 4–5; George Ludlam, "Should Ward Patients have their own Visiting Physician if he be a member of the Staff?" *Hospital World* 1 (1912): 42; W. Gilman Thompson, "The Hospital from the Patient's Point of View," *TAHA* 11 (1909): 161.

13. S.S. Goldwater, "The Medical Staff and its Functions," *TAHA* 8 (1906): 99–100; Goldwater, "The Hospital and the Surgeon," *Modern Hospital* 7 (1916): 374. Goldwater regarded specialism as necessary and laudable and Mt. Sinai itself was a stronghold of special practice. Cf. Joseph Hirsh and Beka Doherty, *The First Hundred Years of the Mount Sinai Hospital of New York, 1852–1952* (New York: Random House, 1952), esp. chap. VII, "The Nineteenth-Century Staff and the Beginnings of Specialization," pp. 76–91.

14. Richard Cabot, *Social Service and the Art of Healing* (New York: Moffat, Yard, 1909), p. 33, cf. pp. 174, 177.

15. F.C. Shattuck, "Specialism, the Laboratory, and Practical Medicine," *BM&SJ* 136 (June 24, 1897): 613; W. Gilman Thompson, "The Relation of the Visiting and House Staff to the Care of Hospital Patients," *National Hospital Record* 9 (1906): 23–24; Henry W. Cattell, "The Relation of the Clinical Laboratory to the Hospital," *National Hospital Record* 5 (1902): 14–15.

16. Adolph Rupp, "Tubbing in Typhoid," *Medical Record* 45 (January 6, 1894): 29.

17. Cf. Barbara G. Rosenkrantz, "Cart before Horse: Theory, Practice, and Professional Image in American Public Health, 1870–1920," *Journal of the History of Medicine* 29 (1974): 55–73.

18. J.A. Hornsby, "The Modern Hospital—A New Entity," *Modern Hospital* 1 (1913): 112–13.

19. Philadelphia Polyclinic Hospital, *AR,* 1907, 10–11.

20. The dispensary was invented in late eighteenth century England. It was an autonomous, free-standing institution, created with the hope of providing an alternative to the hospital in providing medical care to the urban poor. Like most such benevolent institutions, it was soon copied by public spirited Americans. Dispensaries were established in 1786 at Philadelphia, 1791 at New York, 1796 at Boston, and at Baltimore in 1800. By 1874, there were twenty-nine dispensaries in New York, and by 1877, thirty-three in Philadelphia. Their growth was equally impressive in terms of numbers of patients treated. In New York, for example, the city's dispensaries treated 134,069 patients in 1860, roughly 180,000 in 1866, 213,-000 in 1874, and 876,000 in 1900. But by the latter date, hospital outpatient clinics had far outstripped independent dispensaries. Cf. Charles E. Rosenberg, "Social Class and Medical Care in Nineteenth-Century America: The Rise and Fall of the Dispensary," *Journal of the History of Medicine* 29 (1974): 32–54; George Rosen, "The First Neighborhood Health Center Movement—Its Rise and Fall," *American Journal of Public Health* 61 (1971): 1620–37.

21. Most cities and many rural counties employed district or public physicians to treat the dependent poor in their homes. By the end of the century, a good number of urban hospital admissions came as a consequence of referrals from such physicians or from those employed by private dispensaries.

22. Outpatient staff members were frustrated as well by their inability to alter their patients' circumstances. Advice to improve diets or find less strenuous work were as much ironic as practical.

23. Paid positions were often hardest to fill, for these tended to be full time, often in emergency and admission rooms. Positions in specialty clinics, although ordinarily unpaid, were nevertheless more desirable. Those with some family backing or expectations were able to avoid the stable, yet time-consuming and often dead-end salaried positions.

24. The report noted the same experience at other outpatient departments at which they had made inquiries. Executive Committee Minutes, October 31, 1906, NYHA. Cf. L.R.G. Crandon to George Monks, October 15, 1910, Crandon to Paul Thorndike, April 30, 1910, Records of the Surgical Staff, 1906–17, BCH.

25. This refers, of course, to urban practice and to the poor and working classes. It was assumed, at least in theory, that small town and rural practitioners would attend the indigent without charge and the needy at reduced rates or be paid modest fees by county authorities.

26. Some dispensary physicians did use their volunteer posts as a way of meeting and attracting patients who might later consult them privately. A physician's private office address and hours might, for example, be stamped on a dispensary patient's appointment card.

27. At least some contemporaries associated the poor quality of outpatient care with the fact that so many practitioners regarded it as simply a step on the road to inpatient positions. Cf. Editorial, "The Development of Out-Patient Departments," *BM&SJ,* 142 (March 22, 1900): 310–11.

28. During this period, some hospital clinics and dispensaries did, in fact, call for the establishment of evening hours so that clinic services would be available to working people without the sacrifice of a day's pay.

29. The debate surrounding the problem of "dispensary abuse" is extensive and deadeningly repetitious and need not be pursued here. However, it might be noted that it was particularly sharp and divisive among the attending staffs of some of the older and most prestigious hospitals, none more so than the Massachusetts

General. The "Outpatient Department Fees & Abuse" file in the MGH Archives contains a great deal of revealing material, especially responses by staff members to a circular letter of 1893.

30. The superintendent of Philadelphia's Episcopal Hospital complained to his governing board that their experiment of charging fifteen cents a prescription had reduced their patient load and thus, "our source of supply for the wards . . ." Inpatient admissions were down by more than two hundred during the eleven months of the experiment. Henry Sykes to Comm. on Administration, January 9, 1902, Board of Managers Minutes, Episcopal Hospital of Philadelphia Archives (hereafter EHA).

31. E. G. Cutler to Edmund Dwight, November 18, 1893, Pharmacy File, Massachusetts General Hospital Archives (hereafter MGHA). Although reformers tended to emphasize the ill-educated and anti-intellectual (or perhaps anti-authoritarian, the distinction would not have been easily understood at the time) attitudes of urban immigrants, many of these new Americans seem also to have entertained a powerful faith in the "professors" who staffed prestigious hospital clinics.

32. For a systematic exposition of his views, see, Michael M. Davis and Andrew R. Warner, *Dispensaries. Their Management and Development. A Book for Administrators, Public Health Workers, and all Interested in Better Medical Service for the People* (New York: Macmillan, 1918).

33. In 1919, the Boston Dispensary initiated a Health Clinic that provided a complete medical evaluation for a nominal five dollar fee. It included examinations by an ophthalmologist, otolaryngologist, physical diagnosis, and blood and urine tests. Boston Dispensary, *AR*, 1920–21, 13.

34. Cooperative, multispecialist *private* practice organizations became a fashionable reality in the 1920s—most prominently in such widely admired manifestations as the Mayo and Cleveland Clinics. Sinclair Lewis's *Arrowsmith* (1925) provides a scornful picture of one such enterprise.

35. This argument is documented in greater detail in Charles E. Rosenberg, "From Almshouse to Hospital: The Shaping of Philadelphia General Hospital," *Milbank Memorial Fund Q.* 60 (1982): 133–43. Some passages in this chapter have been adapted from this article. On the antebellum history of the Philadelphia Almshouse, see Priscilla Ferguson Clement, *Welfare and the Poor in the Nineteenth-Century City, Philadelphia, 1800–1854* (Rutherford, N.J.: Fairleigh Dickinson University Press, 1985), and for a general account of municipal hospitals, Harry Dowling, *City Hospitals. The Undercare of the Underprivileged* (Cambridge and London: Harvard University Press, 1982).

36. Arthur B. Ancker, "The Municipal Hospital," *Proc. National Conf. Charities and Corrections, 1889,* p. 180.

37. Isaac Ray, *Social Science Association of Philadelphia. Papers of 1873. What Shall Philadelphia Do for Its Paupers?* (Philadelphia: The Association, 1873), cited in Rosenberg, "From Almshouse," p. 134. The paragraph following is adapted from *Ibid*, p. 135, citing the annual report for 1900, pages 8 and 10.

38. In certain areas, most conspicuously neurology, Philadelphia General Hospital's (hereafter PGH) burden of chronic and deteriorated patients made it a natural center for specialized teaching and publication.

39. Kings County was Brooklyn's municipal hospital until the consolidation of the five boroughs in 1898.

40. There is an extraordinarily vivid account of the Long Island Hospital in the testimony offered at an investigation of the hospital in 1903. Boston, *Majority and Minority Reports on Investigation of Boston Almshouse and Hospital at Long Island* (Boston: Municipal Printing Office, 1904). See also David W. Cheever et al., *A History of the Boston City Hospital from its Foundation until 1904* (Boston: Municipal Printing Office,

1906); Morris Vogel, *The Invention of the Modern Hospital, Boston 1870–1930* (Chicago and London: University of Chicago Press, 1980); Brian Gratton, *Urban Elders. Family, Work and Welfare among Boston's Aged, 1890–1950* (Philadelphia: Temple University Press, 1986).

41. This example is drawn from a reading of the Minutes for 1880–85, Board of Commissioners for the City Hospital, RG 29, Charleston City Archives.

42. "President's Address," *Hospital World* 2 (1912): 232. Rural areas had their own persistent problems. Reformers complained in the 1920s that many rural counties provided scandalously inadequate care at poor farms and almshouses little different from their nineteenth-century predecessors.

43. Richard Waterman, *Reports Submitted to the Philadelphia County Medical Society by the Committee on Hospital Efficiency* . . . ([Philadelphia]: Philadelphia County Medical Society, 1914), pp. 7, 5.

44. George P. Ludlam, "President's Address," *TAHA* 8 (1906): 65. Cf. A.J. Ochsner, "Hospital Growth Marks Dawn of New Era," *Modern Hospital* 1 (1913): 1.

45. The best sources documenting the growth of such attitudes and practices are the *National Hospital Record* (published between 1897 and 1915 when it merged into *Modern Hospital*) and TAHA. Revealing as well are the guides to management and design, such as Charlotte Aikens, ed., *Hospital Management: A Handbook for Hospital Trustees, Superintendents, Training School Principals, Physicians, and all who are Actively Engaged in Promoting Hospital Work* (Philadelphia: W.B. Saunders, 1911); John A. Hornsby and R.E. Schmidt, *The Modern Hospital* (Philadelphia: W.B. Saunders, 1913).

46. Secretary, State Board of Charities, to J.W. McLane, Sloane Maternity Hospital, April 13, 1900, Presbyterian Hospital of New York Archives (hereafter PNY).

47. E.A. Vander Veer, "The Importance of a General Hospital in the Education of the Profession and the Public," *Bulletin of the American Academy of Medicine* 12 (1911): 157.

48. E.A. Codman to J.M.T. Finney, December 27, 1915, Codman Papers, HCC. Cf. Susan Reverby, "Stealing the Golden Eggs: Ernest Amory Codman and the Science and Management of Medicine," *BHM* 55 (1981): 156–71.

49. And, in particular, that Codman's end-result system, which was based on the patient reporting their condition on postcards at intervals after the relevant procedure, was itself flawed. S.S. Goldwater to E.A. Codman, December 10, 1913, Codman Papers, HCC.

50. Frank J. Firth, *The Foundation of Hospital Efficiency* (n.p., 1911), pp. 5–6. Increased wages for nonprofessional staff certainly constituted one such cost. Paternalism and better supervision did not guarantee improved performance; a more stable workforce demanded higher salaries.

51. Edward Cowles, "The Relations of the Medical Staff to the Governing Bodies in Hospitals," in John S. Billings and Henry M. Hurd, eds., *Hospitals, Dispensaries and Nursing* (Baltimore: The Johns Hopkins Press, 1894), p. 72; Hurd, "Hospital Organization and Management," *University Medical Magazine* 9 (1896): 492.

52. For a pioneer attempt to rationalize the work of New York's hospitals, see "Considerations to come before the joint meeting of representatives of the different hospitals to convene at no. 8 West 16th," n.d., 1876 File, Papers, Board of Governors, New York Hospital Archives (hereafter NYHA). Philadelphia hospitals had also begun a series of informal meetings on particular issues in the last decades of the century.

53. W.L. Estes, "Hospital Management," *National Hospital Record* 3 (1900): 8–9.

54. By 1911, a New York-based Hospital Bureau of Standards and Supplies functioned as a buying agent for some thirty-five hospitals. Rupert Norton to Board of Trustees, Johns Hopkins Hospital, February 11, 1911, Minutes for Febru-

ary 14, 1911, Johns Hopkins Hospital Archives (hereafter JHH). contains a detailed account of a visit to the Bureau.

55. Alejandra C. Laszlo, "The American Hospital Association: Emergence of a Professional Organization, 1899–1914," unpublished paper. University of Pennsylvania, Dept. of the History and Sociology of Science, 1986.

56. Charles Emerson, "The American Hospital Field," in Aikens, ed., *Hospital Management,* p. 22. The same year, another authority warned against the "needless multiplication of hospitals in a community." The proliferation of those institutions "likely to become a public charge" should be controlled by law. Frank J. Firth, *The Foundation of Hospital Efficiency* (n.p., 1911), p. 9.

57. For an account of MGH and its attempts to answer this problem, see Frederic A. Washburn, *The Massachusetts General Hospital: Its Development. 1900–1935* (Boston: Houghton, Mifflin, 1939), pp. 245–58. The MGH archives contain a scrapbook documenting the background of the Baker Memorial and reactions to it in Boston and elsewhere. See also, C. Rufus Rorem, *The Middle-Rate Plan for Hospital Patients: The First Year's Experience of the Baker Memorial of the Massachusetts General Hospital* (Chicago: Julius Rosenwald Fund, 1931). The Rosenwald Fund commissioned a number of such studies of the middle-income patient at this time.

58. S.S. Goldwater, "The Unfinished Business of General Hospitals," *Medical Record* 73 (1908): 982.

59. Christian R. Holmes, *Modern Hospitals with Special Reference to Our New Municipal Hospital . . .* (Cincinnati: n.p., 1908), p. 8.

60. "Principally these departments are the pathologic and clinical laboratories, the Roentgen-ray department, the morgue and necropsy room, and a competent system of record keeping throughout the whole institution." J.M. Baldy, "Hospital Internship," *JAMA* 67 (1916): 554.

61. Ida Cannon to R.C. Cabot, Box 23, General Correspondence, Cabot Papers, Harvard University Archives.

62. R.C. Cabot, *Case Teaching in Medicine. A Series of Graduated Exercises in the Differential Diagnosis, Prognosis and Treatment of Actual Cases of Disease* (Boston: D.C. Heath, 1906).

63. R.C. Cabot, "Out-Patient Medical Service—The Most Important and Most Neglected Part of Hospital Work," *Hospital World* 2 (1912): 35.

14. Conclusion: The Past in the Present

1. Sex ratios were most disproportionate in large urban municipal and voluntary hospitals. Disparities were not so marked in a growing number of community hospitals founded at the end of the century or at many religious and ethnic institutions. Both social and technical factors, especially antiseptic surgery, made a hospital stay in these institutions less stigmatizing.

2. And to an extent esthetic, removing the patient from the eyes and ears of ward mates.

3. This not entirely complete survey did include mental hospitals. U. S. Dept. of Commerce, Bureau of the Census, *Hospitals and Dispensaries. 1923* (Washington: Government Printing Office, 1925), p. 1; J.M. Toner, "Statistics of Regular Medical Associations and Hospitals of the United States," *TAMA* 24 (1873): 287–333. For a useful discussion of late nineteenth-century hospital growth patterns, see: Jon M. Kingsdale, "The Growth of Hospitals: An Economic History in Baltimore," (Ph.D. diss., Univ. of Michigan, 1981).

4. See the more extended discussion in chapter 13.

5. Medicine was hardly alone in clothing itself in the garb of science—this was an era in which domestic science, library science, and political science, among other disciplines and would-be disciplines, reached self-consciously for "scientific" status and academic acceptance. In the case of medicine, of course, connections with the scientific disciplines was particularly significant and increasingly relevant to care. On the other hand, medicine experienced organizational changes paralleling those undergone by other professions and occupations at the same time, suggesting that its ultimate social form and prerogatives were more than logical and necessary consequences of cognitive change alone.

6. For useful case studies illuminating the economic difficulties of hospitals in the period before 1930, see: David Rosner, *A Once Charitable Enterprise. Hospitals and Health Care in Brooklyn and New York, 1885–1915* (Cambridge, London, New York: Cambridge University Press, 1982) and (on Baltimore) Kingsdale, "The Growth of Hospitals."

7. The growing influence of professional administrators was apparent in politically colored municipal institutions as well as in their private peers. The pattern was apparent in other cultural and benevolent institutions as well where professional managers gradually came to mediate between wealthy directors and the objects of their benevolence. See, for example: Kathleen D. McCarthy, *Noblesse Oblige. Charity and Cultural Philanthropy in Chicago, 1849–1929* (Chicago: University of Chicago Press, 1982).

8. The professionalization of nursing did provide supervisory positions for women, but the great majority of such posts remained subordinate to male superintendents, medical boards, and trustees. In a small minority of women's hospitals, this was not the case and, as we have suggested, the Catholic hospitals also provided a setting in which women could exert a greater degree of real authority. They were insulated by their sex and vocation from the will of medical boards and by their orders from the unfettered control of diocesan administrators.

9. For a useful discussion, see Ernst P. Boas and Nicholas Michelson, *The Challenge of Chronic Diseases* (New York: Macmillan, 1929).

10. For a survey of the hospital's internal architectural history, centering on room and ward arrangements, see John D. Thompson and Grace Goldin, *The Hospital: A Social and Architectural History* (New Haven and London: Yale University Press, 1975). Cf. Adrian Forty, "The Modern Hospital in France and England." In: A. King, ed., *Buildings and Society* (London: Routledge & Kegan Paul, 1980), 61–93.

11. Hospital facilities were seen by contemporary observers to be inadequate particularly in poor or isolated areas, as evidenced by the interest of a number of private foundations in the 1920s and 1930s.

12. The influence of a developing specialism on the hospital and of the hospital on special practice is an extremely important part of hospital history, but one that has been on the whole neglected by historians.

13. New York, Massachusetts, Connecticut, and Pennsylvania, for example, had all found ways to support voluntary hospitals throughout the nineteenth century. For a general discussion, see Rosemary Stevens, " 'A Poor Sort of Memory,': Voluntary Hospitals and Government before the Depression," *Milbank Memorial Fund Q.* 60 (1982): 551–84; Stevens, "Sweet Charity: State Aid to Hospitals in Pennsylvania, 1870–1910," *Bulletin of the History of Medicine* (hereafter *BHM*) 58 (1984): 287–314, 474–95.

14. Hill-Burton did specify conditions, but they seem not to have greatly constrained institutional policies. The intra-institutional effects of externally supported research have been significant but are difficult to evaluate.

15. And the carrying out of that imperative has created economic and bureaucratic interests committed to existing procurement patterns and thus another source of rigidity in both areas.

16. The similarities between for-profit hospitals and the great majority of their not-for-profit peers are at least as significant as their differences. Both are prisoners of the same attitudes, expectations, technology, and funding realities and must pursue a good many parallel strategies.

Index

Academic medicine, 184–89, 208; environmentalist influences in, 312; and hospitals, 211; and patient care, 297

Accreditation, 333–34, 347

Ackernecht, Erwin H., 370n23

Addams, Jane, 298–99, 314–15

Admissions, 22–26, 47, 50, 52, 67; and authority structure, 274–76; and diagnosis, 153, 345; and hospital staffing, 181; and medical education, 207; as physically segregated procedure, 292; to religious hospitals, 113; surgical, 381n30

Admitting privileges, 253, 255, 257

Aged patients, 305–6, 326

Agnew, C. R., 382n45

Aikens, Charlotte A., 411n39

Albany Hospital, 106, 204, 402n4, 408n9

Alcohol, therapeutic use of, 54–55

Alcoholism, 17, 23, 29, 40, 276, 305, 410n27

Alexian Brothers Hospital (Chicago), 110

Almshouses, 4, 15–19, 21, 23, 103, 108, 291, 322, 323, 325, 337, 363n27, 364n43, 421n42; admissions to, 24; apprenticeship in, 61, 62; charity work in, 268; chronic care in, 306, 345; deaths in, 31; foreign-born inmates of, 41, 102; foundlings in, 114; inspections of, 49; length of stay in, 27; location of, 128; medical schools and, 199, 204; nursing in, 214; outdoor physicians to, 66; religious hospitals as alternatives to, 113; rules of, 35; sanitary conditions in, 32; ward designations in, 29, 30; *see also* specific institutions

American College of Surgeons, 329

American Hospital Association, 281, 331

American Medical Association (AMA), 163, 202, 206

Anesthesia, 28, 92, 114, 144, 145, 365n52, 371n39; for private patients, 294

Anesthesiology, 175, 182

Annals of the Poor, 35

Antisepsis, 143–47, 381n32

Appendectomies, 149, 249, 250, 381n25, 405nn45, 49

Apprenticeship, 60–62, 90, 199

Asepsis, 147–50, 242, 245–46, 332, 342, 345

Aspirin, 383n56

Association of Hospital Superintendents, 281